HEALTH INFORMATION EXCHANGE

HEALTH INFORMATION EXCHANGE

Navigating and Managing a Network of Health Information Systems

Edited by

BRIAN E. DIXON MPA, PHD, FHIMSS

Indiana University Richard M. Fairbanks School of Public Health; and the Center for Biomedical Informatics, Regenstrief Institute, Inc., Indianapolis, IN

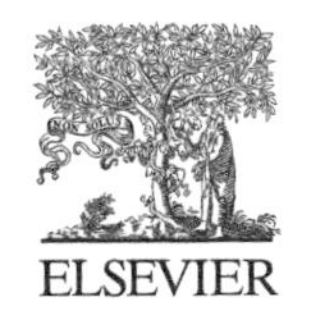

AMSTERDAM • BOSTON • HEIDELBERG • LONDON
NEW YORK • OXFORD • PARIS • SAN DIEGO
SAN FRANCISCO • SINGAPORE • SYDNEY • TOKYO

Academic Press is an imprint of Elsevier

Academic Press is an imprint of Elsevier
125, London Wall, EC2Y 5AS.
525 B Street, Suite 1800, San Diego, CA 92101-4495, USA
50 Hampshire Street, 5th Floor, Cambridge, MA 02139, USA
The Boulevard, Langford Lane, Kidlington, Oxford OX5 1GB, UK

Notices

Knowledge and best practice in this field are constantly changing. As new research and experience broaden our understanding, changes in research methods, professional practices, or medical treatment may become necessary.

Practitioners and researchers must always rely on their own experience and knowledge in evaluating and using any information, methods, compounds, or experiments described herein. In using such information or methods they should be mindful of their own safety and the safety of others, including parties for whom they have a professional responsibility.

To the fullest extent of the law, neither the Publisher nor the authors, contributors, or editors, assume any liability for any injury and/or damage to persons or property as a matter of products liability, negligence or otherwise, or from any use or operation of any methods, products, instructions, or ideas contained in the material herein.

ISBN: 978-0-12-803135-3

British Library Cataloguing-in-Publication Data

A catalogue record for this book is available from the British Library.

Library of Congress Cataloging-in-Publication Data

A catalog record for this book is available from the Library of Congress.

For Information on all Academic Press publications visit our website at http://store.elsevier.com/

Contents

VI

CASE STUDIES IN HEALTH INFORMATION EXCHANGE

List of Contributors

Kelly J. Abrams Canadian Health Information Management Association/Canadian College of Health Information Management, London, Ontario, Canada

Julia Adler-Milstein School of Information, University of Michigan, Ann Arbor, MI

Jennifer M. Alyea Indiana University Richard M. Fairbanks School of Public Health, Indianapolis, IN

Robert Bailey Center for the Advancement of Health IT, RTI International, Research Triangle Park, NC

Paul Biondich Indiana University School of Medicine; and the Center for Biomedical Informatics, Regenstrief Institute, Inc., Indianapolis, IN

Jack Bowie Apelon, Inc., Hartford, CT

David Broyles Indiana University Richard M. Fairbanks School of Public Health, Indianapolis, IN

Ryan Crichton Jembi Health Systems, Cape Town

Caitlin M. Cusack Insight Informatics, Manchester, NH

Monica Daeges Department of Medical Informatics and Clinical Epidemiology, Oregon Health & Science University, and the Pacific Northwest Evidence-Based Practice Center, Portland, OR

Beth Devine Department of Medical Informatics and Clinical Epidemiology, Oregon Health & Science University, and the Pacific Northwest Evidence-Based Practice Center, Portland, OR; University of Washington Centers for Comparative and Health Systems Effectiveness (CHASE) Alliance, Seattle, WA

Brian E. Dixon Indiana University Richard M. Fairbanks School of Public Health; and the Center for Biomedical Informatics, Regenstrief Institute, Inc., Indianapolis, IN; Department of Veterans Affairs, Center for Health Information and Communication, Veterans Health Administration, Health Services Research and Development Service CIN 13-416, Richard L. Roudebush VA Medical Center, Indianapolis, IN

Karen Eden Department of Medical Informatics and Clinical Epidemiology, Oregon Health & Science University, and the Pacific Northwest Evidence-Based Practice Center, Portland, OR

Sue S. Feldman University of South Carolina, Arnold School of Public Health, Columbia, SC

Candace J. Gibson Department of Pathology and Laboratory Medicine, Schulich School of Medicine & Dentistry, The University of Western Ontario, London, Ontario, Canada

Paul Gorman Department of Medical Informatics and Clinical Epidemiology, Oregon Health & Science University, Portland, OR; Department of Medicine, Oregon Health & Science University, Portland, OR; and the Pacific Northwest Evidence-Based Practice Center, Portland, OR

Shaun J. Grannis Indiana University School of Medicine; and the Center for Biomedical Informatics, Regenstrief Institute, Inc., Indianapolis, IN

Steven D. Gravely Partner and Healthcare Practice Group Leader, Troutman Sanders LLP, Richmond, VA, USA

Saira N. Haque Center for the Advancement of Health IT, RTI International, Research Triangle Park, NC

William R. Hersh Department of Medical Informatics and Clinical Epidemiology, Oregon Health & Science University, Portland, OR; Department of Medicine, Oregon Health & Science University, Portland, OR; and the Pacific Northwest Evidence-Based Practice Center, Portland, OR

David Horrocks Chesapeake Regional Information System for our Patients (CRISP), Baltimore, MD

Masoud Hosseini Department of BioHealth Informatics, Indiana University School of Informatics and Computing; and the Center for Biomedical Informatics, Regenstrief Institute, Inc., Indianapolis, IN

Johan Ivar Sæbø Department of Informatics, University of Oslo, Norway

Bob Jolliffe Department of Informatics, University of Oslo, Norway

John P. Kansky Indiana Health Information Exchange, Indianapolis, IN

Andrew S. Kanter Department of Biomedical Informatics, Columbia University, New York, NY; and Intelligent Medical Objects, Inc., Northbrook, IL

Steven Z. Kassakian Department of Medical Informatics and Clinical Epidemiology, Oregon Health & Science University, and the Pacific Northwest Evidence-Based Practice Center, Portland, OR

Keith W. Kelley Indiana Health Information Exchange, Indianapolis, IN

Hadi Kharrazi Johns Hopkins School of Public Health, Department of Health Policy and Management, Center for Population Health IT (CPHIT); and the Johns Hopkins School of Medicine, Division of Health Sciences Informatics, Baltimore, MD

Carl Leitner IntraHealth International, Chapel Hill, NC

Erika G. Martin Nelson A. Rockefeller Institute of Government and Rockefeller College of Public Affairs and Policy, University at Albany, Albany, NY

Barbara Massoudi Center for the Advancement of Health IT, RTI International, Research Triangle Park, NC

Marian S. McDonagh Department of Medical Informatics and Clinical Epidemiology, Oregon Health & Science University, and the Pacific Northwest Evidence-Based Practice Center, Portland, OR

Timothy D. McFarlane Indiana University Richard M. Fairbanks School of Public Health, Indianapolis, IN

Nir Menachemi Indiana University Richard M. Fairbanks School of Public Health, Indianapolis, IN

J. Marc Overhage Cerner Corporation, Kansas City, MO

Miranda Pappas Department of Medical Informatics and Clinical Epidemiology, Oregon Health & Science University, and the Pacific Northwest Evidence-Based Practice Center, Portland, OR

Tim Pletcher Michigan Health Information Network Shared Services (MiHIN); and the Department of Learning Health Sciences, Medical School, University of Michigan, Ann Arbor, MI, USA

Saurabh Rahurkar Center for Biomedical Informatics, Regenstrief Institute, Inc., Indianapolis, IN

Dykki Settle PATH, Seattle, WA

Scott Teesdale InSTEDD

Eric Thieme Faegre Baker Daniels, Indianapolis, IN

Annette M. Totten Department of Medical Informatics and Clinical Epidemiology, Oregon Health & Science University, and the Pacific Northwest Evidence-Based Practice Center, Portland, OR

Joshua R. Vest Indiana University Richard M. Fairbanks School of Public Health; and the Center for Biomedical Informatics, Regenstrief Institute, Inc., Indianapolis, IN

Jonathan Weiner Johns Hopkins School of Public Health, Department of Health Policy and Management, Center for Population Health IT (CPHIT), Baltimore, MD

Susan S. Woods Department of Medical Informatics and Clinical Epidemiology, Oregon Health & Science University, and the Pacific Northwest Evidence-Based Practice Center, Portland, OR; Veterans Affairs Maine Healthcare System, Augusta, ME

Foreword

In the United States, most people receive health care in a variety of locations from a wide variety of health-care providers. In fact, American patients see an average of 18.7 different doctors during their lives, according to a survey conducted by GfK Roper [1]. For patients over 65 years of age, this average increases to 28.4 individual doctors, including primary care, specialists, hospital, and urgent care providers. To coordinate health-care delivery, providers need to communicate with each other. Without coordination, providers may prescribe medications that are contraindicated, duplicate lab tests or procedures, or they may be unaware of critical allergies or diagnoses. Unfortunately, patients are not always able to communicate critical, relevant health information to their providers.

Given the challenges of care coordination, health-care professionals desperately need relevant, timely and comprehensive information about their patients. To that end, physicians, nurses, and allied health professionals spend a significant proportion of their time collecting, processing, managing, and transmitting information across an array of sources that include the biomedical literature, colleagues, referral providers, caregivers, and patients.

Increasingly the capture, management, and sharing of information is facilitated by computers. Over the past two decades, the United States and other nations have developed and implemented electronic health record (EHR) systems in hospitals, clinics, and other care settings. Adoption of EHR systems by 2014 in the United States rose to over 75% among non-federal acute care hospitals and 51% of office-based physicians [2]. Yet while there now exist a plethora of information systems, many are silos unto themselves. In other words, many EHR systems and other forms of health information systems often fail the test of interoperability and only recently has this come to the attention of Congress and the nation.

To address the lack of interoperability among EHR systems, a portion of the American Recovery and Reinvestment Act of 2009 (ARRA) was allocated to states to begin the development of a health information exchange (HIE) infrastructure. HIE networks connect EHR systems together to create longitudinal patient records at the point of care. HIE networks therefore seek solutions to the problem of disparate health-care providers with siloed health records. Such networks, while not exactly a new concept, were challenging for states to formulate given issues with patient consent, competitive health-care systems, lack of technical standards, patient matching, HIE governance, data provenance, and technology costs.

Because of their complexity, HIE networks require highly skilled personnel to design, develop, implement, and manage them. A number of universities and other training programs are rapidly developing courses and curricula to train people to enter the field of health informatics and information management with a specialization in HIE [3].

The editor and authors of this book have organized a tremendous amount of knowledge and lessons on the design, development, implementation, use, evaluation, and management of HIE. The content in this book is comprehensive and will meet the needs of health information technology students as well as existing health IT professionals who seek to learn more about HIE. The insights provided by the case studies are particularly useful, especially for training individuals like myself to manage HIE efforts within a state as well as across a nation.

As the nation moves forward with HIE deployment, this book will surely provide guidance and inspiration for the next generation of health IT leaders who will indeed manage networks of health information systems that will support improvements in managing health information, health-care delivery processes, and outcomes for patients as well as populations.

References

[1] Practice Fusion. Survey: Patients See 18.7 Different Doctors on Average [Internet]. Available from: <http://www.practicefusion.com/pages/pr/survey-patients-see-over-18-different-doctors-on-average.html>; April 27, 2010 [accessed 28.10.15].

[2] DesRoches CM, Painter MW, Jha AK. Health information technology in the United States, 2015: transition to a Post-HITECH world. Robert Wood Johnson Foundation; 2015.

[3] Gibson CJ, Dixon BE, Abrams K. Convergent evolution of health information management and health informatics: a perspective on the future of information professionals in health care. Appl Clin Inform 2015;6(1):163–84.

Laura McCrary Ed.D.
Kansas Health Information Network, Inc.,
Topeka, KS, United States

Acknowledgments

I heartily thank all of the authors of the chapters contained within this book. Countless hours went into the drafting and revising of the material herein, and I thank the authors for sharing their knowledge and wisdom with the world. There would be no book without you.

In addition to the authors, I would like to acknowledge several individuals and organizations for their support in developing this book. I thank Emily Frederick of the Regenstrief Institute for her help in creating and tuning the resolution of images used in several chapters. I also thank Jennifer Williams and Lorinne Banister of the Regenstrief Institute for their help in recruiting and communicating with authors from the OpenHIE collaborative. I am indebted to the entire OpenHIE collaborative for not only agreeing to help coauthor several chapters but also in freely and graciously sharing their collective wisdom and resources on HIE. I am also grateful for all of the support from my colleagues at Indiana University and the Health Services Research & Development Service within the US Department of Veterans Affairs during the many months it took to put the book together.

Finally, I cannot express fully my love and gratitude for my wife Kathryn J. Dixon, M.Ed., and sons, William and Andrew, who supported me as there were several occasions when I had to miss out on family time to write or edit a chapter. Thank you for your endless love and support!

PART I

GETTING STARTED WITH HEALTH INFORMATION EXCHANGE

CHAPTER

1

What is Health Information Exchange?

Brian E. Dixon

Indiana University Richard M. Fairbanks School of Public Health; and the Center for Biomedical Informatics, Regenstrief Institute, Inc., Indianapolis, IN

OUTLINE

LEARNING OBJECTIVES

By the end of this chapter, the reader should be able to:

- Define the concept of health information exchange (HIE)
- Differentiate between the use of HIE as a noun and a verb
- Discuss the evolution of HIE and lessons from early HIE efforts
- Describe various forms of HIE commonly found in the United States
- List and describe the four core components of HIE
- Distinguish between HIE forms in the United States and those in other countries
- Identify the role that HIE plays in support a nation's eHealth strategy.

INTRODUCTION

Medicine, nursing, pharmacy, dentistry, and allied health professions are information-centric occupations [1,2]. Clinicians must navigate a large corpus of knowledge from the biomedical sciences and an endless stream of new facts, new treatments, and new diagnostic tools. Clinicians must further deal with information from an array of disparate sources, which they must process into decisions and prioritized tasks for the clinical team and patient [3–6]. Nonclinical roles must also review and input information about patients and populations to administer health care processes and organizations.

To support health care professionals in managing the array of information available about patients and populations, health systems have adopted and continue to incorporate a variety of information and communications technologies (ICT) into the delivery and administration of health care. Over the past decade, there has been a significant increase in the adoption and use of health ICT systems in the United States and Canada. National surveys in the US estimate adoption of basic electronic health record (EHR) systems to be near 40%, with adoption rates more than doubling from 2008 to 2012 [7–9]. In Canada, EHR adoption among primary care providers doubled from 23% in 2006 to 56% in 2012 [10]. Growth in adoption has been fueled by both policy, such as the Health Information Technology for Economic and Clinical Health (HITECH) Act [11,12] in the United States; Canadian federal investment in Canada Health Infoway and various provincial e-health initiatives [13]; and the belief that these ICT systems can improve the quality, safety, and efficiency of health services and delivery [14–16]. There is similar growth in adoption and use of ICT in other nations as well [17–19].

Although EHR systems and other forms of health ICT have been demonstrated to be effective at improving health care delivery and outcomes, isolated ICT systems cannot maximize health outcomes because health care delivery occurs within the context of a highly complex system. Patients receive care in a variety of care settings. While there exist a number of health systems that organize (and sometimes manage under an umbrella corporation) primary care, inpatient, laboratory, radiology, and pharmacy services, patients have flexibility in where they receive care. Researchers at the Regenstrief Institute found high levels of patient crossover among emergency departments within and between health system networks [20]. Using data from 96 emergency departments representing over 7.4 million visits and 2.8 million patients over a 3-year period, the researchers found that on average 40% of visits involved patients with data at more than one emergency department. At 15 emergency departments, more than half of their encounters involved patients with data in other health system EHR systems. Similar studies find that providers can only access some of their patients' information via their EHR system and therefore ICT systems need to be better connected [21,22]. Such fragmentation of information can occur during specific episodes of care, say when a Veteran is discharged from a non-Veterans hospital to a Veterans home, or over the course of the lifetime as patients receive health care for a wide variety of acute and chronic illness.

Because information exists within ICT "silos" managed by various actors within the health system, patients often become the primary method of information transfer between providers [23]. This is undesirable for many reasons, including but not limited inefficiency and the likelihood for error. For example, a recent study that validated parents' knowledge of their child's vaccination history found discrepancies in 13% of cases between what parents reported and what was recorded in an immunization information system [24]. To alleviate the burden placed on patients and improve efficiency in accessing information critical to care delivery, health systems establish information exchange between ICT systems. Health information exchange (HIE) enables more complete and timely sharing of data and information among ICT systems used in health care delivery, supporting provider and patient access to information when and where it is needed.

The purpose of this book is to provide a robust description of HIE, its various forms, its use around the world, its governance, and its technical design. Because HIE is critical to the success of health care improvement and reform in the United States and around the world, the book aims to inform those in clinical practice, health care administration and information technology about HIE and its role in supporting health systems. This chapter defines HIE then describes the evolution of it within the US health system. This chapter further discusses the rise of HIE in other countries and describes the various forms of HIE found in health systems around the world. The end of the chapter describes the goals and structure of the book, arming the reader with tools for applying the information to their profession.

HEALTH INFORMATION EXCHANGE

HIE is defined as the electronic transfer of clinical and/or administrative information across diverse and often competing health care organizations [25]. In practice, the term HIE is often used both as a *verb* and a *noun*.

HIE as a Verb

As a verb, or action word, HIE refers to movement of data or information electronically among stakeholders in the health care sector. The stakeholders are many in size and shape, including doctors' offices, hospitals, laboratories, payors (eg, insurance companies), pharmacies, urgent care centers, retail-based clinics, home health agencies, long-term postacute care facilities (eg, nursing homes), public health departments, federally qualified health centers, and/or mental health clinics. The information exchanged can range too, from a care plan to a summary of a visit to a laboratory result to a medical history. And while faxes are electronic forms of ICT thus technically HIE, most people tend to conceive of HIE as supporting efforts to move health care organizations away from faxing static, unstructured documents towards the exchange of digital, structured information that can be readily consumed and acted upon by computer systems (eg, semantic interoperability). Yet, as you will come to find out from information and examples in this book, many current forms of HIE occurring all over the world involve the transmission of largely unstructured information in the form of an electronic fax, PDF (Portable Document Format), or a dictated clinical report.

HIE as a Noun

The noun use of HIE refers to an organization, usually a legal corporation, that facilitates information exchange (the verb form) within a network of facilities, community, state, or region. While the exact form and composition of the entity or corporation varies, as you will note from reading the case studies, many communities are organizing HIE activities under an entity that can facilitate the trust, governance, and technical aspects of information sharing within an enterprise, community, state, or nation. This is because HIE involves sharing or transferring sensitive information about a person and most societies in the world value an individual's right to privacy. Therefore HIE occurs within a complex frame of not only multiple health care providers but also legal and regulatory policies that govern how health information should be protected as it is captured, stored, and shared. Sometimes a third-party corporation may be best suited to manage the human, regulatory, and technical aspects of data sharing as opposed to diffusing these responsibilities across a broad group of health care providers who wish to exchange information about their patients. In other instances, it may be a division of a hospital or network of health care facilities that need to facilitate the exchange of information among disparate, standalone ICT systems within an enterprise (eg, large tertiary care hospital, integrated delivery network, group of federally qualified health centers).

How HIE is Used in this Book

In this book we consider HIE principally as a verb, emphasizing the electronic exchange of data or information among various stakeholders within the health care system. However, because HIE is often facilitated in a community, state, or nation by an organization we will also refer to Health Information Organizations (HIOs) when speaking about the noun form of HIE. In putting the book together, we try to be consistent in the use of these two acronyms: HIE and HIO. However, we may occasionally get it wrong or mixed up. Spotting such mix-ups will be good practice for the real-world as you will encounter a variety of uses and terms when reading the sources referenced in the book as well as many other documents that discuss HIE in both the academic and gray literature.

Forms of Organized HIE

While HIE as a verb can exist in a wide variety of forms (eg, secure email of a document from a primary care physician to a specialist, secure file transfer from a hospital to a public health department containing preclinical diagnosis information for patients showing up at an emergency department), organized HIE activities in a geographic community by an HIO generally appears in four forms: Private HIE, Government-facilitated HIE, Community-based HIE, and Vendor-facilitated HIE. In the following sections we examine each form of HIE.

Private HIE

While there still exist many "independent" hospitals and physician practices (eg, management of the hospital or practice is solely performed by the physicians or CEO), many hospitals, physician practices, nursing homes, and even public health clinics operate as part of a larger corporation, referred to often as a health system. These systems can also be referred to by other names, including integrated delivery networks (IDNs) or accountable care organizations (ACOs). Because these health systems are composed of two or more hospitals, physician practices, or other care facilities, they have a need to exchange data and information among the network or group of affiliate organizations.

When a health system interconnects its affiliates, we refer to this as *Private HIE* because the exchange is only within the membership group. For example, the U.S. Department of Veterans Affairs (VA) operates 153 medical centers as well as 909 ambulatory care and community-based outpatient clinics across the United States and its territories. In the early 2000s, the VA interconnected its facilities using a software program referred to as VistaWeb. The software is an Internet-based viewer in which clinicians at the VA medical center in Indianapolis, IN, can access documents such as the discharge summary from the VA medical center in Palo Alto, CA, for a veteran who had a surgery in Palo Alto last year while visiting his grandchildren. This is private HIE, because the VA medical center cannot look up information on facilities outside the VA health system (although this is changing as described elsewhere in the book), only those facilities managed by the VA.

Government-Facilitated HIE

The HITECH Act provided not only eligible US hospitals and providers with incentives for adopting EHR systems but also funding for the Office of the National Coordinator for Health Information Technology (ONC) to stimulate HIE. Since March 2010, ONC has invested over $500 million in state-based HIE programs [26]. To apply for funding from ONC, each state needed to identify a state-designated entity (SDE) to receive and manage HIE efforts within the state. While some states designated entities such as quality improvement organizations or a single HIO within the state, most states elected to designate a state government agency (eg, Governor's office, Medicaid office) to receive and manage the funding given the close ties between HIE and the state's efforts to encourage EHR adoption among Medicaid providers. Although some of the state government agencies redistributed the funds to HIOs within the state to support local HIE efforts, many states created a state-level HIE effort. For example, in Michigan the state created the Michigan Health Information Network (MiHIN) Shared Services which is a collection of shared software and professional services at the state level. Qualified organizations, state agencies as well as private HIEs that demonstrate technical capability and execute the appropriate legal agreements can connect to MiHIN for a number of statewide HIE services such as public health reporting.

Thus when state governments or other publicly funded organizations act as either a statewide HIO or primary facilitator of HIE within state boundaries, we refer to this as government-facilitated HIE. This designation distinguishes these activities which are driven by very public and policy priorities (eg, alignment with Medicaid programs) from the efforts of private HIE which are usually driven by the priorities of a private health system. Government-facilitated HIE efforts are also unique in that they typically operate at a technical level that supports a "network of networks" in which data and information are "pushed" from provider A to provider B at a single point in time. However, the information pushed is not stored in a central data repository or retained by the state HIO. Such a model allows each state to have multiple HIOs that operate independently of the statewide network and focus on community-level HIE activities.

The former Nationwide Health Information Network (now referred to as the eHealth Exchange) is an example of a Government-facilitated HIE. The network was facilitated by the U.S. Federal government, which established a set of HIE services that could be leveraged to enable exchange of information among networks including Private HIE networks (eg, the Veterans Health Administration) and Community-based HIE networks [27]. Often one of the organizations involved in the HIE was a federal agency, such as the Social Security Administration (see Health Information Exchange—The Value Proposition: A Case Study of the US Social Security Administration). However, the network was also used for exchange of data that did not involve the federal government. In 2012, the network became a public–private partnership as the number of nongovernment networks expanded. Therefore today the eHealth Exchange would likely be characterized as a Community-based HIE even though it shares many similarities with the Government-facilitated type.

Community-Based HIE

Community-based HIE involves exchange of data and information among providers and health care organizations that may be marketplace competitors or otherwise unaffiliated, meaning they have no financial relationship with each other. For example, an academic medical center, large hospital system, and group of federally qualified health centers might agree to exchange data for better serving low-incoming populations in an urban area. While they compete in the marketplace, these organizations recognize they are better served through HIE because they routinely observe patient crossover, which can lead to repeating tests and procedures for patients who receive uncompensated care. If each organization became more aware of these patients' history, they might be able to save money while sparing patients from unnecessary care.

Typically community-based HIE efforts are facilitated by an HIO that operates within a specific geographic area (eg, city, county, state, region). Examples of community-based HIE include the Indiana Health Information Exchange in Indianapolis, IN (ihie.org); HealthBridge in Cincinnati, OH (healthbridge.org); and MedVirginia in Richmond, VA (medvirigina.net). Yet there exist national-level networks in which members span multiple, noncontiguous states. A key distinguishing feature of community-based HIE is that the HIO is driven by priorities set by its Board or governance group, which is often composed of Chief Information Officers (CIOs), ICT Directors, or Chief Medical Informatics Officers (CMIOs) at the various organizations that participate in the HIO. Sometimes HIOs can also have Board members from the larger community, including community foundation directors, elected officials, or large employers.

Vendor-Facilitated HIE

An emerging phenomenon is vendor-facilitated HIE, which is a hybrid between Government-facilitated and Community-based HIE. As the name implies, this form of HIE is facilitated by an EHR system vendor such as the Cerner Corporation (Kansas City, MO). Like the Government-facilitated form, the EHR vendor layers a set of HIE services on top of its EHR infrastructure, enabling its customers to send or receive information to other customers of that vendor's EHR system. And like the Community-based form, the vendor services enable exchange of information with hospitals and facilities outside a given integrated delivery network. Unlike a Community-based HIE, the vendor does not typically facilitate the governance structure of the exchange; it simply provides a technical pathway for HIE.

An example of this form of HIE is Care Everywhere™ from Epic Systems (Verona, WI). End users can click an "outside records" button while viewing a patient's chart. The clinician then searches for another institution part of the network (eg, another Epic customer). Once an institution is selected, the provider then searches for the patient within the EHR system of that institution. The provider then enters a reason for the query and completes an authorization form attesting to the need for the release of medical information. Finally, the information from the other EHR is available for viewing.

This form of HIE has been met with distrust because it usually requires the members of the network to be customers of the same EHR system vendor. However, in 2014 Epic announced that customers could also request information from non-Epic customers. Yet connecting to non-Epic customers is said to be more challenging, and non-Epic customers report connecting to Epic-based EHR systems is difficult [28]. Despite criticism, this form of HIE is emerging across a variety of vendor platforms.

Fundamental Components of HIE

Although there exist various forms and types of HIE, fundamentally there are just a few core components to any type of HIE. At a basic level, to conduct HIE, there must exist two health care actors with an established relationship that have a need to send or receive information about a patient or population. These components are illustrated in Fig. 1.1 and discussed later.

Health Care Actors and Relationships

In order for information to be exchanged, there needs to be a reason for conducting the

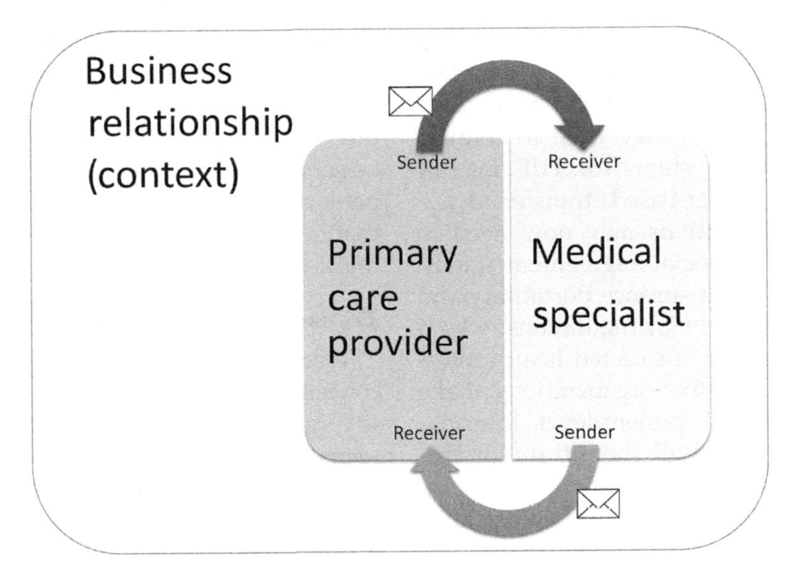

FIGURE 1.1 Graphical representation of the fundamental components of health information exchange. Information is exchanged in transactions between a sender and a receiver, and the exchange of information takes place within the context of a business relationship that governs the sharing of information between the two entities.

exchange. Therefore every form of HIE requires at least two actors who have an established relationship that facilitates HIE. Organizations have numerous, complex relationships to people and other organizations. For example, organizations employ people which creates a social contract in which employees perform duties in exchange for remuneration and other compensation (eg, health benefits, 401k plan). When organizations have relationships with other organizations, they often codify these through contracts or business associate agreements. Physician practices can have relationships with a hospital or health system that outlines things such as patient referrals and physician admitting privileges.

In many cases, the existing relationships between actors in health care provide a foundation for HIE. Suppose that Dr Smith works in his private physician practice on Mondays and Wednesdays and at the hospital outpatient clinic on Tuesdays and Thursdays. When a nurse at the practice calls Dr Smith while he is at the hospital clinic, he can relay information about a patient to the nurse he might be accessing via the hospital EHR system. Now if the nurse at the practice were to access the hospital EHR data directly from her desk without involving Dr Smith, this would probably be facilitated by private HIE, either through a portal into the hospital EHR system or a third-party software that connects the two ICT systems.

In other instances, organizations negotiate a specific data usage agreement (DUA) whereby one organization releases or exchanges data with another organization for an explicit purpose. Consider, for example, a community health system with four acute care hospitals and a long-term care provider with eight nursing homes. Although these organizations perform different health services in the community, they may wish to work together to create efficiencies during transfers of care (eg, which patient is discharged from the hospital to a nursing home). The organizations may enter into a transfer agreement which allows for the general transfer of patients and information when medical needs necessitate a transfer of care. However to improve efficiency, the organizations may wish to connect their respective ICT systems for HIE instead of relying upon paper-based transfer documents. These organizations may now need to execute a business associate agreement pursuant to HIPAA (Health Insurance Portability and Accountability Act of 1996) regulations, which govern the disclosure of protected health information. In doing so, the organizations make explicit what detailed patient-level information each organization will share through HIE between their respective ICT systems.

In either scenario, two or more actors have a relationship that underlies the need for exchange of information about patients or populations. Executing agreements and codifying relationships becomes more complex when there are greater than two actors, and managing many two-way relationships can be challenging. Managing relationships, agreements, and multiple actors is therefore a core function of HIE and HIOs, and the complexities often overshadow the technological methods by which data are exchanged between two or more actors. These challenges and models for facilitating multiple organization HIE are covered in greater detail later in the book.

ICT Systems

HIE as we have defined it necessitates electronic transfer between ICT systems. Therefore ICT systems need technical methods for facilitating exchange of information. In ICT speak, there must be a *sender* and a *receiver*. For example, a laboratory information system (LIS) *sends* lab test results to an EHR system to record the results in a patient's records. Yet an LIS can also *receive* an order to perform a lab test from an EHR system. These electronic transactions provide the technical foundation for HIE. Almost any ICT system in health care can be either a sender or a receiver depending on the scenario. Therefore the potential configuration of technical networks involving ICT is many. Regardless of which ICT systems are involved in HIE or the direction in which information flows, there will be senders and receivers. Several chapters in the book describe in greater detail the technologies that support sending and receiving health information among networks of ICT systems.

Transactions or Messages

Electronic transactions in health care can be conceived of as messages between two people or organizations. In the physical world, messages take the form of envelopes and packages. Envelopes and packages come in all shapes, sizes, and weights. So do electronic transactions. For example, electronically transmitting information that a particular patient has arrived at the clinic and is waiting to see the doctor is akin to putting a single, small piece of paper into a small envelope. Exchanging a discharge summary is like sending a multiple page document in a large envelope. This transaction requires additional "overhead" or structure so that the receiving ICT system can interpret the information inside the envelope. Still greater requirements are needed for the exchange of an MRI scan which includes large, detailed images. A special envelope would be necessary to protect the image from getting bent or damaged in transit. Similarly, ICT systems would require a specialized, structured message and sufficient storage as well as transport capacity for transferring the MRI images. Specialized, structured messages are referred to in the HIE world as technical standards. When ICT systems can send and receive messages, we say they can interoperate or possess interoperability. The book contains several chapters that explain the technical standards that enable the various kinds of messages to be sent and received by health ICT systems.

Content or Payload

Inside of messages are contents—patient demographics, lab results, images. ICT speak sometimes refers to contents as payloads. While in transit from one ICT system to another, the technologies that facilitate the transport do not care about the contents inside the message. However, for the information exchanged to be stored and used by the receiving ICT system (as well as the system's users—humans), ICT systems need methods for understanding the message contents. In HIE we refer to these methods as data standards, which we say create semantic interoperability between ICT systems. This book is full of examples and a couple chapters that illustrate the importance of data standards and the need for semantic interoperability.

EVOLUTION OF HIE

The concept of HIE has been around for more than 25 years. In the 1990s, the John A. Hartford Foundation began a Community Health Management Information System (CHMIS) initiative aimed at improving access to data in support of cost and quality improvement [29]. The idea was to support integrated delivery networks' access to information by engaging health care stakeholders (the members of the network) to electronically exchange transactions that would feed central data repositories. Large investments were made in several states to form what became known as CHINs (Community Health Information Networks). Despite many intellectually supporting the notion of a CHIN [30], most CHINs failed due to a number of reasons, including:

1. Lack of Stakeholder Engagement: Most CHINs did not create shared mission that all stakeholders could rally around. In many markets, the competitive nature overshadowed the weak or poorly conceived mission of the CHIN.
2. Command and Control: Stakeholders, especially providers outside the IDN, often perceived the IDN or health system to be in control of the centralized repository, which bred fear in highly competitive markets. Vendors also "pushed" their proprietary technology platform from the beginning, creating skepticism among the health care executives. A general lack of control ensued and thus no one was really in charge.
3. Unclear Value Proposition: From the beginning, CHIN developers asserted that stakeholders would see benefits after the development and usage of the CHIN. However, stakeholders were not provided with clear evidence or information on the value-add of the CHIN. Quickly the stakeholders lost interest in continuing to finance the CHIN when they could not perceive value to their organization.
4. Infrastructure Woes: Many CHINs aimed to create a large, common data repository into which stakeholders would put claims, encounter data, problem lists, medications, etc. However, the Internet did not yet exist so it was difficult (and expensive) to "wire" all of the stakeholders and create a sufficient infrastructure. Furthermore, the politics of a single data "pot" further exacerbated fears over control.

On the heels of the CHINs, a number of communities began to develop a Local Health Information Infrastructure (LHII). Whereas the CHINs focused on supporting exchange of data to meet the needs of IDNs facilitating managed care, LHIIs focused on clinician-driven, community-wide initiatives focused in scope. For example, providers in the Indianapolis area desired to share information among emergency departments in support of transitions of care [30]. In addition, LHIIs focused on first developing stakeholder engagement rather than jumping directly into discussions around the design of the technical architecture. Emphasis was placed on building trust and establishing a strong, shared vision for what services the LHII would provide and for whom they would be provided. In addition, LHIIs seemed to incorporate a few other factors that resulted in greater success over their CHIN predecessors:

1. Clear Control from a Neutral Third Party: Successful LHIIs engaged a neutral, respected organization to take ownership of community engagement activities. In Indianapolis, it was a health services research organization affiliated with the medical school. In Santa Barbara, CA, it was a regional health plan. These parties helped facilitate dialogue, establish trust among the partners, and mobilize leaders without appearing biased towards a particular vendor, platform or the IDN.
2. Involvement of Public Health: Early LHIIs engaged public health authorities. Sometimes the health department served as the trusted neutral party. In other instances, the LHII simply brought knowledge and experience in coalition building around a health issue to the group.
3. Communication and Change Management: The LHIIs paid particular attention to keeping stakeholders "in the loop," even though it meant many hours of meetings and phone calls for the leadership and managing partner. However, strong communication allowed for reiteration of reasonable expectations and kept committees and volunteers focused.
4. Attention to Legal and Financial Barriers: LHII leadership spent significant time discussing and developing strategies for overcoming both legal issues as well as the plan for sustaining data exchange after a period of initial investment.

Although arguably more successful than the CHINs, many LHIIs also failed to become fully operational or sustain operations [31]. Yet their failures and successes proved to be excellent lessons for the next generation of HIE organizations—the Regional Health Information Organizations (RHIOs). RHIOs emerged about 10 years ago to tackle the very thorny issue of sustainability. Whereas the LHIIs emphasized "local" by engaging stakeholders in a city or county, RHIOs aimed to become regional HIE authorities. The idea was that HIE might not be sustainable on a small scale but would be sustainable with economies of scale across an entire state or group of states. Several RHIOs were funded through grants by the Agency for Healthcare Research and Quality [32–34]. Using the funding, the RHIOs aimed to not only become operational but also develop the business case for HIE [35]. Surveys from the late 2000s by the eHealth Initiative found that over 100 communities reported they were in various stages of developing an RHIO [36,37]. Yet, like many LHIIs, many RHIOs failed for similar reasons as their antecedents [38,39]. As many as 25% of efforts identified in the previous year's survey would simply vanish when community efforts were surveyed the following year.

In the past few years, since the passage of the HITECH Act, HIE has received a large investment from the US government. Funding to create statewide HIE efforts pushed the industry to drop the "R" from RHIO. Furthermore, emerging HIOs began to diversify with respect to form (eg, centralized data repository), technology platform (eg, push, pull), and governance. While some focused on supporting IDNs, others focused on creating "networks of networks" in which HIE could be performed by a wider array of local, regional, and national-level stakeholders. National-level HIE efforts emerged, including the eHealth Exchange [40] that seeks to connect state and regional HIE initiatives with federal government agencies as well as national data networks such as SureScripts, LLC. The landscape changed rapidly, yet the core lessons or principles of the CHINs and LHIIs remain. HIOs must establish value quickly and effectively to stakeholders to generate sustainable revenue streams in order to grow towards achieving a shared vision.

MODELS OF HIE IN THE UNITED STATES

Over the years three models of HIE have been developed and tested in the United States. Early efforts at HIE as described earlier sought to create a **centralized** form whereby data from all hospitals, clinics, and other health care stakeholders are captured and maintained centrally in a single data repository. Later HIEs developed more **federated** models wherein data are captured and maintained separately within disparate hospital, clinic, and other data repositories then queried on demand when they are needed for individual care or a population level analysis. A final form of HIE is **patient controlled** wherein the health system relies upon patients to collect their data as they seek care and share it with future providers using either physical devices or virtual health records.

Centralized

In a centralized model, HIE participants agree to deposit their data, or a copy of their data, into a single, shared health record. The shared EHR is most often instantiated as a monolithic database although other technical implementations have evolved over time (eg, cloud storage). This model entrusts a single custodian, such as the RHIO, to be the steward of the data. Stakeholders agree upon a single method for uniquely identifying patients or clients so that longitudinal health records can be constructed. Similarly, stakeholders agree to use the same codes and identifiers for other data such as lab tests, medication orders, and clinical notes.

The earliest forms of HIE such as the CHINs sought to use the centralized model. While the model has advantages such as a single identifier for a client, normalized terminologies for clinical data and a single source of data about clinical encounters, it also has some limitations. First, centralized models do not scale well. Back in the 1990s, in the days before cloud-based storage, monolithic database management systems did not easily grow beyond a few gigabytes in size. While technically we can scale data storage in the 21st century, centralized models still require a robust architecture in the center of the HIE where the data are stored (eg, at the RHIO). Technical services are necessary to process all of the incoming data and store them in a normalized fashion so they can be used consistently across all of the participants and applications (eg, patient lookup, analytics dashboards). Furthermore, centralized models usually require stakeholder consensus on patient identification and data representation schemes that will be used consistently in the shared health record. This can be politically challenging since each stakeholder will naturally desire to continue to use their own methods for identifying patients and coding clinical services, results and outcomes.

Federated

Whereas centralized models focus on building a shared health record that is centrally maintained by an RHIO, federated models seek to develop a distributed network of health records that are accessed *on demand* or when they are needed for individual care or population analysis. In a federated model, data remain at their source (eg, hospital, clinic) until they are needed. A shared health record is created *virtually* with the help of a **record locator service (RLS)** that centrally links all records for a patient across the various HIE participants that have information on that individual. The RLS is like an enormous card catalogue that guides computer applications and information systems to the information they may be seeking about a patient. While the RLS naturally needs to know some information about patients in order to link their records, the RLS does not store any clinical information about them.

In many ways, federated models are in direct contrast to centralized models, and they evolved as HIE participants became wary of centralizing data in a CHIN. Because of their design, federated models tend to scale better than centralized models because new participants can be added to the network with less effort (it is still not easy). Furthermore, the technical infrastructure to be maintained by the RHIO or data intermediary is more limited making it potentially less costly to maintain a federated model. Yet federated models also have limitations. Queries across the distributed network can be slower than centralized models, because the query must be sent to all nodes on the network and responses must be gathered, reconciled, and normalized or else clinician end users will receive multiple results or documents that must be manually examined akin to reviewing stacks of paper charts. Therefore the applications that consume information from the HIE network must be able to, or remotely call, services that can perform tasks such as data reduction or reconciliation across multiple documents.

Over time there has evolved two subtypes of federated models. The subtype *inconsistent* adheres most to the general definition of federated networks. The data and information systems at the edges of the network are completely independent from one another, and when data are queried they have to be normalized to some degree before they can be digested into an EHR system or rendered for display to a clinical end user. The inconsistency term is used because the data, their structure, and their management are diffuse and vary by the HIE participant. The other subtype is consistent, in which the data are managed in distinct silos but adhere to some common data model prescribed by the HIE intermediary that operates the RLS.

Inconsistent Federated Models

When data are free to be stored and managed using any data schema preferred by the hospital, clinic, or health system that captures them, we refer to this as an inconsistent federated model. This form of HIE scales well because new HIE participants can technically be deployed quickly because the data can be of any size, shape, or variety. However, this model presents a challenge when queried because the services that consume the data must reconcile potentially wildly different data representations and types. Few HIE networks have had success in deploying this model, because they have all realized at some point one must reconcile the messy data generated by health care processes and this is difficult to do unless one can achieve consensus around a common data model [41].

Consistent Federated Models

In this form of HIE, data from each HIE participant are segmented from one another (eg, no monolithic database) yet they are stored using a common data model [42]. The data model prescribes which data are to be available to the HIE network, and it defines *a priori* the relationships between how the data reside in the source EHR or information system and common concepts such as height, weight, and blood pressure, that are to be shared with other HIE participants. In some ways, this model can be perceived as a hybrid approach between the centralized and federated models. This model has been used successfully by a number of HIE networks in the United States, including the Indiana Health Information Exchange and the New York City Primary Care Information Project. The same model has been used successfully for distributing queries across EHR systems in support of quality measurement and research [43,44].

Patient Controlled

In contrast to the centralized and federated models of HIE, in which the principal design is HIE between providers and other health system stakeholders, patient-controlled or "consumer-mediated" forms of HIE have been proposed. In patient-controlled forms of HIE, health care consumers are responsible for either (1) depositing their health records into consumer-controlled data repositories referred to as "health record banks" [45] or (2) downloading their medical records onto secure disk drives or "smart cards" that can be carried with them as they traverse the health system. Because in the United States, patients are provided access to copies of their records under HIPAA, patient-controlled HIE advocates argue that consumers should be able to gather their records and manage them in the same way that individuals manage their bank records and car maintenance logs. Although technical designs exist for both health record bank and health smart card models [46], there have been few trials and pilot projects of them in the United States. While these approaches have an advantage of being patient-centered meaning patients would be in control of their data, critics argue that such models face a number of challenges including cost, sustainability, and scalability similar to other HIE approaches [47].

HIE OUTSIDE THE UNITED STATES

The concept of HIE is not uniquely American, nor does the United States have the largest volumes of HIE activity in the world. There exists quite a lot of exciting HIE activities all over the world [48,49], including low and middle income countries (LMICs). What distinguishes international HIE activities from those in the United States is often the definition or perception of what constitutes HIE. For example, most HIOs in the United States conceive HIE often as a broad set of services or functions that facilitate specific transactions in which information is exchanged for a defined purpose (eg, results delivery, referral, discharge summary). In many countries, HIE is conceived more as a national-level, patient-centric EHR or a longitudinal record of care received by a person over his or her lifetime. Thus many of the HIE functions defined and discussed in the United States occur in other countries through provincial or national health authorities rather than private health systems, and rarely are they defined explicitly as HIE.

In 2014, Adler-Milstein et al. [50] published as comparison of case studies from seven Organisation for Economic Co-operation and Development (OECD) countries: Australia, Canada, Denmark, England, Finland, the Netherlands, and the United States. In each case study, the authors examined how nations defined HIE in addition to telehealth, provider-centric electronic records, and patient-centric electronic records. In four countries (Australia, Canada, England, and the Netherlands), HIE was defined at the national level as a national eHealth record (or Summary Care Record) which centrally holds or links out to data for a given individual over the course of his or her lifetime. Denmark defined HIE as principally a method for securely sharing messages (eg, secure email) between physicians and hospitals; and Finland did not yet have a national definition of HIE. In this same study, the US concept of HIE was defined as all electronic information transactions which supported interactions between health care professionals and organizations for patient care. Although true, this definition in the United States is not quite accurate because it neglects to account for population or public health functions, including but not limited to monitoring of disease burden within a population, prediction of risk for a given disease within a population, and postmarketing surveillance of pharmaceutical treatments.

In 2012, the World Health Organization (WHO) published a National eHealth Strategy Toolkit [51] which supports nation level establishment of a roadmap and action plan for the adoption of health ICT as well as HIE. Although the explicit term HIE is only mentioned a couple times in the "Infrastructure" section, the report nonetheless guides ministries of health towards planning for the exchange of data and information between ICT systems they implement. For example, the WHO suggests that the critical components of a national eHealth environment [51] include:

1. Infrastructure: The foundations for electronic information exchange across geographical and health-sector boundaries. This includes physical infrastructure (eg, networks), core services, and applications that underpin a national eHealth environment.
2. Standards and Interoperability: ICT standards that enable consistent and accurate collection and exchange of health information across health systems and services.

The toolkit and subsequent follow up from the WHO eHealth Technical Advisory Group [52] are driving creation and adoption of national eHealth strategies. Activities in multiple nations supported the development of a Community of Practice (CoP) in which members share knowledge as well as standards-based approaches and reference technologies for facilitating HIE. This initiative, known as OpenHIE (www.ohie.org), seeks "to improve the health of the underserved through the open collaborative development and support of country driven, large-scale health information sharing architectures." Currently OpenHIE has implementations in six nations, including the Philippines, Sierra Leone, Bangladesh, South Africa, Tanzania, and Rwanda (Fig. 1.2).

PURPOSE AND STRUCTURE OF THIS BOOK

The purpose of this book is to cover the landscape of HIE for those in health care

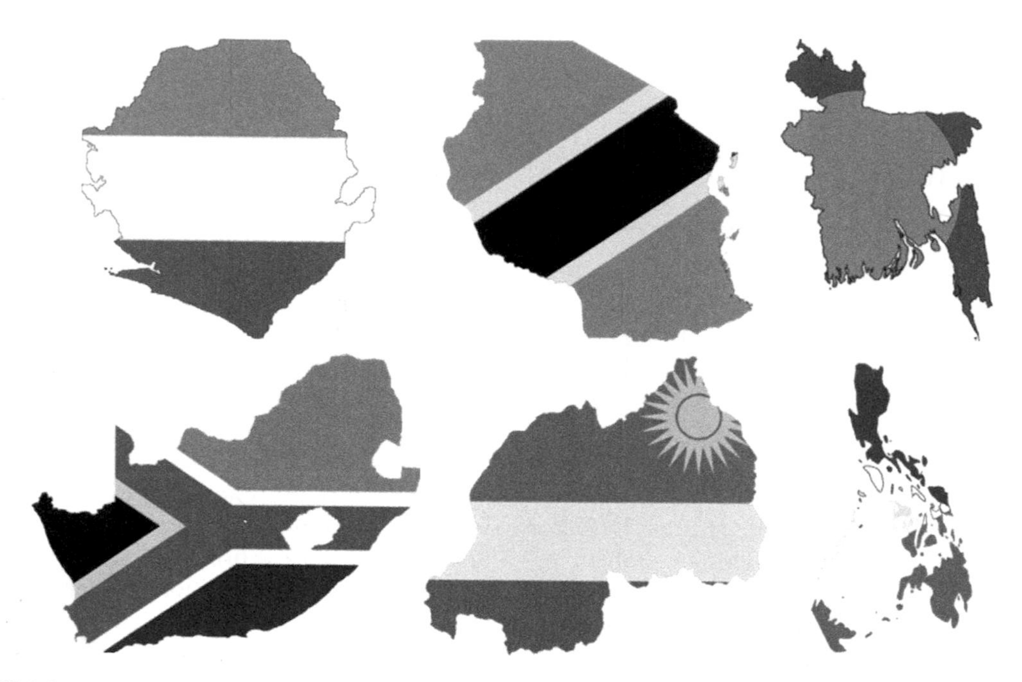

FIGURE 1.2 Graphical representation of the six countries that have implemented or are in the process of implementing OpenHIE components to facilitate HIE within their health systems.

administration, health ICT, and public health. While there exist a number of peer-reviewed articles, whitepapers, and webinars on HIE, to date there has been little comprehensive information on the various dimensions of HIE. As already alluded in this chapter, HIE is much more than simply connecting ICT systems together using hardware and software. The various information sources on HIE to date provide snapshots of these dimensions, analyzing a technical method, legal framework, or governance model. In this book, we put the dimensions together as a reference for those studying or practicing HIE.

This book is divided into multiple sections that provide in-depth coverage of HIE and its dimensions. This first section provides an overview of HIE as a specialized field of study and practice within the larger profession of health ICT or informatics. The following section introduces readers to the organizational and managerial aspects of HIE. Then this book covers the technical aspects in the third section. The fourth section describes the current evidence base for HIE and techniques for evaluating its outcomes, important for growing the evidence base. In the fifth section, this book summarizes and looks ahead to the future of HIE. At the end of the book, the reader will find a collection of case studies in HIE from leading HIOs and researchers that illustrate the various dimensions, forms, and aspects of HIE. At the end of this book, the reader should have a firm grasp on both the complexities involved in HIE and information critical for forging a strategy for developing, implementing, and/or managing HIE activities in their own organization or community.

SUMMARY

Given rapid adoption of ICT systems in health care organizations around the world, it is quickly becoming apparent that HIE is necessary to realize the full value of health ICT. Yet HIE is complex and challenging, requiring not only robust technical standards but also legal, regulatory, and policy frameworks that facilitate (or at least don't prevent) HIE. Exchange of information also requires trust and strong relationships among health care organizations and their leaders. This book provides information on the foundations and nature of HIE as well as guidance on how to manage HIE within a complex environment, be that a health system or nation.

QUESTIONS FOR DISCUSSION

1. Compare and contrast the various forms of HIE. Which form might be most advantageous for an Accountable Care Organization? Which form might be best for a public health agency?
2. Which lesson from the CHINs and LHIIs is most important to modern HIE initiatives?
3. Do the requirements for HIE in "meaningful use" program make building a value proposition for HIE easier or more difficult? Why?
4. Under what conditions would it make sense to use a patient-controlled form of HIE as opposed to a federated or centralized approach?
5. How do the definitions of HIE vary around the world? Why might HIE be implemented differently in a country outside the United States?

References

[1] Krumholz HM. Big data and new knowledge in medicine: the thinking, training, and tools needed for a learning health system. Health Aff (Project Hope) 2014;33(7):1163–70. PubMed PMID: 25006142. Epub July 10, 2014.

[2] McGowan JJ, Passiment M, Hoffman HM. Educating medical students as competent users of health information technologies: the MSOP data. Stud Health

Technol Inform 2007;129(Pt 2):1414–8. PubMed PMID: 17911947. Epub October 4, 2007.

[3] Singh H, Spitzmueller C, Petersen NJ, Sawhney MK, Sittig DF. Information overload and missed test results in electronic health record-based settings. JAMA Intern Med 2013;173(8):702–4. PubMed PMID: 23460235. Epub March 6, 2013.

[4] Markman M. Information overload in oncology practice and its potential negative impact on the delivery of optimal patient care. Curr Oncol Rep 2011;13(4):249–51. PubMed PMID: 21559791. Epub May 12, 2011.

[5] Zeldes N, Baum N. Information overload in medical practice. J Med Pract Manag 2011;26(5):314–6. PubMed PMID: 21595388. Epub May 21, 2011.

[6] Bernard E, Arnould M, Saint-Lary O, Duhot D, Hebbrecht G. Internet use for information seeking in clinical practice: a cross-sectional survey among French general practitioners. Int J Med Inform 2012;81(7):493–9. PubMed PMID: 22425281. Epub March 20, 2012.

[7] Desroches CM, Charles D, Furukawa MF, Joshi MS, Kralovec P, Mostashari F, et al. Adoption of electronic health records grows rapidly, but fewer than half of US Hospitals had at least a basic system in 2012. Health Aff (Project Hope) 2013;32(8):1478–85. PubMed PMID: 23840052. Epub July 11, 2013.

[8] Furukawa MF, Patel V, Charles D, Swain M, Mostashari F. Hospital electronic health information exchange grew substantially in 2008–12. Health Aff (Project Hope) 2013;32(8):1346–54. PubMed PMID: 23918477. Epub August 7, 2013.

[9] Patel V, Jamoom E, Hsiao CJ, Furukawa MF, Buntin M. Variation in electronic health record adoption and readiness for meaningful use: 2008–2011. J Gen Intern Med 2013 PubMed PMID: 23371416. Epub February 2, 2013.

[10] Canada Health Infoway The emerging benefits of electronic medical record use in community-based care Ontario, Canada. : PwC 2013 [cited June 13, 2014]. Available from: http://www.pwc.com/ca/en/healthcare/electronic-medical-record-use-community-based-care.jhtml.

[11] Centers for Medicare and Medicaid Services Meaningful use. Baltimore, MD: Centers for Medicare & Medicaid Services; 2013. [updated Aug 23; cited August 27, 2013]. Available from: https://www.cms.gov/Regulations-and-Guidance/Legislation/EHRIncentivePrograms/Meaningful_Use.html.

[12] Furukawa MF, Poon E. Meaningful use of health information technology: evidence suggests benefits and challenges lie ahead. Am J Manag Care 2011;17(12) SP76a-SP. PubMed PMID: 22216771. Epub June 27, 2012.

[13] Canada Health Infoway. Progress in Canada [cited June 13, 2014]. Available from: https://www.infoway-inforoute.ca/index.php/progress-in-canada.

[14] Whipple EC, Dixon BE, McGowan JJ. Linking health information technology to patient safety and quality outcomes: a bibliometric analysis and review. Inform Health Soc Care 2013;38(1):1–14. PubMed PMID: 22657387. Epub June 5, 2012.

[15] Blaya JA, Fraser HS, Holt B. E-health technologies show promise in developing countries. Health Aff (Project Hope) 2010;29(2):244–51. PubMed PMID: 20348068. Epub March 30, 2010.

[16] Bates DW, Gawande AA. Improving safety with information technology. N Engl J Med 2003;348(25):2526–34. PubMed PMID: 12815139. Epub June 20, 2003.

[17] Kyratsis Y, Ahmad R, Holmes A. Technology adoption and implementation in organisations: comparative case studies of 12 English NHS Trusts. BMJ Open 2012;2(2):e000872. PubMed PMID: 22492183. PMCID: 3329608. Epub April 12, 2012.

[18] Lewis T, Synowiec C, Lagomarsino G, Schweitzer J. E-health in low- and middle-income countries: findings from the Center for Health Market Innovations. Bull World Health Organ 2012;90(5):332–40. PubMed PMID: 22589566. PMCID: 3341696. Epub May 17, 2012.

[19] Abraham C, Nishihara E, Akiyama M. Transforming healthcare with information technology in Japan: a review of policy, people, and progress. Int J Med Inform 2011;80(3):157–70. PubMed PMID: 21292546. Epub February 5, 2011.

[20] Finnell JT, Overhage JM, Grannis S. All health care is not local: an evaluation of the distribution of emergency department care delivered in indiana. AMIA Annu Symp Proc 2011;2011:409–16. PubMed PMID: 22195094. PMCID: 3243262. Epub December 24, 2011.

[21] Schoen C, Osborn R, Squires D, Doty M, Pierson R, Applebaum S. New 2011 survey of patients with complex care needs in eleven countries finds that care is often poorly coordinated. Health Aff (Project Hope) 2011;30(12):2437–48. PubMed PMID: 22072063. Epub November 11, 2011.

[22] Hammond WE, Bailey C, Boucher P, Spohr M, Whitaker P. Connecting information to improve health. Health Aff (Project Hope) 2010;29(2):284–8. PubMed PMID: 20348075. Epub March 30, 2010.

[23] Gaglioti A, Cozad A, Wittrock S, Stewart K, Lampman M, Ono S, et al. Non-VA primary care providers' perspectives on comanagement for rural veterans. Mil Med 2014;179(11):1236–43. PubMed PMID: 25373047. Epub November 6, 2014.

[24] MacDonald SE, Schopflocher DP, Golonka RP. The pot calling the kettle black: the extent and type of errors

in a computerized immunization registry and by parent report. BMC Pediatr 2014;14:1. PubMed PMID: 24387002. PMCID: 3880846. Epub January 7, 2014.

[25] Dixon BE, Zafar A, Overhage JM. A framework for evaluating the costs, effort, and value of nationwide health information exchange. J Am Med Inform Assoc 2010;17(3):295–301. PubMed PMID: 20442147. PMCID: 2995720. Epub May 6, 2010.

[26] Office of the National Coordinator for Health Information Technology State Health Information Exchange Cooperative Agreement Program. Washington, DC: U.S. Department of Health & Human Services; 2014. [updated April 14, 2014; cited May 7, 2015]. Available from: http://healthit.gov/policy-researchers-implementers/state-health-information-exchange.

[27] Department of Health & Human Services,.US Nationwide Health Information Network (NwHIN) [cited February 21, 2013]. Available from: http://www.healthit.gov/policy-researchers-implementers/nationwide-health-information-network-nwhin; 2013.

[28] Leventhal R. KLAS report: epic to non-epic data sharing is real, but challenging. Healthcare Informatics 2014 [cited May 19, 2015]. Available from: http://www.healthcare-informatics.com/news-item/klas-report-epic-non-epic-data-sharing-real-challenging.

[29] Rubin RD. The community health information movement: where it's been, where it's going O'Carroll PW, Yasnoff WA, Ward ME, Ripp LH, Martin EL, editors. Public health informatics and information systems: Springer-Verlag; 2002. p. 595–616.

[30] Lorenzi NM. U.S. Department of Health and Human Services Strategies for creating successful local health information infrastructure initiatives. Washington, DC: Assistant Secretary for Policy and Evaluation; 2003.

[31] Miller RH, Miller BS. The Santa Barbara county care data exchange: what happened? Health Aff (Project Hope) 2007;26(5):w568–80. PubMed PMID: 17670775. Epub August 3, 2007.

[32] Nocella KC, Horowitz KJ, Young JJ. Against all odds: designing and implementing a grassroots, community-designed RHIO in a rural region. J Healthc Inf Manag 2008;22(2):34–41. PubMed PMID: 19266993. Epub March 10, 2009.

[33] Frisse ME, King JK, Rice WB, Tang L, Porter JP, Coffman TA, et al. A regional health information exchange: architecture and implementation. AMIA Annu Symp Proc 2008:212–6. PubMed PMID: 18999138. PMCID: 2655967. Epub November 13, 2008.

[34] Dixon BE, Welebob EM, Dullabh P, Samarth A, Gaylin D. Summary of the Status of Regional Health Information Exchanges (RHIOs) in the United States. Rockville, MD: Agency for Healthcare Research and Quality; 2007. [May 15, 2009]. Available from: http://healthit.ahrq.gov/portal/server.pt/gateway/PTARGS_0_3882_813237_0_0_18/Summary%20of%20the%20Status%20of%20Regional%20Health%20Information%20Exchanges.pdf.

[35] Poon EG, Cusack CM, McGowan JJ. Evaluating healthcare information technology outside of academia: observations from the national resource center for healthcare information technology at the Agency for Healthcare Research and Quality. J Am Med Inform Assoc 2009;16(5):631–6. PubMed PMID: 19567800. PMCID: 2744713. Epub July 2, 2009.

[36] eHealth Initiative Results of 2009 Survey on health information exchange: state of the field. Washington, DC: eHealth Initiative; 2009. [cited March 22, 2010]. Available from: http://www.ehealthinitiative.org/results-2009-survey-health-information-exchange.html.

[37] eHealth Initiative. The State of Health Information Exchange in 2010: Connecting the Nation to Achieve Meaningful Use Washington, DC; 2010 [cited September 29, 2010]. Available from: http://ehealthinitiative.org/uploads/file/Final%20Report.pdf.

[38] Adler-Milstein J, Bates DW, Jha AKUS. Regional health information organizations: progress and challenges. Health Aff (Project Hope) 2009;28(2):483–92. PubMed PMID: 19276008. Epub March 12, 2009.

[39] Adler-Milstein J, McAfee AP, Bates DW, Jha AK. The state of regional health information organizations: current activities and financing. Health Aff (Project Hope) 2008;27(1):w60–9. PubMed PMID: 18073225. Epub December 13, 2007.

[40] Healtheway. Home 2012 [cited February 6, 2013]. Available from: http://www.healthewayinc.org/.

[41] Overhage JM, Ryan PB, Reich CG, Hartzema AG, Stang PE. Validation of a common data model for active safety surveillance research. J Am Med Inform Assoc 2012;19(1):54–60. PubMed PMID: 22037893. PMCID: 3240764. Epub November 1, 2011.

[42] Zafar A, Dixon BE. Pulling back the covers: technical lessons of a real-world health information exchange. Stud Health Technol Inform 2007;129(Pt 1):488–92. PubMed PMID: 17911765. Epub October 4, 2007.

[43] Klann JG, Murphy SN. Computing health quality measures using informatics for integrating biology and the bedside. J Med Internet Res 2013;15(4):e75. PubMed PMID: 23603227. PMCID: 3636801. Epub April 23, 2013.

[44] Klann JG, McCoy AB, Wright A, Wattanasin N, Sittig DF, Murphy SN. Health care transformation through collaboration on open-source informatics projects: integrating a medical applications platform, research data repository, and patient summarization. Interact J Med Res 2013;2(1):e11. PubMed PMID: 23722634. PMCID: 3668611. Epub June 1, 2013.

[45] Yasnoff WA, Shortliffe EH. Lessons learned from a health record bank start-up. Methods Inf Med 2014;53(2):66–72. PubMed PMID: 24477917. Epub January 31, 2014.

[46] Kardas G, Tunali ET. Design and implementation of a smart card based healthcare information system. Comput Methods Programs Biomed 2006;81(1):66–78. PubMed PMID: 16356586. Epub December 17, 2005.

[47] Cimino JJ, Frisse ME, Halamka J, Sweeney L, Yasnoff W. Consumer-mediated health information exchanges: the 2012 ACMI debate. J Biomed Inform 2014;48:5–15. PubMed PMID: 24561078. Epub February 25, 2014.

[48] Park H, Lee SI, Hwang H, Kim Y, Heo EY, Kim JW, et al. Can a health information exchange save healthcare costs? Evidence from a pilot program in South Korea. Int J Med Inform 2015 PubMed PMID: 26048738. Epub June 7, 2015.

[49] Geissbuhler A. Lessons learned implementing a regional health information exchange in Geneva as a pilot for the Swiss national eHealth strategy. Int J Med Inform 2013;82(5):e118–24. PubMed PMID: 23332387. Epub January 22, 2013.

[50] Adler-Milstein J, Ronchi E, Cohen GR, Winn LA, Jha AK. Benchmarking health IT among OECD countries: better data for better policy. J Am Med Inform Assoc 2014;21(1):111–6. PubMed PMID: 23721983. PMCID: 3912720. Epub June 1, 2013.

[51] World Health Organization National eHealth strategy toolkit. Geneva, Switzerland: World Health Organization and International Telecommunication Union; 2012.

[52] World Health Organization. eHealth Technical Advisory Group 2015 [cited March 29, 2015]. Available from: http://www.who.int/ehealth/tag/en/.

CHAPTER

2

Health Information Exchange as a Profession

Candace J. Gibson[1]*, Kelly J. Abrams*[2] *and Tim Pletcher*[3]

[1]Department of Pathology and Laboratory Medicine, Schulich School of Medicine & Dentistry, The University of Western Ontario, London, Ontario, Canada [2]Canadian Health Information Management Association/Canadian College of Health Information Management, London, Ontario, Canada [3]Michigan Health Information Network Shared Services (MiHIN); and the Department of Learning Health Sciences, Medical School, University of Michigan, Ann Arbor, MI, USA

OUTLINE

LEARNING OBJECTIVES

By the end of the chapter the reader should be able to:

- Describe the different types of professionals needed to establish and work with electronic health records and link them in a health information exchange.
- Understand the current supply and demand for individuals in the eHealth workforce.
- Describe the routes for education, training, and credentialing of these professionals.
- Describe the specific roles and functions of health information exchange professionals.

INTRODUCTION

Great strides have been made in deploying and implementing electronic medical records (EMR)/patient records within physicians' offices [1–4] and health facilities [5–7] over the past decade. Practices that are part of an integrated delivery system or share resources with other clinicians have higher rates of EMR adoption, use of multifunctional health information technology (HIT), electronic health information exchange (HIE), and electronic access for patients [8], yet a high percentage of primary care physicians still reported that they did not routinely receive timely information from specialists or hospitals [1]. In 2012, nearly 6 in 10 hospitals actively exchanged electronic health information with providers and hospitals outside their organization, an increase of 41% since 2008 [7]. EHR adoption and HIE participation were associated with significantly greater hospital exchange activity, but exchanges with providers outside the organization and exchanges of clinical care summaries and medication lists remained limited [7]. We are still a long way from the goal of a truly interactive system in which many of these currently "siloed" systems become interoperable and fully able to exchange information securely and efficiently.

The Health Information Technology for Economic and Clinical Health (HITECH) Act of 2009, enacted as part of the American Recovery and Reinvestment Act (ARRA), was intended to promote the adoption and "meaningful use" of HIT and provide needed resources to build the national HIT infrastructure. HITECH provided incentives for EHR adoption, strengthened privacy, and security provisions of the Health Insurance Portability and Accountability Act (HIPAA) of 1996, provided technical assistance through regional extension centers and funded HIE communities [9,10]. In addition, the Patient Protection and Affordable Care Act (ACA) of 2010 fostered payment and delivery system reforms, with an increased focus on the patient-centered medical home, accountable care organizations (ACOs), and through the Health Center Network grants, support of the adoption and meaningful use of certified EHR technology and quality-improvement strategies in federally qualified health centers [10,11]. These policy initiatives and payment reforms are accelerating HIE by creating new data exchange options, defining standards for interoperability, and creating payment incentives for information sharing across organizational boundaries [7,8].

As we move past the tipping point and simple replacement of the paper record to a critical mass of electronic records and users, we increasingly run into a barrier due to the lack of adequately trained personnel. To realize fully operational EHRs and HIEs and their benefits, industry requires health professionals who are familiar with technology and information systems; data and information standards and interoperability across platforms; human factors and process engineering; and technology adoption and user-supporting mechanisms; methods of reengineering and project management; privacy and security of personal health information; the management of health information through its lifecycle; and the use of health data for optimization of health care delivery [12].

This chapter will outline the human resources needed to put an HIE in place and ensure that data are available for meaningful use and health system improvement. The chapter will provide an overview of the various types of eHealth workers needed, explain each profession's skill set and knowledge base, and define the new roles in HIE. Learning outcomes or competencies have been delineated by various professional associations and/or credentialing bodies. These competencies will be briefly presented along with the current credentials and their certifying bodies. A national human resources strategy is suggested to address the current shortage of skilled workers and to develop a long-term strategy for education and training of the necessary eHealth personnel to ensure the quality of health data collected, its security and confidentiality, interoperability of health information systems, and to manage and maintain health information organizations (HIOs) and exchanges in the future.

THE NATURE OF eHEALTH PROFESSIONALS: THEIR COMPETENCIES, ROLES, AND WORK

Who Are the eHealth Professionals?

Eysenbach [13] has defined eHealth as "an emerging field in the intersection of medical informatics, public health and business, referring to health services and information delivered or enhanced through the Internet and related technologies." He further describes the term as not only the information and communication technologies (ICTs), but the way of thinking and commitment to a networked community (be it local, regional, or global) to improve health care. Thus eHealth refers to the application of informatics concepts, methods, and tools to the health system and the people (providers, administrators, patients, and families) involved in it. As such, eHealth refers to the work of health informaticians, health information managers, health information technologists, and HIE professionals, as well as others [13].

Health Informaticians (HI Professionals)

Health informatics (HI) is the discipline that researches, formulates, designs, develops, implements, and evaluates information-related concepts, methods, and tools (eg, ICT) to support clinical care, research, health services administration, and education. Health informaticians are eHealth professionals who have become competent in the discipline of HI and thus deploy and use methods (eg, planning, management, analytic, and procedural) and tools (eg, information and communications systems) in support of health system processes. Generally speaking, health informaticians qualify for this designation by completion of a bachelor's degree in HI or another field, and/or an advanced degree in HI, or by achieving professional certification (eg, CPHIMS). HI professionals also exist within clinical specialties (eg, medicine, public health, nursing, dentistry, and pharmacy) and may have completed advanced informatics training following clinical education and/or several years of clinical practice. Samplings of HI job roles include health application designer or developer, change manager/workflow redesigner, data analyst, chief informatics officer, program evaluation specialist [12,14].

Health Information Managers (HIM Professionals)

Health Information Management (HIM) professionals are members of the eHealth team trained in the discipline of HIM [15,16]. The Canadian Health Information Management Association (CHIMA) defines HIM as the discipline that focuses on health care data and the management of health care information, regardless of the medium and format [15]. The American Health Information Management Association (AHIMA) defines health information management as the body of knowledge and practice that ensures the availability of health information to facilitate real-time health care delivery and critical health-related decision making for multiple purposes across diverse organizations, settings, and disciplines [16].

Research and practice in HIM address the nature, structure, and translation of data into usable forms of information for the advancement of health and health care of individuals and populations. HIM roles are described as health information managers, clinical data specialists, patient information coordinators, data quality managers, information security manager, data resource administrator, and research and decision support specialist. The HIM practice domains also broadly include planning (administration, policy development, information governance, and strategic planning), informatics, and HIT [12,15].

Health Information Technologists (HIT or HICT Professionals)

Health information technologists may have a computer science or engineering background and are familiar with ICT (including hardware and software), information systems and networks, and programming. HIT professionals are trained in one or more technical areas that may include systems (eg, operating system, database, programming languages, software engineering, and development) and applications software (eg, productivity tools, departmental information systems, and office systems), hardware, communications and networking, biomedical engineering, and in a variety of methods or procedures such as project management, security, risk management, and process engineering [12,14].

Health Information Exchange Specialists (HIE Professionals)

HIE, as defined in Chapter 1, is "the electronic transfer of clinical and/or administrative information across diverse and often competing health care organizations." The nature and size of these organizations are quite variable (eg, hospitals, physician's offices, laboratory systems, community care centers, mental health centers) as well as the information transmitted (eg, a discharge summary, care plan, laboratory results, and medication list). An HIO refers to "an organization that facilitates information exchange within a network of facilities, community, state, or region" ensuring the protection and security of personal health information as it is shared across multiple health care providers.

Although several of the professionals already discussed may possess the skills and knowledge to work in an HIO, specific certification programs for HIE professionals extend beyond the technical, legal, and regulatory requirements for data and information governance. These programs include content specific to HIE planning, information architecture and stewardship, the use of new technologies to integrate and exchange data between and among organizations, personal health records, telehealth and home monitoring, and other exchanges of electronic information among organizations [17]. Within an HIO, there may also be health informaticians, health information managers, as well as additional support staff providing necessary business, financial, public relations, and privacy and security skills.

eHEALTH PROFESSIONALS—SUPPLY AND DEMAND

The US Bureau of Labor Statistics [18] collects specific information for "medical records and health information technicians" that are largely RHIA and RHIT positions related to HIM; coding and categorizing patient information for insurance reimbursement purposes, and for databases and registries; and to maintain patients' medical and treatment histories mainly within health facilities. These jobs are expected to grow at a rate of 22% over the next 10 years (2012–2022) or 41,000 individuals—a rate much higher than the average for all occupational categories included in the US Bureau of Labor Statistics database. An estimated 186,300 people are currently employed in the "medical records and health information technicians" category.

Additional HI and HIM expertise is also part of a separate category, "medical and health services managers." The medical and health services managers' category includes labor statistics representing those employed as managers of HIM or HIT services, health information analysis or decision support, and health care administrators defined as those "who plan, direct, and coordinate medical and health services in health care facilities, including hospitals and nursing homes, and group medical practices." This category again is expected to experience a far greater growth rate than the average for all job categories. Medical and health services managers held about 315,500 jobs in 2012, and a growth rate of 23% or 73,300 jobs is expected [19].

Categories within the area of information technology such as computer network systems analyst (25% growth), information security analysts (37%), computer and information systems managers (15%), computer network architect (15%), and database administrator (15%) are all expected to grow at rates well above the average (of 14% over the 10-year projection period). Overall employment in computer systems design and related services has grown rapidly in recent years, even during the economic downturn in 2008, and is projected to continue to grow much faster than the average for all industry occupations (eg, software developers, systems at 72% and software developers, applications at 57%). Workers in the major occupation groups in this industry earn high wages, and most individuals enter the workforce with at least a bachelor's degree [20].

Two recent Canadian HI-HIM human resource sector studies forecast a similar shortfall of up to 12,000 skilled individuals in the eHealth field over the next 5 years [21,22]. In the 2014 study, the two areas of major concern are information technology and HIM. Within the HIM profession alone, 44.5% of all certified HIM professionals in Canada are 50 years or older and expected to retire within the next 5–10 years necessitating a minimum replacement demand of 718 HIM professionals over the next 5 years.

Based on the current replacement rate of HIM professionals in Canada (approximately 300 per year become certified), Canada is already falling short of new entrants to the profession by approximately 418 individuals per annum. When both the growth and skills shortage numbers are included, the number of HIM professionals required increases to 1124 per annum, a projected shortage of 824 people per year. Unless the forecast job vacancies are filled and the existing workforce retrained, the report paints a dire picture of unexpected delays, cost over-runs, and risks to patient safety and care [22,23].

A target figure for eHealth professional needs/supply in the United States has been based on rough estimates of ongoing implementation of electronic records within hospitals and physicians' offices. An analysis of about 5000 hospitals using the Healthcare Information Management Systems Society (HIMSS) Analytics Database [24,25] found an overall staffing ratio of 0.142 IT full time equivalents per hospital bed and, extrapolating to all hospital beds in the United States, an estimated workforce size of 108,390 FTE. It was estimated that to achieve a fully EMR with shared data contributing to an electronic health record (EHR), a total of 149,174 IT FTE would be needed or an increase in supply of 40,784 HIT personnel.

An additional study, looking at the estimated workforce for deployment of the nationwide health information network (NHIN) and implementation of electronic records for the 400,000 practicing physicians who do not have them, estimated the need for another 7600 FTEs. For the 4000 hospitals that still needed EHRs, another 28,600 specialists and about 420 other professionals were needed to build the infrastructure in communities to interconnect all these systems [26].

The only environmental scan on HIE/HIO human resources to date, the white paper issued by HIMSS and AHIMA based on the results of a 2012 survey on "Trends in Health Information Exchange Organizational Staffing" reiterates the need to pay attention to the staffing needs of HIOs [27, p. 5].

> Many initiatives are underway at the federal, state and local levels, and in the private sector, to foster and enable interoperable electronic health information exchange, most of which is facilitated through Health Information Exchange Organizations or Networks (HIO). Significant focus is placed on the governance, business models, policies, standards and technical infrastructure required for long-term sustainability; however, little attention is focused on the staffing of HIOs. This is an unfortunate oversight—even the most well-designed HIO cannot operate in a silo. It is therefore essential to consider current and future staffing needs of these organizations.

The HIMSS and AHIMA workgroup noted three roles as particularly important to HIEs:

- HIM and exchange specialists,
- health information privacy and security specialists, and
- programmers and software engineers.

The majority (86%) of respondents to the HIMSS and AHIMA survey had a staff of 25 people or less with the greatest number of staff employed in technology positions, followed by operations. Roles within the technology category included: security, data integration, data integrity, connectivity, data quality/compliance, payment processing, technical project management, software application support, business intelligence, specification/design/coding or testing, and help desk/support [26, p. 17]. The most prevalent technical roles were software applications support, help desk support, and data integration. Operations roles were dominated by marketing/sales/PR (related to a source of income and sustainability for the HIE), executive management roles, project management, and administrative assistant roles. Fewer positions were filled for privacy and security (but likely to be onsite rather than outsourced) and HIM [26, p. 20]. Organizations used a variety of staffing mixes including full-time and part-time employees, job sharing, onsite contractors, and outsourcing.

Future staffing needs again were heavily focused on technical staff (eg, data integration, help desk, data integrity, connectivity, software support, business intelligence, data quality, and technical project management) and operations (eg, executive management, marketing/sales, and finance). Technology skills are an ongoing need among all HIOs [26, p. 23]. Over half (58%) of organizations were hiring positions at the bachelor's level with areas of specialization in finance, accounting, HIM, HIT, business, provider relations, computer science, or IT; and the predominant credential sought was that of project management professional followed by CPHIMS and RHIA. Even while stating that the most common staffing challenge was a lack of available qualified candidates, few respondents were involved with the federally funded HITECH Workforce Development Program either through partnerships with one of the educational development consortia (usually a community college) and use of interns in the training programs, or hiring of HITECH graduates (only 12%).

In a follow-up survey of C-suite executives in 16 HIOs, a growth within these organizations just within the elapsed 2-year time span was noted, with a shift in staffing numbers of participating organizations from 50 or less in 2012 to greater than 400 (in more than half) in 2014 and a broader range of participants beyond hospital and physician practice (eg, payers, EMS, long-term care, nursing homes, behavioral health centers, and state public health) [28]. IT still represented over half of the staff and within this category three problem areas identified in the first survey—data integrity, connectivity, and data integration—were further explored.

Participants in the survey reported the following experiences in hiring and recruiting for these positions:

- difficulty finding project management experience specific to HIEs,
- extended periods of time needed to find qualified candidates who had both a cultural and technical fit to the organization, and
- lack of a system for networking with peers to identify qualified candidates [28].

SKILLS AND TRAINING OF eHEALTH PROFESSIONALS

Outside of the long-standing accredited programs and credentialing in HIM through the professional associations AHIMA and CHIMA [14–16], training programs for e-Health and/or HI professionals are relatively new and, at the best, producing well under the number of graduates needed to address the projected demand [25,26]. Each year about 3000 new graduates enter the HIM profession. In Canada, roughly 100 students graduate every year from HI programs and only 250–300 graduates from HIM programs. These numbers are not enough to provide the thousands needed for EHR and HIE implementation in the short term. They are increasingly insufficient to meet long-term demands for the development, operation, and management of the health information infrastructure in nations around the world and for the ongoing work with EHRs and HIOs and meaningful use of health information.

Current Credentials Offered

A number of certifications in eHealth fields are available and often sponsored through a recognized professional college or commission (eg, Canadian College of Health Information Management, Commission on Certification for Health Informatics and Information Management) or professional association (eg, AHIMA, HIMSS) or state certifying body (Table 2.1). Certification distinguishes an individual as competent and knowledgeable in a specific area, adds credibility to the profession, and offers some assurance to employers that these individuals have demonstrated proficiency and possess a broad base of knowledge by undertaking studies in an accredited educational program and/or passing a rigorous national examination. Certification demonstrates a commitment to ongoing professional development and maintenance of certification.

In some instances, the criteria for eligibility to write the credentialing examination require graduation from an accredited program. Accreditation is a voluntary process that educational programs participate in as a means to demonstrate to the public and potential students that a program meets or exceeds stated standards of educational quality. AHIMA developed an accreditation program for medical record programs in 1943, and currently the Commission on Accreditation for Health Informatics and Information Management Education (CAHIIM) is recognized by the Council for Higher Education Accreditation. Program accreditation by CAHIIM is necessary

TABLE 2.1 Health Information Certifications—Credentials Offered

Credential Designation	Competency Area	Curriculum Standard	Training or Degree Required
HIM CERTIFICATIONS THROUGH CCHIIM			
Registered Health Information Technician—RHIT	Health Information Management (HIM): The skills cover health data management; health statistics, biomedical research, and data quality; health services organization and delivery; information technology and systems; and organizational resources.	Standards and interpretations for Accreditation of Associate Degree Programs in Health Information Management (CAHIIM)	Associate/Diploma From a CAHIIM-accredited program
Registered Health Information Administrator—RHIA	HIM: follows the HIM Profession Core Model [30, 31]. See HIM Profession Core Model [44] Functional components include: data/information analysis, transformation, and decision support; information dissemination and liaison; health information resource management and innovation; information governance and stewardship; and quality and patient safety	Standards and interpretations for Accreditation of Baccalaureate Degree Programs in Health Information Management (CAHIIM)	Baccalaureate degree From a CAHIIM-accredited program
Certified Coding Associate—CCA		AHIMA-approved coding certificate program	Entry level; minimum high-school level diploma + 6 months experience or completion of an AHIMA-approved coding certificate program
Certified Coding Specialist—CCS		Focus on more experienced coder in inpatient setting	Two or more years of coding experience…
Certified Coding Specialist—CCS-P		Focus on more experienced coder in ambulatory care and outpatient setting	Two or more years of coding experience…
Certified Health Data Analyst—CHDA		Knowledge to acquire, manage, analyze, interpret, and transform health care data into accurate, consistent, and timely information and to communicate with individuals and groups at multiple levels	Associate degree + 5-y experience; RHIT + 3-y experience, or a baccalaureate or master's degree + 1-y experience

(*Continued*)

TABLE 2.1 *Continued*

Credential Designation	Competency Area	Curriculum Standard	Training or Degree Required
Clinical Documentation Improvement Practitioner—CDIP		Experience in CDI guidance, knowledge of documentation requirements relative to compliant coding and billing, in addition to EHR functionality to support documentation capture.	RHIA or RHIT or CCS/ CCS-P or RN, MD, DO + 2 yr experience in CDI OR associate degree + 3 yr experience
Certified Healthcare Privacy and Security—CHPS	Competence in designing, implementing, and administering comprehensive privacy and security protection programs in all types of health care organizations.		Baccalaureate + 4 years of experience; RHIA + 2 years of experience or advanced graduate degree + 2 years of experience; RHIT + 4 years of experience; associate + 6 years of experience
Certified Healthcare Technology Specialist—CHTS (formerly HIT Pro)	Assess workflows, select hardware and software, work with vendors, install and test systems, diagnose IT problems, and train practice staff on systems.	Assess competency in clinical/ practitioner consultant; practice workflow and IM redesign; implementation manager; implementation support specialist; technical/ software support staff; trainer	No formal eligibility requirements; completion of one of the Workforce Development programs or work experience
Certified Health Information Management Professional—CHIM Offered by the Canadian College of Health Information Management (CCHIM)	Health Information Management (includes coding and classifications; privacy, security, and confidentiality; and analysis and business intelligence)	LOHIM (Version 3) Designates learning outcomes required in eight domains (biomedical sciences; Canadian health care system; HIM; analysis and business intelligence; privacy, confidentiality and access; information systems and technology; management; ethics and practice)	College/Diploma Baccalaureate degree From a CCHIM accredited program
HI CERTIFICATION THROUGH HIMSS			
Certified Associate in Healthcare Information and Management Systems—CAHIMS	Health informatics Health information systems	Knowledge of health IT and management systems. The CAHIMS credential is designed to be a career pathway to the CPHIMS credential. Content outlined in: CAHIMS Candidate Handbook and Application, May 2015	Undergraduate degree with <5 years of related experience

(*Continued*)

TABLE 2.1 *Continued*

Credential Designation	Competency Area	Curriculum Standard	Training or Degree Required
Certified Professional in Healthcare Information and Management Systems—CPHIMS	Health informatics Health information systems	Covers general health care and technology areas as well as in-depth knowledge of health IT systems, including analysis, design, selection, implementation, support, maintenance, testing, evaluation, privacy, and security. Content outlined in: CPHIMS Candidate Handbook and Application, May 2015	Undergraduate degree with 5 years of related experience (3 years in health care); graduate degree with 3 years' experience (2 years in health care)
CPHIMS-CA Administered by COACH; developed in conjunction with HIMSS—Canadian version	Health informatics Health information systems	Competency and the skills, knowledge and abilities to perform safely and effectively in a broad range of Canadian practice settings.	Undergraduate degree with 5 years of related experience (3 years in HI); graduate degree with 3 years' experience (2 years in HI)
OTHER HI-RELATED CREDENTIALS AND CERTIFICATION ORGANIZATIONS			
Certified Professional in the EHR—CPEHR	Electronic health records	Completion of outlined curriculum (Table 2.2).	Administered through Health IT Certification
Certified Professional in Health Information Exchange—CPHIE	Health information exchange	Completion of outlined curriculum (Table 2.2).	Administered through Health IT Certification
Certified Professional in Health Information Technology—CPHIT	Health information technology	Plans for, selects, implements and manages health information technology. Can identify emerging technology trends and their impact on health information exchanges, and lead teams from planning through management of health information projects.	Administered through Health IT Certification
Computing Technology Industry Association (CompTIA) — Healthcare IT Technician	Healthcare IT systems	Skills and knowledge needed to implement, deploy and support healthcare IT systems in clinical settings that range from individual practices to healthcare facilities. Covers a variety of topics, including regulatory rules and requirements, organizational behavior, IT best practices and operations, medical business operations and security topics.	

(*Continued*)

TABLE 2.1 *Continued*

Credential Designation	Competency Area	Curriculum Standard	Training or Degree Required
HealthCare Information Security and Privacy Practitioner—HCISPP (Administered through ISC^2—membership body of certified information and software security professionals worldwide)	Health care industry Regulatory environment Privacy and security Information governance and risk management Information risk assessment Third party risk management	Fundamental knowledge and experience in security and privacy controls that protect personal health information.	Must have a minimum of 2 years of experience in one domain of the HCISPP credential that includes security, compliance and privacy. Legal experience may be substituted for compliance. Information management experience may be subtitled for privacy. SHOULD have 1 year of the 2 years of experience in the health care industry.

for eligibility for the AHIMA/CCHIIM professional HIM Certification Exams and CAHIIM accredits programs in HIM at the associate, baccalaureate, and master's level and in HI at the masters level [14,16]. Required curriculum in these programs has been established by a number of subject matter experts in the field, industry leaders, and educators for HIM and HI [29–32].

Well-defined competencies for HIE are still in their infancy, and distinctions in HIE versus the longer standing HIM and HI professionals are still being identified and clarified [17,27,28].

Within HIM, CCHIIM administers two certifications: Registered Health Information Administrator (RHIA) and Registered Health Information Technician (RHIT) (Table 2.1).

Individuals who hold the RHIA credential are experts in managing patient health information and medical records, administering computer information systems, collecting and analyzing patient data, and using classification systems and medical terminologies. They have comprehensive knowledge of medical, administrative, ethical and legal requirements, and standards related to health care delivery and the privacy of protected patient information.

Professionals holding the RHIT credential ensure the quality of medical records by verifying their completeness, accuracy, and proper entry into computer systems. RHITs use computer applications to assemble and analyze patient data. They often specialize in coding diagnoses and procedures in patient records for reimbursement and research.

A number of specializations and advanced coding certifications are also offered by AHIMA including Coding Associate (CCA), Coding Specialist (CCS), and a physician-based coding specialist (CS-P). Specialty certifications and training programs are offered in health data analysis (CHDA); clinical documentation improvement (CDIP); health care privacy and security specialist (CHPS); and health care technology specialist (CHTS). The advanced and specialized certifications offered by AHIMA require (1) prior training through an HIM program at the college, baccalaureate, or masters level; (2) prior certification in HIM at RHIT or RHIA levels; (3) certification in a variety of health professions (eg, RN, MD, PhD, and DO) plus related work experience; or (4) an associate level degree and various years of related experience (Table 2.1).

Within the field of HI, there are two credentials, Certified Professional in Healthcare Information and Management Systems (CPHIMS) and Certified Associate in Healthcare

Information and Management Systems (CAHIMS), offered in the United States, with a Canadian extension, CPHIMS-CA, offered in Canada through the HIMSS (Table 2.1). CAHIMS certification is designed for emerging professionals within the industry (5 years or less of experience) who demonstrate knowledge of health IT and management systems. CPHIMS professionals demonstrate mastery of knowledge considered important to competent practice in the health care information and management systems field. The certification covers general health care and technology areas as well as in-depth knowledge of health IT systems, including analysis, design, selection, implementation, support, maintenance, testing, evaluation, privacy, and security with a focus on the administration and management of IT systems used in health care environments.

Health IT Certification, LLC, is a professional organization that provides training and certification for professionals charged with planning, selecting, implementing, and managing EHR and HIT systems, as well as those who are involved with creation and management of HIEs (CPHIE; Table 2.1). Health IT Certification has made several arrangements with Regional Extension Centers in the United States to train staff and physician practices and with community colleges to offer online HIT and EHR courses and certification exams.

Beyond core courses in HIT, the CPHIE acquires additional training in technology and policy elements specific to the exchange of health information including considerations of HIE architecture and the NHIN; use of remote technologies for home monitoring and telehealth; and specific policy issues related to data stewardship and information governance. The impact and connectivity of personal health records are also considered (Table 2.2).

Workforce Development in the United States

The US government, through ARRA, released millions of dollars to universities and colleges to train 50,000 health IT professionals

TABLE 2.2 Health IT Certifications—Curricular Content

Certification	CPHIT	CPEHR	CPHIE
Core Content	Overview of Health IT		
	Legal and Regulatory Aspects of Health IT		
	Goal Setting and Change Management for Health IT		
	Workflow and Process Improvement for Health IT		
Track-Specific Content	Health IT Technology/Privacy and Security	Data Management and Clinical Documentation	Goals and Governance
	Principles of Health IT Project Management	Patient Safety: CPOE, e-Rx, BC-MAR	HIE Architecture
	Managing HIT Return on Investment	Health IT for Health Reform	Data Stewardship
	HIT System Selection	Interoperability	Personal Health Records
	HIT Implementation Support	Clinical Decision Support	Telehealth and Home Monitoring
	Health Information Exchange	Health Information Exchange in EHR	Nationwide Health Information Network

as part of its $2 billion strategy to achieve widespread meaningful use of health care IT and provide for the use of an EHR for each person in the United States. Funds were administered in the Information Technology Professional in Health Care Program (the "Workforce Program") developed through the Office of the National Coordinator for Health Information Technology (ONC). In April 2010, four programs were initiated:

- The Community College Consortia to educate Information Technology Professionals in Health Care ($68 million to five consortia supporting approximately 81 community colleges to establish or improve nondegree health IT training programs designed to be completed within 6 months).
- A program of assistance for university-based training ($32 million to nine colleges and universities to create or expand health IT training programs focused on roles that required a higher level of training—master's degrees or certificates of advanced training)
- Curriculum development centers ($10 million to five universities) for development of modules and curriculum content that could be shared across educational institutions.
- A competency examination—the HIT Pro examination ($6 million to North Virginia CC to fund the design and initial competency exams in health IT for individuals who completed one of the CCC programs).

Did the Program Accomplish What it Intended to do?

An evaluation of all four workforce development programs conducted by the NORC at the University of Chicago indicates that the program was at least partially successful in that it trained 1704 students through the university programs, 19,733 students through the college programs, and administered 9500 HIT Pro exams (as of end of December 2013 at the time of survey). Among the university- and college-trained students, about two-thirds were employed in health IT or health IT-related positions 6 months after program completion [33]. Curricular materials developed for the program were generally found to be useful by schools, and programs were able to choose which elements they wanted to include in their courses. Some concerns were noted about the quality of the materials but these improved with revised versions and later releases of the material [33]. All 20 course components are now freely available through the HI Forum online (released under a Creative Commons Attribution-NonCommercial-Share Alike 3.0 Unported License) [34].

Many employers were either unaware of the ONC workforce program or skeptical that a 6-month training period alone could provide the skills needed for employability. Within the workforce program, schools that established relationships with employers for student placements and hands-on experience were better able to support students in finding employment after graduation [33].

The HIT Pro exams evaluate the competency of health IT professionals to assess workflows, select hardware and software, work with vendors, install and test systems, diagnose IT problems, and train practice staff on systems. By 2012 the number of HIT Pro exams administered was lower than expected, largely due to a lack of awareness by employers and little emphasis placed on the exam by the colleges (for instance, it was not a graduation requirement). Examinations were then provided free of charge, and individuals could sit for more than one exam leading to an increase in exam requests (9500 by the end of December 2013). Responsibility for the examination has now passed to AHIMA, and the name of the certification was changed to Certified Healthcare Technology Specialist (CHTS). The CHTS credential is now offered through CCHIIM as one of their advanced certification exams (Table 2.1).

DEFINING AND EXECUTING A FUTURE STRATEGY FOR eHEALTH AND HIE PROFESSIONALS

The ONC has recently awarded seven universities with close to a million dollars each to update the curricular materials developed through the original workforce development program and to add four new areas of content relevant for improved health care delivery: population health, care coordination, new care delivery and payments models, and value-based care [35]. "In addition to updating training materials, the goal of this program is to train 6000 incumbent health care workers to use new health information technologies in a variety of settings including: team-based care environment, long-term care facilities, patient-centered medical homes, accountable care organizations, hospitals and clinics" [35].

Additional research into workforce development programs through ONC [33] and others is still needed to identify and define the "skills and experience required to meet the demands and advance the profession of both current and future HIOs." Talent is critical to leveraging opportunities and advantages afforded by electronic records and the exchange of health information in improving health care delivery and integration of care, health outcomes, cost savings, and patient satisfaction. A national human resources strategy is needed to address the current shortage of skilled workers and to develop a long-term strategy for education and training of eHealth personnel necessary to ensure the continued quality of health data collected, its security and confidentiality, and to manage and maintain the systems and data in the future.

Labor statistics beyond the categories currently available are needed; a category of eHealth workers and/or work should be monitored and tracked. In addition the ONC Health IT Workforce Development Program needs to continue to support HIOs in addressing their skilled workforce needs, particularly in the three areas that have been identified as critical:

- health information management and exchange specialists,
- health information privacy and security specialists, and
- programmers and software engineers [27,28].

In many instances, existing health professionals in the domains of informatics and/or information management are able to transition into roles supporting HIE.

EMERGING TRENDS

Current certifications in HIE will take time to become known to employers and the advantages of credentialed employees versus noncredentialed employees is still to be determined. In many instances employers are looking for individuals who can fulfill multiple roles so that narrowly defined certifications or credentials may not be desirable. The proliferation of certifications, subtle differences in their curriculum and competencies are confusing to potential employers and students alike. Many of these programs are short-term and offered online with limited opportunities for hands-on experience that develops true expertise and competency in a given task or skill.

We have previously argued that within the fields of HI and HIM, there is a convergence of knowledge, skills, and roles that will shape the training of future health information professionals and shape the programs being offered [14]. We are already seeing a number of "merged" or "balanced" programs in health informatics and information management (HIIM), such as Conestoga College's Bachelor of Applied Health Information Science program that provides education in both HI and HIM [36] and whose graduates are eligible to sit the Canadian HIM credentialing exam; Louisiana

Tech University has a HIIM department that offers a HIIM Bachelors and HI Masters [37]; and the University of Tennessee Health Science Center offers a combined bachelors and post-graduate HIIM program [38].

Although most people currently working within HIOs are entering at the baccalaureate level, professional associations are moving towards masters level preparation as the new level of entry for these highly skilled professions who are dealing with greater complexity in the workplace [39]. In its Vision 2016 whitepaper, AHIMA outlines the need for positions requiring new skills and experience with EHR technology, project management, team leadership, data analytics, or strategic planning and by 2016 recommends the transition to "a stage where HIM professionals at an advanced level of practice are master's degree prepared upon entry into the work force" [39]. AMIA has joined CAHIIM as an organizational member to initiate the establishment of a separate informatics accreditation council that will revise Accreditation Standards for Masters' degree programs in HI [40].

Short-term certification programs in HIE, EHR, Privacy and Security, Decision Support, or Data Analytics may have their greatest value in providing more in depth information and knowledge to post-baccalaureate trainees who already have a rudimentary foundational knowledge of informatics and information management. We are seeing this trend in some HIIM programs and departments, including the University of Illinois at Chicago [41] and the Indiana University School of Informatics and Computing [42], which offer undergraduate degrees in HIM and graduate degrees that focus on HI. Many of these existing programs are accredited through CAHIIM so that their graduates can sit for the national RHIA examination. It may not be necessary, or desirable, to accredit all health information certificate programs but, at the very least, curriculum should follow some generally agreed-upon and necessary curricular competencies.

SUMMARY

Although great progress has been made over the past decade in introducing the EHR in health care facilities and physicians' offices, many systems remain siloed, and movement towards a fully integrated electronic network and HIE has been slow. Hampering the implementation of the technical infrastructure is the lack of adequate eHealth professionals who can not only assist in deployment of systems but who can also work with the information that they contain and who can be instrumental in the establishment of standards for capture, transmission, and sharing of health data. The previous workforce development program from ARRA provided an initial impetus to develop and define the needed competencies and to educate a portion of the estimated 50,000 eHealth workers, but further work is needed on the definition of HIE competencies and skills, and the continued provision of eHealth professionals. Development of training programs for individuals interested in building HIE skills can be stand-alone (eg, certification in HIE) or as additional post-graduate training for other eHealth professionals (eg, HIMs, HIs, and HITs). There is a continued need for additional training to clinical health professionals (eg, physicians, nurses, and pharmacists) in informatics and information management skills who will be working with electronic records as well as HIE. The newly introduced subspecialty in "clinical informatics" will provide specialized training to physicians and opening up of certification opportunities for non-MDs is being considered [43].

Given the state of the workforce and training options for HIT and HIE professionals, a national strategy for eHealth human resources is needed in every country for monitoring both supply and demand for these crucial health care workers. We need to be able to better track those individuals who work in eHealth, above and beyond the current labor statistics monitoring HIMs alone, and in monitoring supply of individuals through current training and/or educational programs.

QUESTIONS FOR DISCUSSION

1. In which roles within a hospital, clinical or health system would knowledge and/or expertise in HIE be useful?
2. Describe how HIE specialists might interact with or support operations within a national health system. How about an individual hospital or clinic?
3. What knowledge and skills might be important for HIE specialists to develop over time to complement the larger eHealth workforce?
4. What kind of ongoing professional certification or development might be necessary for HIE specialists to seek as they mature in their careers?

References

[1] Schoen C, Osborn R, Doty MM, Squires D, Peugh J, Applebaum S. A survey of primary care physicians in 11 countries, 2009: perspectives on care, costs, and experience. Health Aff 2009;28(6):w1171–83.

[2] Schoen C, Osborn R, Squires D, Doty M, Rasmussen P, Pierson R, et al. A survey of primary care doctors in ten countries shows progress in use of health information technology, less in other areas. Health Aff 2012;31(12):2805–16.

[3] Hsiao CJ, Hing E. Use and characteristics of electronic health record systems among office-based physician practices: United States, 2001–2012. : National Center for Health Statistics; 2012. Data Brief 111, Available at: <http://www.cdc.gov/nchs/data/databriefs/db111.pdf> [Accessed December 18, 2012].

[4] National physician survey. National physician survey: backgrounder. Available at: <http://nationalphysiciansurvey.ca/wp-content/uploads/2014/12/NPS-backgrounder-2014-EN-r.pdf>; 2014.

[5] Charles D, Gabriel M, Furukawa MF. Adoption of electronic health record systems among U.S. non-federal acute care hospitals: 2008–2013, ONC Data Brief, no. 16. Washington, DC: Office of the National Coordinator for Health Information Technology; 2014.

[6] Gabriel M, Jones EB, Samy L, King J. Among critical-access hospitals progress and challenges: implementation and use of health information technology. Health Aff 2014;33(7):1262–70. http://dx.doi.org/10.1377/hlthaff.2014.0279.

[7] Furukawa MF, Patel V, Charles D, Swain M, Mostashari F. Hospital electronic health information exchange grew substantially in 2008–12. Health Aff (Project Hope) 2013;32(8):1346–54. Epub August 7, 2013.

[8] Audet A-M, Squires D, Doty MM. Where are we on the diffusion curve? Trends and drivers of primary care physicians' use of health information technology. Health Serv Res 2014;49(1 Pt 2):347–60. Published online December 21, 2013. http://dx.doi.org/10.1111/1475-6773.12139.

[9] HITECH Act 2009. HITECH Act excerpts from ARRA with Index. Available at: <http://healthit.gov/sites/default/files/hitech_act_excerpt_from_arra_with_index.pdf>.

[10] HealthIT.gov. Health IT Legislation and Regulations. Last updated: Friday, March 27, 2015. At: <http://healthit.gov/policy-researchers-implementers/health-it-legislation>.

[11] HealthIT.gov. Policymaking, Regulation, & Strategy. Last updated: Thursday, September 25, 2014. Available from: <http://www.healthit.gov/policy-researchers-implementers/health-it-legislation-and-regulations>.

[12] Gibson CJ, Covvey HD. Demystifying E-health human resources Medical Information Science Reference Kabene SM, editor. Human resources in healthcare, health informatics and healthcare systems. Hershey, PA: IGI Global; 2010.

[13] Eysenbach G. What is e-health? J Med Internet Res 2001;3(2):e20. http://dx.doi.org/10.2196/jmir.3.2.e20.

[14] Gibson CJ, Dixon B, Abrams K. Convergent evolution of health information management and health informatics—a perspective on the future of information professionals in health care. Appl Clin Inf 2015;6(1):163–84.

[15] Crook G, Abrams K, Arnold GB. Ch 2: the health information management profession Abrams K, Gibson C, editors. Fundamentals of health information management (2nd ed.). Ottawa, ON: CHIMA, CHA Press; 2013.

[16] Brodnick MS. The health informatics and information management professional Abdelhak M, Hanken MA, editors. Health information: management of a strategic resource (5th ed.). St. Louis: Elsevier Saunders; 2016.

[17] Health IT Certification (nd). CPHIT, CPEHR, CPHIE and CPORA Overview. Available from: <http://www.healthitcertification.com/overview.html>.

[18] Bureau of Labor Statistics, U.S. Department of Labor, Occupational Outlook Handbook, 2014–15 Edition, Medical Records and Health Information Technicians. Available from: <http://www.bls.gov/ooh/healthcare/medical-records-and-health-information-technicians.htm> (published January 8, 2014; cited May 22, 2015).

[19] Bureau of Labor Statistics, U.S. Department of Labor, Occupational Outlook Handbook, 2014–15 Edition, Medical and Health Services Managers. Available from: <http://www.bls.gov/ooh/management/medical-and-health-services-managers.htm> (published January 8, 2014; cited May 22, 2015.

[20] Csorny L. Careers in growing field of information technology services Beyond the Numbers: Employment and Unemployment, vol. 2 : U.S. Bureau of Labor Statistics; 2013.9. Available from: <http://www.bls.gov/opub/btn/volume-2/careers-in-growing-field-of-information-technology-services.htm>.

[21] O'Grady J. Health informatics and health information management: human resources report [Internet]. Toronto: Prism Economics and Analysis; 2009. Available from: <http://www.ictc-ctic.ca/wp-content/uploads/2012/06/ICTC_HI-HIMReport_EN_11-09.pdf>.

[22] Prism Economics and Analysis Health informatics and health information management: human resources outlook 2014–2019. Toronto, ON: Prism Economics and Analysis; 2014.

[23] Schick S. Canada faces widespread e-health skills shortage. : IT World Canada; 2009. Available at: <http://www.itworldcanada.com/article/canada-faces-widespread-e-health-skills-shortage/40533#ixzz3bGCmMXy9>.

[24] Hersh W. Who are the informaticians? What we know and should know. J Am Med Inform Assoc 2006;13:166–70. http://dx.doi.org/10.1197/jamia.M1912.

[25] Hersh W, Wright A. What workforce is needed to implement the health information technology agenda? Analysis from the HIMSS Analytics™ database. AMIA Annu Symp Proc 2008 2008;2008:303–7.

[26] Department of Health and Human Services (DHHS): Assistant Secretary for Planning and Evaluation, 2007. Nationwide Health Information Network (NHIN) Workforce Study: Final Report <http://aspe.hhs.gov/sp/reports/2007/NHIN/NHINReport.shtml>.

[27] AHIMA/HIMSS HIE Technology Staffing Workgroup, 2013. Trends in health information exchange organizational staffing, AHIMA/HIMSS HIE staffing model environmental scan. Available at: <http://www.himss.org/ResourceLibrary/genResourceDetailPDF.aspx?ItemNumber=31182>.

[28] AHIMA/HIMSS HIE Technology Staffing Workgroup, 2014. Trends in health information exchange organizational staffing: part 2: A deeper look at staffing challenges. Available from: <http://www.himss.org/ResourceLibrary/genResourceDetailPDF.aspx?ItemNumber=34412>.

[29] CHIMA, 2010. Learning outcomes for health information management, version 3.0. ISBN: 978-0-9783332-1-8.

[30] AHIMA Foundation. 2015. Academic curricula competencies. Available at: <http://www.ahimafoundation.org/education/curricula.aspx>.

[31] CAHIIM 2015. Curriculum requirements. Available from: <http://www.cahiim.org/him/curriculumrequirements.html>.

[32] CAHIIM 2015. Curriculum requirements: 2014 Health Informatics Master's Degree Curriculum Requirements. Available from: <http://www.cahiim.org/hi/curriculumrequirements.html>.

[33] Lowell K. Final Report. Evaluation of the information technology professionals in health care ("Workforce") program—summative report. Chicago, IL: NORC at University of Chicago; 2014.

[34] Health Informatics Forum. 2015. Health informatics forum massive open online course (MOOC). Available from: <http://www.healthinformaticsforum.com/MOOC>.

[35] HealthIT.gov (2015) Workforce development programs. Available from: <http://www.healthit.gov/providers-professionals/workforce-development-programs> [Accessed August 18, 2015].

[36] Conestoga College. Applied health information science (Bachelor of) (Co-op). Program details. Available from: <http://www.conestogac.on.ca/fulltime/1131C.jsp>.

[37] Louisiana Tech University. Department of Health Informatics & Information Management. Available from: <http://him.latech.edu/>.

[38] The University of Tennessee Health Science Center. Health Informatics & Information Management. Available from: <http://www.uthsc.edu/health-professions/him/index.php>.

[39] AHIMA 2007. VISION 2016: A blueprint for quality education in health information management. American Health Information Management Association, Chicago, IL. Available from: <http://library.ahima.org/xpedio/groups/public/documents/ahima/bok1_035517.pdf>.

[40] AMIA 2014. AMIA joins CAHIIM to lead informatics program accreditation. Available from: <https://www.amia.org/news-and-publications/press-release/amia-joins-cahiim-lead-informatics-program-accreditation>.

[41] University of Illinois at Chicago. Masters in Health Informatics & Health Information Management Degrees. Available from: <http://healthinformatics.uic.edu/>.

[42] Indiana University-Purdue University Indianapolis. School of Computing and Informatics. Department of BioHealth Informatics. Available from: <http://soic.iupui.edu/departments/biohealth/>.

[43] Detmer DE, Lumpkin JR, Williamson JJ. Defining the medical subspecialty of clinical informatics. JAMIA 2009;16:167–8.

[44] Cassidy BS. Teaching the future: an educational response to the AHIMA core model. J AHIMA 82 2011;10:34–8. Available from: <http://library.ahima.org/xpedio/groups/public/documents/ahima/bok1_049268.hcsp?dDocName=bok1_049268>.

PART II

ORGANIZATIONAL ASPECTS OF MANAGING HEALTH INFORMATION EXCHANGE

CHAPTER

3

Drivers and Barriers to Adoption: Towards the Last Mile

Saurabh Rahurkar[1], *Brian E. Dixon*[2] *and Nir Menachemi*[3]

[1]Center for Biomedical Informatics, Regenstrief Institute, Inc., Indianapolis, IN
[2]Indiana University Richard M. Fairbanks School of Public Health; and the Center for Biomedical Informatics, Regenstrief Institute, Inc., Indianapolis, IN [3]Indiana University Richard M. Fairbanks School of Public Health, Indianapolis, IN

OUTLINE

LEARNING OBJECTIVES

By the end of this chapter the reader should:

- Identify and list major initiatives as well as stakeholders that play a role in the adoption of health information exchange (HIE)
- Report the current levels of HIE adoption in the United States as well as globally
- Understand the salient barriers to HIE adoption

- Describe historic and current efforts taken to address barriers to HIE adoption and generally promote adoption and implementation
- Discuss the role of policy in shaping HIE adoption and utilization
- List and describe emerging trends influencing the adoption and use of HIE.

INTRODUCTION

A consistent thread in US health policy over the past decade has been a focus on the need to adopt health information technology (HIT) and connect HIT systems through health information exchange (HIE). The primary motivation or reason for this focus is a belief that HIT and HIE systems can improve the quality of health care. Therefore it is worthwhile to briefly discuss two seminal reports by the Institute of Medicine (IOM) that played a pivotal role in stimulating the advent of HIT in the United States. The first report, *To Err is Human*, was released in 1999 and reported that up to 98,000 people died each year due to medical errors which included medication errors, surgical errors, and other errors such as incorrect diagnoses [1]. The report emphasized the role played by poorly designed care delivery systems that created an environment that was conducive to committing errors by otherwise competent clinicians.

In 2001, the IOM released a second report which played an instrumental role in the shift towards HIT [2]. Entitled *Crossing the Quality Chasm*, this report marks a major milestone in the national quality movement. Specifically, the report provided a formal definition of quality of care as consisting of six main components (Fig. 3.1). First, high quality care is focused on *patient safety*, ie, it is free from harmful effects such as those associated with medical errors. High quality care is both *effective* and *efficient*, ie, it is evidence based and does not result in a prodigal use of resources. Additionally, in order to be of high quality, care needs to be *timely*,

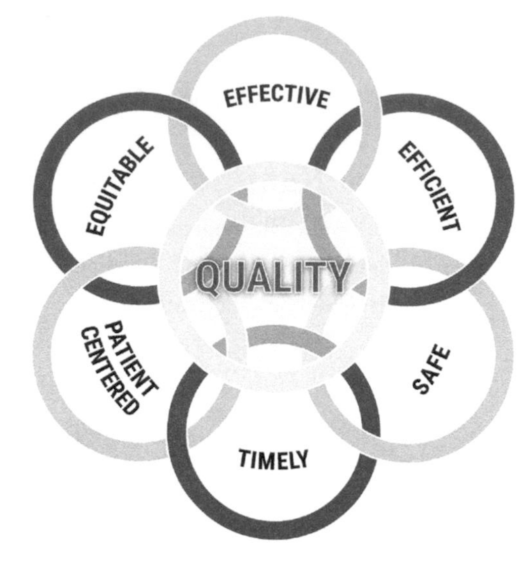

FIGURE 3.1 The six dimensions of high quality care. *Adapted from the Institute of Medicine [2].*

patient centered, and *equitable* so as to address extant disparities. Most importantly, the report argued that HIT addresses all six components of quality of care, and the report called for the adoption of HIT as a means to improve health care quality in the United States.

Following the IOM reports, health policy discussions, including the State of the Union address by President George W. Bush in 2004 calling for all Americans to have electronic health records by 2014, shifted to include HIT adoption. Furthermore, reports by the Center for IT Leadership emphasizes that the maximum benefit from HIT adoption could only be achieved through widespread exchange of data [3]. This expanded the policy discussions to include HIE as a critical component of the American roadmap towards the Triple Aim of improving the quality of and satisfaction with patient care while improving the health of populations and reducing the per capita cost of health care [4,5].

The push to adopt HIE was further bolstered by research that identified specific instances in medical decision making or clinical workflow where HIT or HIE could help avoid errors. For example, researchers at Brigham's and Women's Hospital suggested that HIE could eliminate up to 18% of patient safety errors generally and as much as 70% of adverse drug events by delivering appropriate information to providers during decision-making processes [6]. Additional research on HIE and its potential impact on quality, safety, as well as costs continues to emerge [7]. A recent reevaluation of the IOM estimates of medical error indicates that between 210,000 and 400,000 Americans die each year due to preventable medical errors [8]. Continued lapses in quality of care and estimates that medical errors cost the US health system approximately $980 billion only bolster the argument in the favor of adoption [9].

This chapter begins by orienting the reader to the HIE marketplace and examining the landscape of information sharing and interoperability activities in the United States as well as globally. Next, we present factors that have been linked as impediments to adoption of HIE, followed by an overview of efforts directed at addressing these barriers. In the final section, we briefly examine emerging trends in HIE.

LANDSCAPE OF THE HIE MARKETPLACE

In this section, we first examine the state of HIE in the United States and globally. First, we look at HIE as a verb (refer to the chapter: What is Health Information Exchange?) by examining the prevalence of HIE across various sectors of the health care ecosystem. Next, we look at HIE as a noun (also defined in the chapter: What is Health Information Exchange?) and focus on the growth of HIE organizations. Evaluating HIE trends from the perspective of general availability and use as well as the organizations that are facilitating HIE presents a deeper understanding of the multifaceted nature of HIE adoption.

Adoption of HIE Functionalities

About the time of President Bush's 2004 State of the Union address calling for EHR adoption, no information on the electronic exchange of data between hospitals and other health care providers was routinely captured. However, given estimates in 2003 regarding the adoption of EHR systems at 27% of providers, it is likely that HIE adoption was significantly less than 25% [10]. Over time, national surveys began to ask questions annually about the adoption of both EHR systems and functionality as well as HIE between various health system actors.

As of 2014, 76% of all nonfederal acute care hospitals (referred to as "hospitals" henceforth) in the United States participated[1] in HIE, representing an 85% increase from 2008 prior to the passage of the Health Information Technology for Economic and Clinical Health (HITECH) Act [11,12]. Of these hospitals, 69% exchanged laboratory results with other hospitals and providers outside their system [11,12]. About two-thirds of hospitals shared radiology reports (65%) and clinical care summaries (64%) with all types of providers (other hospitals and clinics) outside their system [11,12]. Finally, 58% of hospitals shared medication histories with outside system providers [11,12]. These data and other recent studies consistently demonstrate

[1] HIE participation was defined as electronically exchanging laboratory results, radiology reports, clinical care summaries, or medication lists with ambulatory care providers or hospitals outside their organization

upward trends in the adoption of both EHR systems and HIE among hospitals. Yet HIE with providers outside an integrated delivery network (eg, Community-based HIE and Government-facilitated HIE) lag behind the adoption of Private HIE.

HIE trends among office-based physicians differ from those of hospitals. Whereas almost 40% office-based physicians exchanged health information electronically with any providers—within or outside their system, only about 13% did so with outside providers [13]. Considerable variation was found among physicians regarding the various HIE-related capabilities. For example, in 2013, while almost 83% of physicians had the capability to order prescriptions electronically, only 39.1% had the capability to electronic report to immunization registries [13]. These rates however only represent capabilities and not actual exchange of health information. Increases have been reported in rates of electronic prescriptions (eRx), which involves electronically transmitting a prescription from a clinic to a pharmacy. As of 2014, close to 70% of all prescriptions were sent electronically, representing a more than a 14-fold increase since 2008 [11,14].

Among independent and hospital laboratories, two-thirds of all laboratories reported the capability to share structured test results electronically with providers [15]. Of those with the capability to electronically exchange data, one in five (20%) did not do so. Of all test results processed by laboratories, 58% were sent to providers electronically [15]. Electronic exchange of tests results between labs and public health departments has also increased dramatically in the past decade. In 2005, only eight state health departments had the capacity to receive electronic lab reports. This increased to 48 in 2014 with 62% of total laboratory reports received by state health departments reported to be transmitted electronically [16].

Growth in the Number of HIE Organizations

In 2004, there were nine operational HIE organizations in the United States [17], then referred to as RHIOs (see chapter: What is Health Information Exchange?). Like HIE functionalities, significant growth in the number of HIE organizations has occurred in the decade since. As of 2014, the eHealth Initiative identified 125 HIE organizations, which consisted of 74 community-based HIEs, 26 private HIEs, and 25 Government-facilitated HIEs [18]. There has been similar expansion within HIE organizations, including the following large HIE initiatives in the United States:

- The Indiana Network for Patient Care (INPC), managed by the Indiana HIE in partnership with the Regenstrief Institute, is one of the largest and oldest community-based HIEs in the United States [19]. The INPC grew from just a handful of hospitals in the early 2000s to more than 25,000 physicians, 93 hospitals, 110 clinics and surgery centers, public health departments and other health care organizations securely exchanging over 2 million transactions daily in 2014 [20,21].
- Kaiser Permanente (KP)—the largest not-for-profit integrated health care delivery system in the United States —operates and maintains an EHR system called *KP HealthConnect* and facilitates private HIE across its network. Overall, participation consists of over 600 medical offices and 37 hospitals, and connects providers across 8 states [22].
- As of 2015, the Surescripts Health Information Network, a private HIE, connected over 1000 hospitals and 800,000 health care professionals across the United States averaging about 16 million eRx transactions a day [23].
- The eHealth Exchange, originally established by the U.S. Office of the National Coordinator for HIT in 2004 through a program called the Nationwide Health Information Exchange

or NwHIN [24], established operations with two entities in 2009. As of 2015, the eHealth Exchange included participants from all 50 states, including 30% of all US hospitals, 10,000 medical groups, 8200 pharmacies, and over 900 dialysis centers [25,26]. Additionally, the eHealth Exchange also connects 101 state HIEs and 4 federal agencies—the Veterans Health Administration, U.S. Department of Defense, U.S. Social Services Administration, and the U.S. Centers for Medicare and Medicaid Services [27].

International Growth in the Adoption of HIE

Adoption of HIE internationally is more difficult to assess due to lack of published evidence and few representative surveys on HIE. Many developed nations, especially in Europe, have some level of HIE adoption based on data from the Commonwealth Fund [28]. Efforts to exchange data in developed countries appear to be similar to those in the United States: transmission of data between hospitals and general practitioners as well as specialists. Yet as pointed out by Adler-Milstein et al. [28], definitions of HIE vary by country.

HIE in other parts of the world is more difficult to assess. In the Middle East, papers from diverse countries such as Israel and Iran suggest there is emerging infrastructure in various locations that is at least supporting pilot projects that aim to advance HIE between hospitals, clinics, and ministries of health [29–32]. Some Israeli studies have even discussed HIE within the national HMO (health maintenance organization) network as far back as 2004. In low- to middle-income countries (LMICs), there has also been some level of HIE adoption. Efforts, though, in many LMICs have focused on laying the foundation for a robust eHealth infrastructure that will eventually support HIE. Yet there do exist working implementations of HIE in the following nations: South Africa, Rwanda, Sierra Leone, Tanzania, Bangladesh, and the Philippines [33].

Barriers to Adoption

Although there is great potential for HIE to improve health care delivery and outcomes, there has been resistance to its adoption among nations, organizations, and individual providers. Research on the implementation and adoption of HIE among providers has identified several challenges that warrant discussion. The following factors have consistent evidence in the literature for being barriers to the adoption and implementation of HIE:

- **Costs:** Adoption and implementation of HIE often requires large up-front investment of time and money by a provider or health system [34–37]. These costs include those related to hardware, software, labor and technical assistance costs, as well as the indirect costs associated with loss of productivity in the initial phase following implementation. In addition to start-up costs, providers have to account for recurrent costs associated with HIE. These ongoing costs include those related to maintenance expenses, as well as those related to connectivity such as membership or subscription fees and transaction fees. Further, the commonly theorized benefits from HIE such as reduction in medical errors, reduced diagnostic and imaging tests are accrued primarily by payers (eg, insurance carriers), and providers may potentially lose revenue generated by extraneous services utilization. Overall, these factors present an uncertainty from the perspective of gaining a positive return on investment for the decision to participate in HIE (see chapter "Business Planning: Towards Sustainability" for a full discussion of HIE value).
- **Resources:** HIE implementation is dependent on the availability of numerous resources in

addition to funding sources. These include technical or human resources, infrastructure, and availability of time. Providers routinely indicate their facilities lack the hardware, software, or network connectivity required for HIE. Even when an infrastructure is present, providers suggest it is insufficient for efficient (eg, fast) exchange of data. Furthermore, a lack of sufficiently trained human resources knowledgeable in HIE presents a bottleneck to adoption of HIE. In addition, providers often resist adoption due to a perception that HIE leads to increases in physician and administrative workload.

- **Privacy:** Stakeholders consistently express concern regarding the privacy and confidentiality of data captured, stored, and shared via HIE [34–38]. While federal law in the United States provides a core set of regulations that govern confidentiality, privacy, and security of data in HIT and HIE systems, laws in the 50 states vary and can be more restrictive making HIE complex and challenging. For example, some states require patients to give consent before their data can be exchanged by an HIE while other states only require the ability for patients, who so desire, to remove themselves from the HIE. In addition to varying and complex regulations, up to 75% patients report in surveys being "somewhat" to "very concerned" regarding the privacy of their health data [38]. Patients' concerns are legitimate and need to be addressed by health care providers as well as HIEs, because unauthorized breaches of health information are reported on a weekly basis in addition to breaches of databases that contain financial data. Chapter "Privacy, Security, Confidentiality, and Transparency: Towards Trust" contains a detailed discussion of privacy, security, and confidentiality of data in the context of HIE.
- **Interoperability:** EHR systems have historically been silos unto themselves, thus lacking interoperability [4,34,37–39]. Therefore providers and health care organizations consistently ask the federal government as well as international authorities to create and/or dictate the use of technical standards by EHR vendors to facilitate interoperability. Complaints by providers about the absence of standards, as well as the complexity of available standards, have been an excuse, by some, to avoid adoption of HIE. While limited, adoption of available standards has grown over time. Yet interoperability is limited, which makes it an important issue for HIEs to address. An assessment of available and emerging technical standards, as well as their adoption, is presented in chapter "Standardizing and Exchanging Messages."
- **Competition:** Competition has traditionally been a salient barrier to adoption of HIE with vendors and providers in highly competitive markets refusing to share data with competitors [34,37–39]. Even when they shared data, stakeholders limited the type and amount of data shared [37]. Given that the financial benefits of data exchange are principally accrued by payers, sharing data with competitors, especially as new models of care such as accountable care organizations emerge in the marketplace, could put a hospital or physician practice at financial risk.

Drivers of Adoption

Although there are barriers, there also exist two significant forces that drive the market to adopt and use HIE. First, there is a natural force in the market that seeks to exchange data electronically now that many organizations have transitioned from paper charts to EHR systems. Recall from chapter "What is Health Information Exchange?" that data are fragmented in the health care system and providers have an inherent need to access patient information, no matter where it might be stored, when making clinical decisions. The rise of EHR systems naturally breeds a desire to access other institutions' HIT systems.

Yet a much larger force is driving adoption of HIE in most nations. Federal governments in both the United States and globally are directly tackling the aforementioned barriers through policy, which is having a direct effect on adoption of HIE. As previously mentioned, then President George W. Bush challenged America to adopt EHR systems by the year 2014. While we are not yet at 100% adoption, the aforementioned figures demonstrate significant progress. The President followed his State of the Union address with several policies that stimulated adoption of EHR systems as well as HIE among hospitals.

President Bush, via executive order, established the Office of the National Coordinator for HIT (ONC) as a division within the U.S. Department of Health and Human Services (HHS) following his address to Congress. He then charged the ONC with coordinating the adoption of HIT across the federal government and private sector through public–private partnerships. While the initial focus of the ONC was on EHR, eRx, computerized provider order entry (CPOE), and clinical decision support (CDS) systems, the ONC quickly advanced the agenda for HIE. This was due, in part, to reports and urging from private sector actors. For example, the Markle Foundation, which established a public–private collaborative in 2002 called *Connecting for Health* [40], created a *Common Framework* in 2006 that identified barriers to widespread sharing of health information and prioritized key policy and technical aspects that needed to be addressed to promote interoperability [36].

Leaders at HHS, ONC, Markle, and the eHealth Initiative along with several academic medical centers and private IT consulting firms then launched the formation of a NwHIN to connect private HIEs, community-based HIEs, and federal agencies to bring HIE to scale in the United States [41,42]. Over several years, national HIE efforts culminated into a set of policies, technical specifications, and implementation guides that provided a foundation for nationwide HIE. In parallel, the U.S. Agency for Healthcare Research and Quality (AHRQ), also part of HHS, funded several statewide initiatives aimed at cultivating HIE at that level [43,44]. While successful, these efforts by HHS were not enough to create a tipping point in which providers overwhelmingly sought to create and adoption HIE.

Arguably the tipping point came following the passage of HITECH in 2009 and the Patient Protection and Affordable Care Act (PPACA) in 2010. While the earlier efforts by HHS created a pathway for others to follow, these policies create sufficient incentives to overcome the aforementioned barriers while leading others down the path. These policies specifically address barriers of cost, resources, privacy, and competition.

HITECH principally promotes adoption of HIT by creating incentives for the *meaningful use* (MU) of EHR systems by eligible hospitals and providers. Through the U.S. Centers for Medicare and Medicaid Services (CMS), HITECH provisions financial incentives to certain eligible hospitals and providers, specified in the law, which can demonstrate criteria established through administrative rule-making processes part of the MU program. To date CMS has outlined criteria for three stages with incentives offered through 2019 followed by penalties for providers who do not adopt certified EHR technology or meet MU criteria. Each successive stage of the program, informed by experts and comments from the industry, adds increasingly advanced capabilities to both the EHR technology and the use of that technology by eligible hospitals and providers. By the first quarter of 2015, CMS had distributed $28.1 billion through the MU program [45]. These dollars mediate the cost of adopting EHR systems and connecting those systems together via HIE technologies.

Criteria relevant to HIE, defined in Stage 2 of the MU program (the active stage in effect at the time of writing), are summarized in Table 3.1. These criteria create a *floor* or minimum level of adoption. While many providers

TABLE 3.1 Summary of Core HIE-Related Criteria in Stage 1 and Stage 2 of the Meaningful Use Program

Health Outcomes Policy Priority	Meaningful Use Objective	Meaningful Use Measure	HIE Implication
STAGE 1			
Improving quality, safety, efficiency and reducing health disparities	Use CPOE for medication, laboratory, and radiology orders directly entered by any licensed health care professional who enters orders into the medical records per state, local, and professional guidelines	More than 30% of medication orders created by the EP or authorized providers of the eligible hospital's or CAH's inpatient or emergency department during the EHR reporting period are recorded using CPOE	Potential HIE implication
	Implement drug–drug and drug–allergy interaction checks	The EP/EH/CAH has enabled this functionality for the entire EHR reporting period	Potential HIE implication
	Implement one clinical decision support rule and the ability to track compliance with the rule	Implement one clinical decision support rule	Potential HIE implication
	EPs only: Generate and transmit permissible discharge prescriptions electronically (eRx)	Requires EPs to transmit 40% of all permissible prescriptions to be transmitted using a certified EHR	Potential HIE implication
	Defined CQMs under meaningful user definition: reporting of clinical quality measures to the CMS or the states	Requires EHR to import, export, and submit CQMs electronically	Potential HIE implication
	Incorporate clinical lab test results into the EHR	Requires more than 55% of all clinical lab tests to be incorporated into the EHR structured data	Potential HIE implication
Engage patients and families in their health care	EPs only: Provide patients the ability to view online, download, and transmit their health information within the EHR reporting period (4 business days of the information being available to the EP)	Requires provision of online access to 50% of all unique patients seen by the EP to health information during the EHR reporting period subject to EP's discretion to withhold certain information	Potential HIE implication
	Provide patients the ability to view online, download, and transmit their health information within 4 business days of the information being available to the EP	More than 50% of all unique patients seen by the EP during the EHR reporting period are provided timely (within 4 business days after the information is available to the EP) online access to their health information subject to the EP's discretion to withhold certain information	Potential HIE implication
	Provide patients the ability to view online, download, and transmit information about a hospital admission	More than 50% of all patients who are discharged from the inpatient or emergency department of an eligible hospital or CAH have their information available online within 36 h of discharge	Potential HIE implication
Improve care coordination	Capability to exchange key clinical information (eg, problem list, medication list, medication allergies, diagnostic test results), among providers of care and patient authorized entities electronically	Performed at least one test of the certified EHR technology's capacity to electronically exchange key clinical information	Explicit HIE implication

(*Continued*)

TABLE 3.1 *Continued*

Health Outcomes Policy Priority	Meaningful Use Objective	Meaningful Use Measure	HIE Implication
STAGE 2			
Improving quality, safety, efficiency, and reducing health disparities	Use CPOE for medication, laboratory, and radiology orders directly entered by any licensed healthcare professional who enters orders into the medical records per state, local, and professional guidelines	More than • 60% of medication, • 30% of laboratory, and • 30% of radiology orders created by EP or authorized providers of eligible hospitals or CAH's inpatient and ED during the EHR reporting period	Potential HIE implication
	Generate and transmit permissible prescriptions electronically (eRx)	More than • 50% of all Rx or • All Rx written by the EP and queried for drug formulary and transmitted electronically using certified EHR	Potential HIE implication in terms of exchanging health information
	EP: Record the following: • Preferred language • Sex • Race • Ethnicity • Date of birth EH/CAH: In addition to the above record: • Date and preliminary cause of death in the event of mortality in the EH or CAH	More than 80% of all unique patients seen by the EP or admitted to the EH's or CAH's inpatient or emergency department during the EHR reporting period have demographics recorded as structured data	Potential HIE implication
	Record and chart changes in vital signs: • Height/length • Weight • Blood pressure (age 3 and over) • Calculate and display BMI • Plot and display growth charts for patients 0–20 years, including BMI	More than 80% of all unique patients seen by the EP or admitted to the eligible hospital's or CAH's inpatient or emergency department during the EHR reporting period have blood pressure (for patients age 3 and over only) and height/length and weight (for all ages) recorded as structured data	Potential HIE implication
	Use clinical decision support to improve performance on high priority health conditions	1. Implement 5 CDS interventions related to 4 or more CQMs at a relevant point in patient care for the entire EHR reporting period. Absent 4 CQMs related to an EP, eligible hospital or CAH's scope of practice or patient population, the CDS interventions must be related to high priority health conditions. It is suggested that one of the 5 CDS interventions be related to improving healthcare efficiency. 2. The EP, EH, or CAH has enabled and implemented the functionality for drug and drug–allergy interaction checks for the entire EHR reporting period.	Potential HIE implication

(*Continued*)

TABLE 3.1 *Continued*

Health Outcomes Policy Priority	Meaningful Use Objective	Meaningful Use Measure	HIE Implication
	Incorporate clinical lab test results into Certified EHR Technology as structured data	More than 55 % of all clinical lab tests results ordered by the EP or by authorized providers of the eligible hospital or CAH for patients admitted to its inpatient or ED during the EHR reporting period whose results are either in a positive/ negative affirmation or numerical format are incorporated in Certified EHR Technology as structured data.	Potential HIE implication
	Generate lists of patients by specific conditions to use for quality improvement, reduction of disparities, research, or outreach	Generate at least one report listing patients of the EP, eligible hospital, or CAH with a specific condition	Potential HIE implication
	EP only: Use clinically relevant information to identify patients who should receive reminders for preventive/follow-up care and send these patients the reminder, per patient preference	More than 10% of all unique patients who have had two or more office visits with the EP within the 24 months before the beginning of the EHR reporting period were sent a reminder, per patient preference when available	Potential HIE implication
	EH/CAH only: Automatically track medications from order to administration using assistive technologies in conjunction with an electronic medication administration record (eMAR)	More than 10% of medication orders created by authorized providers of the EH's or CAH's inpatient or ED during the EHR reporting period for which all doses are tracked using eMAR	Potential HIE implication
Engage patients and families in their health care	EP only: Provide patients the ability to view online, download, and transmit their health information within 4 business days of the information being available to the EP	**1.** More than 50% of all unique patients seen by the EP during the EHR reporting period are provided timely (within 4 business days after the information is available to the EP) online access to their health information subject to the EP's discretion to withhold certain information **2.** More than 5% of all unique patients seen by the EP during the EHR reporting period (or their authorized representatives) view, download, or transmit to a third party their health information	Potential HIE implication
	EH/CAH only: Provide patients the ability to view online, download, and transmit information about a hospital admission.	**1.** More than 50% of all patients who are discharged from the inpatient or emergency department of an EH or CAH have their information available online within 36 h of discharge. **2.** More than 5% of all patients (or their authorized representatives) who are discharged from the inpatient or emergency department of an EH or CAH view, download or transmit to a third party their information during the reporting period.	Potential HIE implication

(*Continued*)

TABLE 3.1 *Continued*

Health Outcomes Policy Priority	Meaningful Use Objective	Meaningful Use Measure	HIE Implication
	EP only: Provide clinical summaries for patients for each office visit.	Clinical summaries provided to patients or patient-authorized representatives within 1 business day for more than 50% of office visits.	Potential HIE implication
	Use Certified EHR Technology to identify patient-specific education resources and provide those resources to the patient	Patient-specific education resources identified by CEHRT are provided to patients for more than 10% of all unique patients with office visits seen by the EP during the EHR reporting period. More than 10% of all unique patients admitted to the eligible hospitals or CAH's inpatient or emergency departments are provided patient-specific education resources identified by Certified EHR Technology	Potential HIE implication
	EP only: Use secure electronic messaging to communicate with patients on relevant health information	A secure message was sent using the electronic messaging function of Certified EHR Technology by more than 5% of unique patients (or their authorized representatives) seen by the EP during the EHR reporting period	Potential HIE implication
Improve care coordination	The EP, EH, or CAH who transitions their patient to another setting of care or provider of care or refers their patient to another provider of care provides a summary of care record for each transition of care or referral	1. The EP, EH, or CAH that transitions or refers their patient to another setting of care or provider of care provides a summary of care record for more than 50% of transitions of care and referrals 2. The EP, EH, or CAH that transitions or refers their patient to another setting of care or provider of care provides a summary of care record for more than 10% of such transitions and referrals either (1) electronically transmitted using CEHRT to a recipient or (2) where the recipient receives the summary of care record via exchange facilitated by an organization that is a NwHIN Exchange participant or in a manner that is consistent with the governance mechanism ONC establishes for the nationwide health information network 3. An EP, EH, or CAH must satisfy one of the two following criteria: (1) conducts one or more successful electronic exchanges of a summary of care document with a recipient who has EHR technology that was developed designed by a different EHR technology developer than the sender's EHR technology, (2) conducts one or more successful tests with the CMS designated test EHR during the EHR reporting period	Strong HIE implication

(Continued)

TABLE 3.1 *Continued*

Health Outcomes Policy Priority	Meaningful Use Objective	Meaningful Use Measure	HIE Implication
Improve population and public health	Capability to submit electronic data to immunization registries or immunization information systems except where prohibited, and in accordance with applicable law and practice	Successful ongoing submission of electronic immunization data from Certified EHR Technology to an immunization registry or immunization information system for the entire EHR reporting period	Potential HIE implication
	EH/CAH only: Capability to submit electronic reportable laboratory results to public health agencies, except where prohibited, and in accordance with applicable law and practice	Successful ongoing submission of electronic reportable laboratory results from Certified EHR Technology to public health agencies for the entire EHR reporting period	Explicit HIE implication
	Capability to submit electronic syndromic surveillance data to public health agencies, except where prohibited, and in accordance with applicable law and practice	Successful ongoing submission of electronic syndromic surveillance data from Certified EHR Technology to a public health agency for the entire EHR reporting period	Potential HIE implication
	Ensure adequate privacy and security protections for personal health information	Protect electronic health information created or maintained by the Certified EHR Technology through the implementation of appropriate technical capabilities	Explicit HIE implication

EP, eligible professionals; EH, eligible hospital; CAH, critical access hospitals.

may only be able to achieve the floor, other providers will operate at a higher level or possess more advanced EHR and/or HIE functionality. For example, Stage 2 requires eligible hospitals to electronically deliver "more than 55 percent of all clinical lab test results ordered by an authorized provider … for patients admitted to its inpatient or emergency department." Many hospitals that have fully implemented interfaces between their lab information systems and their EHR systems will likely exchange upwards of 80–90% of lab results. Yet the regulations set a bar for others to work towards. These criteria focus resources within health systems to implement HIE technologies that are necessary to meet the MU criteria.

In addition to addressing the cost and resource barriers by providing financial incentives for adoption of activities involving HIE, HITECH further addressed interoperability and privacy barriers. Beyond funds for CMS incentives, HITECH allocated funds for the advancement of technical standards. For example, ONC received funding for what it calls the Standards & Interoperability (S&I) framework, which aims to create best practices for interoperability [46]. More than half a billion US dollars were also allocated to state government designated entities to create HIE infrastructure in all 50 states and territories. Moreover, HITECH supported the creation of Regional Extension Centers as well as Beacon communities to provide technical assistance and model the possibilities for what a connected, interoperable health information infrastructure might do for quality and safety of care. Finally, under the Workforce Development Program, HITECH created a highly skilled HIT workforce to support providers in the adoption and implementation as well as in achieving meaningful use of an EHR system. Finally, HITECH modified prior federal law referred to as the Health Insurance Portability and Accountability Act (HIPAA) of 1996. These changes are discussed at length in chapter "Privacy, Security, Confidentiality, and Transparency: Towards Trust," but essentially they expanded protections for the privacy and security of health information as it is captured, stored, managed, and shared by both health care providers and HIE organizations.

Finally, we examine the impact thus far of the PPACA. The PPACA is helping to align provider, patient, and payer interests by making major changes to reimbursement policies. Whereas existing fee-for-service payment models reward providers for the "volume" of care they provide (eg, ordering unnecessary or redundant tests could result in higher fees collected for these services), the PPACA focuses more on "value" by rewarding providers for higher quality care that is more patient centric and less costly. This shift from volume to value forces providers to identify ways to prevent costly hospitalizations and direct patients toward care settings most cost-effective as a way to earn higher reimbursement rates. Moreover, the new payment models now utilizes routinely collected patient satisfaction data to help determine providers' reimbursement amounts. Thus, providers are able to earn higher fees when their patients are more satisfied. Ultimately, under the new models of care, providers are required to take on more financial risk for the prevention of costly health services utilization, assuring adequate patient satisfaction, and clinically managing patients appropriately such that they are routed to the most efficient use of resources. Being able to coordinate patient care under this new payment model requires HIE to be successful. The case study "Use of HIEs for Value-Based Care Delivery: A Case Study of Maryland's HIE" illustrates how the HIE in the State of Maryland is supporting a range of population health management services to support providers' transition to new models of care delivery.

Internationally, countries are moving towards the adoption of HIE as a component of their eHealth Strategy. As discussed in chapter "What is Health Information Exchange?", the World Health Organization (WHO) encourages member states to develop and implement integrated eHealth strategies to advance care delivery and public health. Many nations are seeking to formulate their national strategies, yet it will likely be a decade or more before some of them can achieve broad scale HIE.

Throughout the book, we present examples of efforts in several countries. While these tend to be small steps towards HIE, they are important ones because they (1) align with the nation's overall eHealth strategy and (2) they establish a foundation upon which the nation can build in the future. Some experts believe that a few of these nations might eventually leapfrog the United States in HIE in the same way many adopted cellular infrastructures and mobile phones long before the Americans.

EMERGING TRENDS

In this section, we briefly discuss three emerging trends that are likely to have an impact on HIE adoption in the coming years. First, we examine the fervor in health care around *Big Data* and how it is likely to drive adoption of HIE. Second, we discuss the challenge of unstructured data in parallel with the rise of *natural language processing* as a method for mitigating this challenge. Finally, we discuss an important challenge of *information blocking* and the proposed action by the U.S. federal government to curtail it.

Within the last 3–5 years, two major initiatives have begun to unfold in the United States. First, the IOM issued a series of reports on what it calls the *Learning Health System*

(LHS). Second, the White House and Congress launched a campaign for *precision medicine*. Both of these initiatives requires collection, management, and use of extremely large-scale data sets, otherwise known as *Big Data*. To date, Big Data have demonstrated utility in monitoring seasonal outbreaks as well as predicting their spread [47–50]. They have further shown promise in predicting healthcare utilization and monitoring drug safety [51,52]. Data-driven health care is the cornerstone for both the IOM and White House initiatives. Yet to effectively capture, store, manage, and make use of Big Data, the nation will require a robust HIE infrastructure to move data and transform it to information and knowledge. The drive to deliver CDS at scale through these initiatives could add additional fuel to push adoption of HIE.

A challenge facing HIE is unstructured data, otherwise referred to as free text because it represents typed notes from clinicians and other health workers. Today a strong majority of clinical data are generated in the form of a note written by a physician, nurse, or other health worker. Making computers understand or interpret the contents of these unstructured data is a challenge, therefore making it a challenge for HIEs which are largely in the business of exchanging and doing something with clinical data.

An increasingly used innovation in HIT is *Natural Language Processing* (NLP) which can be applied to parse or interpret unstructured data. NLP is the method by which IBM's Watson technology can answer *Jeopardy* questions. If similarly applied to health care notes, it may be possible to transform unstructured data into a series of structured observations about a patient, which could be stored and shared within an HIE. Therefore HIEs might become more involved in NLP development as well as implementation as health care providers increasingly seek to get more value out of HIE infrastructures.

In the early period of HIE implementation, it was observed that numerous entities sought to control electronic health information and limit its availability and use. This was evidenced in the form of numerous complaints received by the ONC [53]. The ONC termed this behavior on the part of the stakeholders, *information blocking*. According to the ONC, "Information blocking occurs when persons or entities knowingly and unreasonably interfere with the exchange or use of electronic health information [53]."

Three definitive criteria must be met in order to identify information blocking: **Interference** in the form of an act or course of conduct that impedes authorized persons or entities from accessing health information, the decision to engage in this practice must be **willful** and with the stakeholder's **knowledge**, and this conduct should be such that there is **no reasonable justification** to interfere with the access to authorized personnel.

It is vital to differentiate information blocking from interference with access for legitimate reasons such as patient safety, privacy and security concerns, or potential to improve patient health care. Reasons for interference should be thoroughly scrutinized to differentiate them from any of the barriers discussed in the previous sections before such behavior is categorized as information blocking. Information blocking is a complex issue and while some of the precipitating factors are well understood, efforts are ongoing to identify and understand others.

When present, however, information blocking presents a serious problem. In addition to interfering with effective HIE, it adversely affects aspects of health care such as clinical decision making, and the safety, quality, and effectiveness of care provided to patients. It also presents an impediment to patient engagement by preventing access to health care that may be used by consumers to make informed decisions about their health and health care [53]. Finally, information blocking presents a barrier to advances in biomedical and public health resource which depends on the ability to analyze information from numerous sources to enable data-driven health care.

SUMMARY

HIE has been linked to benefits in healthcare utilization, health care costs, and coordination of care. Moreover, major changes to how hospitals and other providers are reimbursed are increasing the need for seamless exchange of clinical data. HIE is now considered an important prerequisite for a modern health care system. However, most HIEs are still in their early developmental stage. In fact, as an organization type, HIEs need further maturation which will involve innovations and technology that are expected to continue to evolve. As more and more providers adopt HIE, and more data is exchanged leading to the creation of ever larger data sets, opportunities open up to truly unleash the potential of improving the quality and cost of care. Benefits accrued from these developments may eventually address shortcomings that have plagued the health care system in the United States. Globally, HIEs have the potential to strengthen and transform health systems that are similarly facing challenges.

QUESTIONS FOR DISCUSSION

1. What has been the role of government in the adoption of health information technologies including HIE? What should it be?
2. Which meaningful use incentives within the United States are most likely to influence health systems to adopt HIE? How about providers? Is there is a difference between these two groups?
3. What is the adoption of HIE like outside the United States? What are some reasons for greater or lesser levels of adoption?
4. Which emerging trend will have the greatest impact on HIE adoption? Why?
5. What additional activities should governments, including ministries of health, be doing to encourage the adoption and use of HIE?
6. Which barriers to adoption of HIE are unlikely to be solved by governmental health policy? How might these barriers be addressed?

References

[1] Institute of Medicine Kohn LT, Corrigan JM, Donaldson MS, editors. To Err is human: building a safer health system. Washington, DC: The National Academies Press; 1999.

[2] Institute of Medicine Crossing the quality chasm: a new health system for the 21st century: National Academies Press; 2001.

[3] Walker J, Pan E, Johnston D, Adler-Milstein J, Bates DW, Middleton B. The value of health care information exchange and interoperability. Health Aff (Millwood); 2005; Suppl Web Exclusives:W5-10-W5-8. PubMed PMID: 15659453.

[4] Dixon BE. A roadmap for the adoption of e-Health. e-Service J 2007;5(3):3–13.

[5] Berwick DM, Nolan TW, Whittington J. The triple aim: care, health, and cost. Health Aff (Millwood) 2008;27(3):759–69. PubMed PMID: 18474969.

[6] Kaelber DC, Bates DW. Health information exchange and patient safety. J Biomed Inform 2007;40(Suppl. 6):S40–5. PubMed PMID: 17950041.

[7] Rahurkar S, Vest JR, Menachemi N. Despite the spread of health information exchange, there is little evidence of its impact on cost, use, and quality of care. Health Aff (Millwood) 2015;34(3):477–83. PubMed PMID: 25732499.

[8] James JT. A new, evidence-based estimate of patient harms associated with hospital care. J Patient Saf 2013;9(3):122–8. PubMed PMID: 23860193.

[9] Andel C, Davidow SL, Hollander M, Moreno DA. The economics of health care quality and medical errors. J Health Care Finance 2012;39(1):39–50. PubMed PMID: 1095371694; 23155743.

[10] Bates DW. Physicians and ambulatory electronic health records. Health Aff (Millwood) 2005;24(5): 1180–9. PubMed PMID: 16162561.

[11] Office of the National Coordinator for Health Information Technology. Update on the Adoption of Health Information Technology and Related Efforts to

Facilitate the Electronic Use and Exchange of Health Information. The Office of the National Coordinator for Health Information Technology, Office of the Secretary, United States Department of Health and Human Services, Services USDoHaH; 2014.

[12] Swain M, Charles D, Patel V, Searcy T. Health Information Exchange among U.S. Non-federal Acute Care Hospitals: 2008–2014. ONC Data Brief. 2015;24:1–12.

[13] Furukawa MF, King J, Patel V, Hsiao CJ, Adler-Milstein J, Jha AK. Despite substantial progress in EHR adoption, health information exchange and patient engagement remain low in office settings. Health Aff (Millwood) 2014;33(9):1672–9. PubMed PMID: 25104827.

[14] Gabriel MH, Swain M. E-prescribing trends in the United States. Washington, DC: Office of the National Coordinator of Health Information Technoogy; 2014.

[15] Swain M, Patel V. Health information exchange among clinical laboratories. Washington, DC: Office of the National Coordinator for Health Information Technology; 2014.

[16] Wu L, Abbey R, Daniel J, Danie J, Hieisey-Grove D, Murray M, et al. Health IT for Public Health Reporting and Information Systems. Washington, DC: Office of the National Coordinator for Health Information Technnology; 2014.

[17] Overhage JM, Evans L, Marchibroda J. Communities' readiness for health information exchange: the National Landscape in 2004. J Am Med Inform Assoc 2005;12(2):107–12. PubMed PMID: 15561785. PMCID: 551542.

[18] Snell E. eHealth Initiative Survey: HIEs lacking in interoperability Online: healthitsecurity.com; 2014 [cited August 1, 2015]. Available from: <http://healthitsecurity.com/news/ehealth-initiative-survey-hies-lacking-in-interoperability>.

[19] McDonald CJ, Overhage JM, Barnes M, Schadow G, Blevins L, Dexter PR, et al. The Indiana network for patient care: a working local health information infrastructure. An example of a working infrastructure collaboration that links data from five health systems and hundreds of millions of entries. Health Aff (Millwood) 2005;24(5):1214–20. PubMed PMID: 16162565.

[20] Schleyer T, K.L., editor. Big data in healthcare: The Indiana Network for Patient Care. Informatics: "Big Data" uses and challenges in the life sciences. Indiana Government Center; 2014.

[21] Indiana Health Information Exchange. Indiana Network for Patient Care, ihie.org: Indiana Health Information Exchange. Available from: <http://www.ihie.org/indiana-network-for-patient-care>; 2015 [cited July 24, 2015].

[22] Kaiser Permenente. Kaiser Permanente Share: Connectivity, kaiserpermanente.org: Kaiser Permenente. Available from: <http://share.kaiserpermanente.org/total-health/connectivity/>; 2013 [cited July 24, 2015].

[23] Surescripts. Surescripts : About us surescripts.com: Surescripts. Available from: <http://surescripts.com/about-us/why-choose-surescripts>; 2015 [cited July 24, 2015].

[24] Office of the National Coordinator for Health Information Technology. What is the NHIN? In: Office of the National Coordinator for Health Information Technology, Department of Health and Human Services, editors. healthit.gov: Office of the National Coordinator for Health Information Technology; 2009.

[25] Slabodkin G. eHealth Exchange Claims Title of Largest U.S. HIE Network. In: Goedert J, editor: HealthData Management; 2015.

[26] The Sequoia Project. About The Sequoia Project sequoiaproject.org: The Sequoia Project; 2015 [cited 2015 07/20/2015]. Available from: <http://sequoiaproject.org/ehealth-exchange/about/>.

[27] The Sequoia Project. The Sequoia Project—Participants sequoiaproject.org: The Sequoia Project. Available from: <http://sequoiaproject.org/ehealth-exchange/participants/>; 2015 [cited July 20, 2015].

[28] Adler-Milstein J, Ronchi E, Cohen GR, Winn LA, Jha AK. Benchmarking health IT among OECD countries: better data for better policy. J Am Med Inform Assoc 2014;21(1):111–6. PubMed PMID: 23721983. PMCID: 3912720.

[29] Ben-Assuli O, Shabtai I, Leshno M. Using electronic health record systems to optimize admission decisions: the Creatinine case study. Health Informatics J 2014 Apr 1. PubMed PMID: 24692078.

[30] Ben-Assuli O, Shabtai I, Leshno M, Hill S. EHR in emergency rooms: exploring the effect of key information components on main complaints. J Med Syst 2014;38(4):36. PubMed PMID: 24687240.

[31] Nirel N, Rosen B, Sharon A, Blondheim O, Sherf M, Samuel H, et al. The impact of an integrated hospital-community medical information system on quality and service utilization in hospital departments. Int J Med Inform 2010;79(9):649–57. PubMed PMID: 20655276.

[32] Hosseini M, Ahmadi M, Dixon BE. A service oriented architecture approach to achieve interoperability between immunization information systems in Iran. AMIA Annu Symp Proc 2014;2014:1797–805. PubMed PMID: 25954452. PMCID: 4419958.

[33] OpenHIE. Our work online: ohie.org. Available from: <https://ohie.org/#ourwork>; 2013 [cited August 1, 2015].

[34] Adler-Milstein J, Bates DW, Jha AKUS. Regional health information organizations: progress and challenges. Health Aff (Millwood) 2009;28(2):483–92. PubMed PMID: 19276008. Epub March 12, 2009.
[35] Dixon B, Miller T, Overhage M. Barriers to achieving the last mile in health information exchange: a survey of small hospitals and physician practices. J Healthcare Inf Manag 2013;27(4):55–8.
[36] Markle Foundation. The common framework: overview and principles. Markle Foundation; 2006.
[37] Vest JR, Gamm LD. Health information exchange: persistent challenges and new strategies. J Am Med Inform Assoc 2010;17(3):288–94. PubMed PMID: 20442146. PMCID: Pmc2995716. Epub May 6, 2010.
[38] Fontaine P, Ross SE, Zink T, Schilling LM. Systematic review of health information exchange in primary care practices. J Am Board Fam Med 2010;23(5):655–70. PubMed PMID: 20823361.
[39] Vest JR. More than just a question of technology: factors related to hospitals' adoption and implementation of health information exchange. Int J Med Inform 2010;79(12):797–806. PubMed PMID: 20889370. Epub October 5, 2010.
[40] Markle Foundation. Health 2002. Available from: <http://www.markle.org/health>.
[41] Rishel W, Rielhl V, Blanton C. Summary of the NHIN prototype architecture contracts. Washington, DC: U.S. Department of Health and Human Services; 2007.
[42] Gravely SD, Whaley ES. The next step in health data exchanges: trust and privacy in exchange networks. J Healthc Inf Manag 2009;23(2):33–7. PubMed PMID: 19382738.
[43] Agency for Healthcare Research and Quality. State and Regional Demonstration Projects Rockville, MD: ahrq.gov. Available from: <http://healthit.ahrq.gov/ahrq-funded-projects/state-and-regional-demonstration-projects>; 2009 [cited June 24, 2015].
[44] Banger AK, Dullabh P, Eichner J, Kissam S. Lessons learned from AHRQ's State and Regional Demonstrations in Health Information Technology. (Prepared by RTI International, under Contract No. HHSA2902009000027i) Rockville, MD: Contract No: AHRQ Publication No. 10-0075-EF.
[45] Centers for Medicare and Medicaid Services. Medicare & Medicaid EHR Incentive Programs. February 10, 2015.
[46] Office of the National Coordinator for Health Information Technology. Standards & Interoperability (S&I) Framework: www.siframework.org. Available from: <http://wiki.siframework.org/Frequently+Asked+Questions+%28FAQs%29>; 2010.
[47] Carneiro HA, Mylonakis E. Google trends: a web-based tool for real-time surveillance of disease outbreaks. Clin Infect Dis 2009;49(10):1557–64. PubMed PMID: 19845471.
[48] Cho S, Sohn CH, Jo MW, Shin SY, Lee JH, Ryoo SM, et al. Correlation between national influenza surveillance data and google trends in South Korea. PLoS One 2013;8(12):e81422. PubMed PMID: 24339927. PMCID: 3855287.
[49] Cook S, Conrad C, Fowlkes AL, Mohebbi MH. Assessing Google flu trends performance in the United States during the 2009 influenza virus A (H1N1) pandemic. PLoS One 2011;6(8):e23610. PubMed PMID: 21886802. PMCID: 3158788.
[50] Hulth A, Rydevik G, Linde A. Web queries as a source for syndromic surveillance. PLoS One 2009;4(2):e4378. PubMed PMID: 19197389. PMCID: 2634970.
[51] White RW, Horvitz E. From health search to healthcare: explorations of intention and utilization via query logs and user surveys. J Am Med Inform Assoc 2014;21(1):49–55. PubMed PMID: 23666794. PMCID: 3912725.
[52] White RW, Tatonetti NP, Shah NH, Altman RB, Horvitz E. Web-scale pharmacovigilance: listening to signals from the crowd. J Am Med Inform Assoc 2013;20(3):404–8. PubMed PMID: 23467469. PMCID: 3628066.
[53] Office of the National Coordinator for Health Information Technology. Report on Health Information Blocking. Washington, DC: The Office of the National Coordinatior for Health Information Technoogy, Department of Health and Human Services; 2015.

CHAPTER

4

Engaging and Sustaining Stakeholders: Towards Governance

Keith W. Kelley[1], Sue S. Feldman[2] and Steven D. Gravely[3]

[1]Indiana Health Information Exchange, Indianapolis, IN

[2]Arnold School of Public Health, University of South Carolina, Columbia, SC

[3]Partner and Healthcare Practice Group Leader, Troutman Sanders LLP, Richmond, VA, USA

OUTLINE

INTRODUCTION

Governance in the context of health information exchange (HIE) refers to the establishment and oversight of a common set of behaviors, policies, and standards that enable trusted, electronic HIE among a set of participants [1]. Before data can be shared, the parties involved must establish a governing body with a set of broad and representative stakeholders.

The *governing body* defines what data will be shared, how they will be shared, and under what circumstances they will be shared. The governing body creates a *governance framework* to ensure compliance with legal, technical, and operational requirements related to the protection, use, and disclosure of protected health information (PHI). Data sharing agreements codify the policies and procedures established by the governing body. These elements are essential for competing health care organizations to agree to share data. As outlined in Figure 4.1, a governance framework begins with the formation of a governing body, which creates policies and procedures and establishes a series of data sharing agreements.

As the volume and type of data exchanged expands, the importance of governance grows. The governance framework must be able to scale, sustain, and respond over time. A governance framework requires active engagement with participating organizations to establish transparency and achieve consensus. Governance is important for all types of health information organizations (HIOs; defined in chapter: What Is Health Information Exchange?), but it is more critical as membership diversity, approved use cases, and the geographic footprint of the HIO expands. Due to the complexities associated with large exchanges consisting of several competing and diverse organizations, this chapter will focus on regional, state, and nationwide HIOs.

GOVERNING BODY

The HIO governing body serves several key functions:

- It embodies the governance principles of the HIO for all those who are involved in exchanging information using the HIO's technology infrastructure;
- It provides a forum for ideas to be discussed, questions asked, and policies debated;
- It demonstrates the ongoing commitment of the key stakeholders to the HIO through their continued participation on the governing body;
- It presents a "public face" for the HIO which is important as governments consider the correct level of oversight and the public decides whether to trust electronic data exchange; and
- It reinforces the message that the policies of the HIO need to be followed because they will be enforced if necessary.

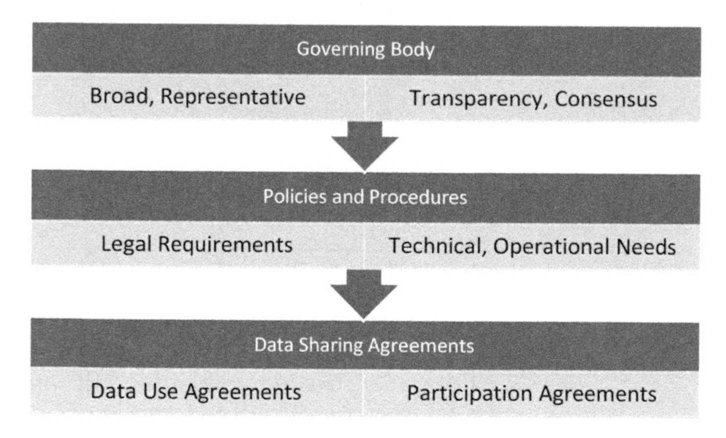

FIGURE 4.1 A governance framework for health information exchange.

When the HIO identifies the stakeholders whom will make up the governing body, it is important to have a body that is large and diverse enough to be representative of the stakeholders engaged in HIE, but not so large that efficiency and effectiveness are compromised. More importantly, this governing body must be responsive to stakeholder, environmental, state, and federal changes. Once these members are identified, they will establish bylaws or organizational policies, such as how often to meet, what establishes a quorum, and who are the officers. They will also need to be apprised of federal, state and, sometimes, local laws that govern health data use so that they can develop policies and procedures that are in accordance with those laws.

The governing body is responsible for managing governance for the HIO. The governing body is different than the HIO Board of Directors although the same health care organizations may be represented in both groups. An HIO Board of Directors holds the HIO leadership accountable for its operational performance and financial sustainability. It provides oversight to ensure proper management controls are in place. A governing body establishes and maintains policies and procedures regarding data management and use. The governing body should have broad representation from all stakeholder groups participating in the exchange.

Disparate health data organizations need a governing body to begin health data exchange. As Figure 4.2 shows, actions of a governing body are not a singular action, but rather a repetitive process of defining and redefining policies and procedures that scale with health data exchange operations.

The governing body serves as a trusted agent on behalf of all stakeholders to achieve consensus regarding data use and data access. The decisions must strike an effective balance between making data available and proper security controls. For example, consider the following data access request that occurred at a regional HIE.

> A group of primary care physicians and specialists would like approval to access a care summary from the exchange without a patient registration transaction, which is the approved use case. Instead, they would like to self-attest to a patient relationship to access a care summary. They would only do this for their patients, and they understand they could be subject to audit to ensure that they weren't accessing patients who did not belong to them. This request was brought to the governing body three years ago, and it was declined. However, the physicians feel strongly that approval will improve patient care.

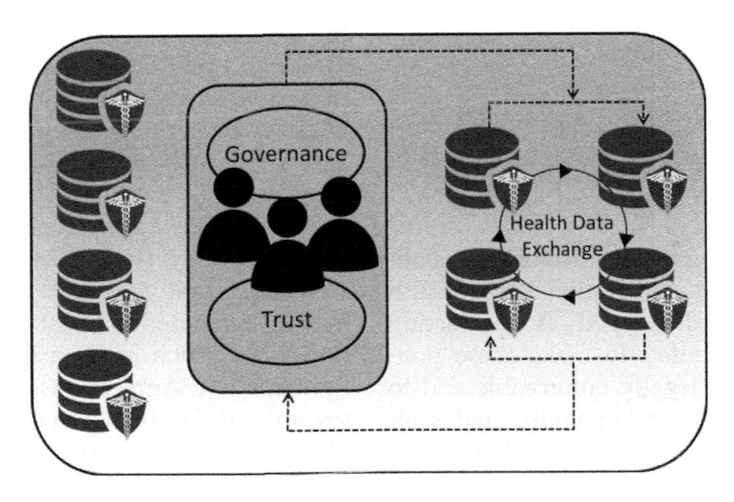

FIGURE 4.2 A representation of the health data exchange governance and trust process.

PARTICIPANTS

Who should be a part of the governing body? As discussed above, the governing body should be representative of the stakeholders engaged in data exchange. Yet, while each participant should have a voice in HIE governance, not every participant needs to have a formal vote or seat on the governing body. Several HIOs use governance models in which participants (eg, each organization engaged in HIE) elect representatives to the governing body. The governing bodies then represent various classes or types of participants. Common participant types include the following:

- Health systems, such as integrated delivery networks or accountable care organizations;
- Hospitals, including community, critical access, and for-profit;
- Physician practices of all sizes;
- Behavioral health providers, including independent psychiatrists and mental health centers;
- Long term post-acute care organizations, such as nursing homes;
- Laboratories, including hospital-based or independent labs;
- Radiology centers;
- Public health agencies;
- Insurance companies; and
- Quality improvement organizations.

POLICIES AND PROCEDURES

Once the governing body is established, policies and procedures for operationalizing health data exchange are developed. A contracting structure is implemented to make these policies and procedures legally enforceable and to ensure accountability, sustainability, and scalability. Elements include setting definitions, establishing permitted purposes of the data, subsequent data use, participation, consent, and data protection (eg, security, privacy).

Table 4.1 provides a high-level outline of what the policies and procedures should address. Each area is defined, and the table further provides examples of policies and procedures.

DATA SHARING AGREEMENTS

Data sharing agreements must be specific enough to constrain the use of shared data to specific use cases. However, such agreements also need to be flexible enough to incorporate new use cases as they are approved or modified. Creating these agreements is not easy in the early stages of establishing HIE. For this reason, formal governance may be deferred as the exchange develops and the use cases are being defined and approved. As policies are developed and procedures are defined, formal governance processes should also develop. Formal contracting agreements provide the necessary controls and protections for all participating stakeholders.

Governance describes how data are handled, shared, used, and secured. It creates a mechanism for monitoring compliance with the policies and procedures of the exchange. The HIO must be trusted to provide information to improve the safety, efficiency, and effectiveness of patient care. For this reason, trust agreements are critical to successful governance programs.

HIOs create a set of contractual documents, referred to as *trust agreements* because they engender trust amongst the parties involved in the agreements. Trust agreements include documents such as Data Use Agreements and Participation Agreements. Table 4.2 provides several types of trust agreements used by HIOs. The table outlines the components of each agreement type and provides definitions.

TABLE 4.1 Policies and Procedures by Area of Governance

Area of Governance	
Policy	**Procedure**
PERMITTED PURPOSES	
Use for the purposes of payment, treatment, operations, public heath reporting, meaningful use, SSA disability determination, research, system audits, ACO management, etc.	• Each participant is responsible for ensuring that data requested are for a permitted purpose • Each participant organization is responsible for auditing and monitoring usage
PERMITTED USERS	
Types of participants as well as the types of users and the type of access (based on the permitted purposes) each user has, what actions the user can perform with that access. Participants include hospitals, physician offices, laboratories, free-standing same-day surgery centers, public health clinics, ACOs, long term post-acute care facilities, etc. Users include physicians, nurses, nurse practitioners, clinical researchers, billing personnel, etc. Access types includes payment, treatment, operations, public health reporting, etc. User actions includes sending information, obtaining information, reading information, etc.	• To enforce roles-based access, each participant can assign each user a role consistent with a standardized role code (eg, SNOMED) • Each participant is responsible for ensuring that permitted users are appropriate and that unauthorized users are not requesting data • Each participant organization is responsible for auditing and monitoring each permitted user
SUBSEQUENT USE OF INFORMATION RECEIVED THROUGH THE HIO	
Policies around reuse promote trust. Common subsequent use policies establish if the information is: read-only without reuse, retained without reuse unless patient authorization is received, retained and reused for only the original purpose, or retained with reused governed by applicable law	• Participants are responsible for ensuring that record retention policies and procedures are followed • If applicable law requires that participant obtain a patient consent or authorization before it reuses or re-discloses information, then it is the responsibility of participant to obtain this consent or authorization prior to such use or re-disclosure
MINIMUM REQUIREMENTS FOR PARTICIPATION	
Minimum participation levels mitigate participation for the purpose of receiving information without equally providing information and ensure data exchange will ensue. Examples of minimum participation levels include: exchanging only with each other, exchanging for like purposes (eg, treatment only), a minimum number of transactions, laboratory results routing, etc.	• Participants are responsible for monitoring compliance related to the agreed upon minimum requirements. Monitoring can be accomplish through central auditing, reports of noncompliance from requesting participants, or self-reporting
CONSENT AND AUTHORIZATION EXPECTATIONS	
Consent and authorization are different in that consent is a general form allowing use and disclosure of health information, whereas authorization is a specific form allowing use and disclosure of specific health information for specific purposes. Consent policies are around establishing opt-in or out-out policies and can have varying degrees of granularity, whereas authorization policies are around what information will be provided to an organization, such as the U.S. Social Security Administration who uses clinical data from medical records for disability determination	• Depending on the granularity of the consent, the participant is responsible for ensuring that only consented to data are exchanged
PRIVACY AND SECURITY REQUIREMENTS	
Privacy and security requirements are well-established by HIPAA. However, stakeholders frequently use privacy and security policies as a mechanism to bring these requirements to the forefront. These include areas such as virus protection, password complexity and security, establishing stakeholder privacy and security requirements, etc. Additional information on privacy and security can be found in chapter "Privacy, Security, and Confidentiality: Toward Trust"	• The participant is responsible for monitoring compliance and mitigating and managing breaches • The participant is responsible to adhere to breach response and reporting requirements by applicable law • The participant is responsible for ensuring risk management, auditing and incident procedures, password management, data backup and disaster recovery plan are current at all times

TABLE 4.2 Types, Definitions, and Components of Data Sharing Agreements

Types of Agreements	Definitions	Components
Data Use Agreement	Data Use Agreement (DUA): A covered entity may use or disclose a limited data set if that entity obtains a DUA from the potential recipient. This information can only be used for: Research, Public Health, or Health Care Operations A limited data set is protected health information that excludes direct identifiers of the individual or of relatives, employers, or household members of the individual [3]	• Establishes what the data will be used for, as permitted above. The DUA must not violate this principle • Establishes who is permitted to use or receive the limited data set • Provides that the limited data set recipient will: – Not use the information in a matter inconsistent with the DUA or other laws – Employ safeguards to ensure that this does not happen – Report to the covered entity any use of the information that was not stipulated in the DUA – Ensure that any other parties, including subcontractors, agree to the same conditions as the limited data set recipient in the DUA – Not identify the information or contact the individuals themselves
Business Associate Agreement	A business associate is a person or entity that performs certain functions or activities involving the use or disclosure of protected health information on behalf of, or provides services to, a covered entity. A covered entity's contract or other written arrangement with its business associate must contain the elements specified at 45 CFR 164.504(e) [4]	• Describes the permitted and required uses of protected health information by the business associate • Provides that the business associate will not use or further disclose the protected health information other than as permitted or required by the contract or as required by law • Requires the business associate to use appropriate safeguards to prevent a use or disclosure of the protected health information other than as provided for by the contract
Data Use and Reciprocal Support Agreement	The DURSA (Data Use Reciprocal Support Agreement) is the legal, multiparty trust agreement that is entered into voluntarily by all entities, organizations, and federal agencies that desire to engage in electronic health information exchange with each other using an agreed upon set of national standards, services, and policies developed in coordination with the office of the National Coordinator for Health IT (ONC) in the U.S. Department of Health and Human Services [5]	Multiparty agreement that specifies: • Participants actively engaged in health information exchange • Privacy and security obligations • Requests for information based on a permitted purpose • Duty to respond • Future use of data received from another participant • Respective duties of submitting and receiving participants • Autonomy principle for access • Use of authorizations to support requests for data • Participant breach notification • Mandatory nonbinding dispute resolution • Allocation of liability risk
Participation Agreement	Designed to ensure that participants comply with the data sharing policies and procedures, participation Agreements spell out the terms of the relationship, including the roles, rights, and responsibility of each party as they pertain to the initiative [6]	May include or reference one or more of the above-named agreements

Adapted from Ref. [2].

GOVERNANCE KEY SUCCESS FACTORS

Governance builds trust, scales to accommodate new stakeholders, and adapts to change. Steady and important progress can be achieved by HIOs as they incorporate the key elements.

Trust

It is said that it takes years to build trust and seconds to lose it. This saying holds true for HIE. Health care organizations must have a high confidence of trust that the HIO will be good stewards of their data. This is becoming more critical as the frequency and size of data breaches continues to grow. Some forming HIOs identify a tipping point when health care organizations acknowledge they should not compete on the data; rather, they should compete on *what they do with* the data. By agreeing to share their data, they are also agreeing to trust the HIO to manage it effectively. Effective governance builds trust among participants, and it must always be a top priority.

Scale

The success of an HIO hinges on its ability to securely send and receive clinical data to a variety of stakeholders to support payment, treatment, and operations. Data governance becomes more complex as more organizations participate, especially among diverse stakeholders. For example, a governance framework may need to account for the needs of health plans, which are different than a health care provider. The HIO may also adopt new use cases, including public health, population health, and research. The governance framework should be able to expand to support a variety of use cases.

While data governance exists in single health care organizations and integrated delivery networks, the governance requirements are more complex for HIOs. As the exchange grows beyond state lines and incorporates new types of health care organizations, the governance structure must scale to meet these new demands. For example, as the Indiana Health Information Exchange (IHIE) grew from a central Indiana focus to a statewide focus, its governance needs evolved. The representation expanded to include health care leaders throughout the state. Consensus-based decisions needed to account for the needs of small rural facilities in addition to large urban-based hospital systems.

Flexibility

Sharing information has become more common due to federal legislation and health care reform. HIE improves care coordination, creates efficiencies to reduce medical errors and improve clinical outcomes, and provides support for accountable care organizations. As new uses of HIE are identified, the data governance model must be flexible to adapt to these changes. The contracting structure must also be flexible to accommodate changes through the governance mechanism.

The governance model must be prepared to respond to environmental changes. When the HIPAA Omnibus Rule was finalized, many HIEs needed to make governance adjustments. For example, a change in the administrative rule prohibits information from being shared with a health plan at the patient's request if the patient self pays. If an HIE's governance model had previously allowed sharing data with health plans, the data use policy must be revised to adhere to the HIPAA final rule.

GOVERNANCE CHALLENGES

Enterprise, regional, state, and nationwide HIOs have some common governance challenges. For example, all exchanges must

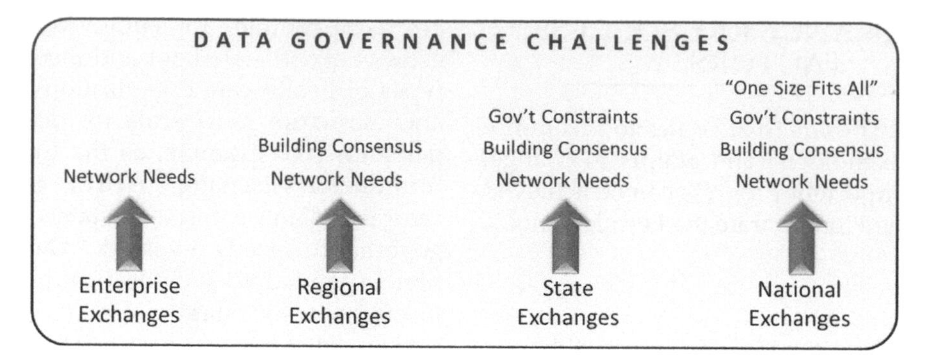

FIGURE 4.3 Data governance challenges at various levels of health information exchange.

convince stakeholders to place the network needs for data sharing above the needs of the individual participating organizations. However, some governance challenges are unique. Only a nationwide exchange organization must address the "one size fits all" challenge of establishing governance that works equitably across all stakeholders in the country. Thus, it is difficult to develop a single-governance structure for all types of exchanges. Figure 4.3 illustrates four governance challenges and each type of HIE to which they apply.

Enterprise Exchange Challenges

Enterprise HIOs, referred to as Private HIEs (see definition in chapter: What Is Health Information Exchange?), have basic governance needs. Since participating organizations belong to the same enterprise (eg, integrated delivery network) or are closely affiliated (eg, an independent practice association), they generally agree on data governance. The primary challenge is to place the network needs of the exchange above the interests of each participating organization (eg, hospital, clinic).

Regional Exchange Challenges

Regional HIOs, referred to as community-based HIEs (see definition in chapter: What Is Health Information Exchange?), typically include competing health care organizations, which adds a level of complexity to governance. Because the participating organizations compete, they will likely have different opinions about data management and use by the HIO. They might also have different interpretations of legal requirements and how much risk is acceptable.

In addition to placing network needs above the interests of each organization, regional HIOs have the difficult task of building consensus among participants. Achieving consensus can be difficult between large urban and small rural organizations. It can also be challenging between health care providers and commercial health plans. Large regional HIOs have sophisticated governance needs, especially if they cross state lines or include diverse health care organization types. Most large regional HIEs establish formal governance structures to serve the needs of its stakeholders. Mature HIEs have evolved these structures over many years and there is variability in their governance models. This is to be expected because there is variability in the business models of HIOs.

Many regional exchanges struggle to establish a robust governance structure. If the network extends across state lines, there may be conflicting state laws. For example, patient consent laws may be different between neighboring states. Differences in state laws must be identified and addressed in a way that participating state laws can support. One approach to address this is through legislative changes. Some regional exchanges have successfully convinced state government to update certain legislation to enable new use cases. However, this can be time consuming and is not always successful. Another challenge is managing conflicts between nationwide governance structures and regional governance structures. These conflicts are only beginning to surface, but it is anticipated that more conflicts will arise.

State HIO Challenges

State HIOs or government-facilitated HIE (see definition in chapter: What Is Health Information Exchange?) have similar governance needs of regional HIOs with an important difference. Because a state HIO is associated with state government, it adds a new layer of complexity associated with state government regulations and laws. The network needs of the exchange may be constrained by state government policies or processes, and it may be difficult to achieve consensus among stakeholders when the exchange is directed by a state government agency.

Stakeholders demand a high level of trust that there will be reciprocal stewardship of patient data that are accessed, used, shared, and reused. When the focus is on state level HIO, consideration must be given to private organizations, such as health systems, as well as public agencies, such as the Department of Health or Medicaid agencies. Therefore, acknowledging that there are multiple levels of data governance to be addressed when trust agreements are developed, this is accomplished with careful consideration of all participating public and private organizations.

Nationwide Exchange Challenges

Like the other types of exchanges, nationwide HIOs, like the eHealth Exchange, have governance challenges related to network needs, consensus building, and government influence. Nationwide exchanges have the most complexity because they must deal with the differences of all state laws, the diversity of all health care organizations, and a desire to have a single governance structure that works for the entire nation. Gaining support for a "one size fits all" governance solution is arduous when much of health care is managed locally and regionally. If important decisions about sharing health data are made nationally, there may be unintended consequences that create problems in parts of the country. For example, in Indiana there is a robust clinical and claims repository that has been standardized and normalized. It is a unique asset that does not exist in much of the country. How would a nationwide governance structure make decisions regarding this unique asset?

Each state can create laws regarding the sharing of health data. For example, most states have created patient consent laws that are not consistent across the country [7]. Until differences in state laws regarding HIE are addressed, a nationwide governance structure will be constrained to use cases where they can avoid conflicts between state laws. For example, consider how the ability to conduct nationwide reporting of infectious diseases might be impacted by differing state laws regarding what kind of health data can and cannot be shared and under what circumstances. Figure 4.4 shows the public health information supply chain, illustrating how data flow up from local health departments, state health agencies, and the national Centers for Disease Control and Prevention (CDC). The figure also illustrates that individual health care organizations and HIOs have relationships at all levels of the public health system. The ability of CDC to act in

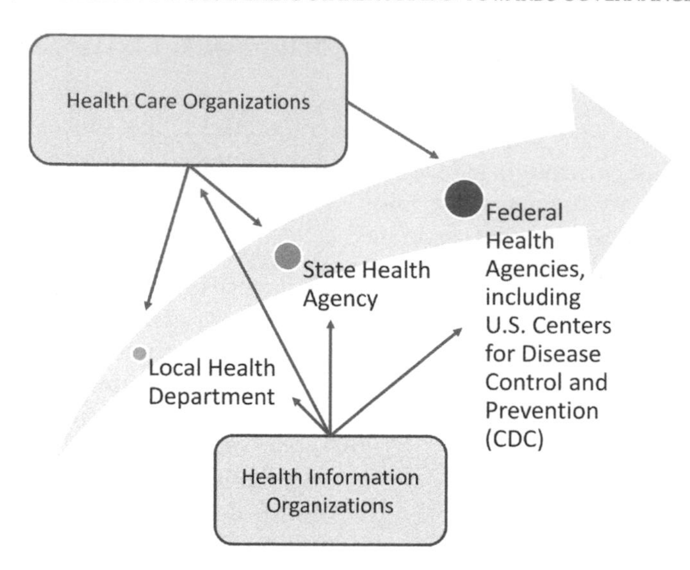

FIGURE 4.4 The flow of public health information in the United States.

the best interest of the public with comprehensive surveillance and alerts becomes incomplete when just one state has laws limiting data sharing or restricting data use.

To encourage consistent approaches to public health reporting, the Standards and Interoperability (S&I) Framework issued guidelines regarding three public health domain use cases as examples of HIE for Stage 1 of the meaningful use program.[1] The guidelines pertain to the following areas of public health recording:

1. Capability to submit electronic *syndromic surveillance* data to public health agencies and actual transmission according to applicable law and practice.
2. Capability to submit electronic data to *immunization* registries of Immunization Information Systems and actual submission in accordance with applicable law and practice.
3. Capability to submit *electronic data on reportable* (as required by state or local law) *lab results* to public health agencies and actual submission in accordance with applicable law and practice.

Although the guidelines seek to harmonize data sharing efforts, they are subject to applicable law and practice, meaning that health data exchange will differ from state to state. Furthermore, because health care organizations and HIOs have independent relationships with the various levels of public health, clear and consistent pathways for data sharing are challenging given the technical capacity and HIE engagement among the various public health agencies in a given state or region.

One benefit of creating a nationwide governance structure is to replace hundreds of point to point and multiparty governance arrangements in regional and state exchanges. However, the complexities of establishing a nationwide governance model has been difficult to achieve. In 2014 the Office of the National Coordinator (ONC) published a Program Information Notice (PIN) regarding governance. The good

[1] The S&I Framework is a public–private collaborative focused on tools, services, and guidance to facilitate functional HIE (http://wiki.siframework.org/).

news is that it attracted substantial feedback; however, much of it was unfavorable and some questioned the federal government's role in governance.

REGIONAL HIO GOVERNANCE EXAMPLE: INDIANA NETWORK FOR PATIENT CARE

Regional HIOs come in many different shapes and sizes. Some operate within a single state while others cross the borders of several states. Some are sponsored by communities while others have roots in large integrated delivery networks or payers. This is important when thinking about governance because it is natural for those who sponsor HIE activity to seek a substantial role in governance of the activity. Developing a successful HIO takes a lot of work, money, and time which is the scarcest resource of all. It is perfectly logical for those who commit the resources to develop an HIO to seek a substantial role in governance. This is about more than simply wanting to control their investment, it reflects a deep commitment by these sponsors to promote expansive data sharing and interoperability.

The principles of sound governance that have guided the development of eHealth Exchange apply equally to regional HIE initiatives. This means that the governing body should be representative of key stakeholders whether or not those stakeholders have invested in capital in the HIO, should operate in a transparent manner for all those involved, should remain responsive to the concerns of those who participate in the HIO.

In the mid-1990s the Regenstrief Institute created one of the first HIE governance bodies, called the Indiana Network for Patient Care (INPC), which is now facilitated by IHIE. The governance structure was originally created to serve the Indianapolis market and a few use cases. Over the past 20 years, the scope expanded to include health care organizations across the state and dozens of use cases. See *Case Study 1* in this book for additional information about the INPC.

STATE HIO EXAMPLE: CONNECTVIRGINIA

This HIO began as a state-level HIO funded by a grant from ONC. The Virginia Department of Health (VDH) served as the grant recipient and conducted a competitive bidding process to select a contractor to implement the HIO. One of the contractor's responsibilities was to develop a governance model for ConnectVirginia. VDH wanted to be certain that the governing body was credible and broadly representative of all stakeholders. Therefore, the initial governing body was selected by the Virginia Secretary of Health and Human Services and the State Health Commissioner with input from key stakeholders. The Secretary of Health served as the chairperson of the initial governing body which included representatives of the following:

- Health systems, both not-for-profit and for-profit
- Teaching hospitals
- The Virginia Health Information Technology Advisory Council
- Physicians
- The Virginia Regional Extension Center funded by ONC
- Federally Qualified Health Centers
- The State Health Commissioner

The ConnectVirginia governing body chose to conduct its meetings in public with advance notice that complied with the Virginia regulations applicable to public bodies. This assured that the governance was open and transparent. The board had the legal authority to convene into executive session and did so when necessary to address personnel issues and other matters that were especially sensitive. However, this was rare and, generally, all deliberations and decisions of the governing body were conducted in public. This not only helped assure that diverse input was received but also provided credibility for the governing body. In fact, the model was so effective that this approach has continued even after the grant funding ended in February 2014.

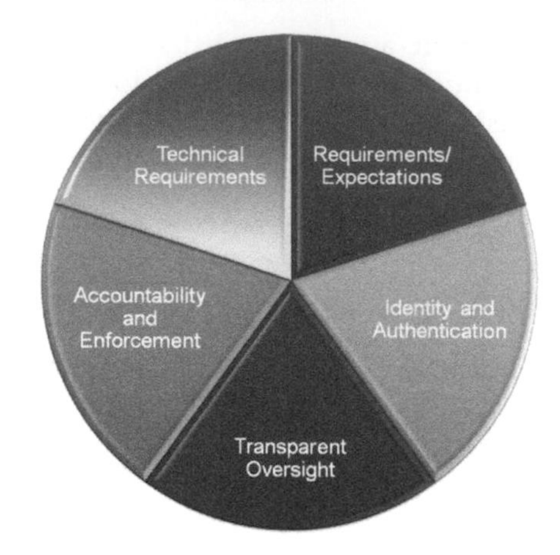

FIGURE 4.5 Universal trust framework developed by the eHealth Exchange.

NATIONWIDE HIO GOVERNANCE EXAMPLE: eHEALTH EXCHANGE

The vision of fully interoperable electronic health records was first articulated as early as the 1980s.[2] eHealth Exchange (formerly known as the Nationwide Health Information Network or NwHIN) was designed as a "network of networks" to enable the exchange of health information between a diverse range of stakeholders including HIOs, integrated delivery networks (IDNs), federal and state government agencies, and health plans. eHealth Exchange was founded on the principal that "point-to-point" data sharing agreements, in which two data sharing organizations negotiate a specific data sharing agreement to support the sharing of specific types of data, are not scalable on a national level.

The eHealth Exchange model of a network of networks where a wide variety of organizations can share health information safely and securely using a common trust framework is preferred over the point-to-point model. The common trust framework includes both technical requirements to enable data sharing and policy requirements that govern the use and disclosure of data sharing. Developing a common trust framework for the NwHIN was very challenging from both a technical and policy perspective. It became clear during the NwHIN Trial Implementation sponsored by ONC that a common trust framework would have to be created from whole cloth. ONC established national work groups charged with developing specific components of the trust framework. The effort of these work groups resulted in a universal trust framework, depicted in Figure 4.5, which was ultimately endorsed by the HIT Policy Committee in 2010.

Technical specifications, while essential for electronic health systems to communicate, are not sufficient to support widespread interoperability. There are many reasons why this is true. Some organizations consider health data to be proprietary information, some health care provider organizations fear losing a competitive advantage by sharing health data, and others are simply too fearful of liability for data breach. It became clear that widespread interoperability would not happen unless there was a set of data use policies that governed the use of the HIE technology, that all participants in the network agreed to comply with the policies,

[2] The workgroup for Electronic Data Interchange was formed in 1991 by the secretary of HHS to promote the use of Health IT to improve the quality, cost, and efficiency of health care delivery. There were years of discussion at the national level leading up to the formation of WEDI.

and that there was a means to enforce those policies in the event of noncompliance. The conundrum was how to create a common trust framework that would be legally binding in the absence of a comprehensive federal legislative or regulatory scheme. This was complicated by the fact that the legal framework which did exist consisted primarily of data privacy laws, such as HIPAA and state laws, which were often contradictory.

ONC recognized this challenge and created a national workgroup to develop a data sharing trust agreement that would support the NwHIN's model of network to network data sharing. ONC named this trust agreement the Data Use Reciprocal Support Agreement (DURSA).[3] The DURSA has since become the foundational legal document of the eHealth Exchange and a model for HIE data sharing networks generally. The DURSA is a multiparty legally binding agreement that identifies key requirements that every organization participating in eHealth Exchange agrees to follow. However, it is more than that, it also embodies the policy framework that undergirds the eHealth Exchange.

The DURSA memorializes the set of core data sharing principles on which all eHealth Exchange participants agreed. These principles address how the eHealth Exchange can be used (Permitted Purposes), by whom it can be used (Participants and Permitted Users), the level of use that is required of each Participant to maintain a healthy data sharing community (minimum level of participation), respect for the rights of Participants (autonomy principle), requirements for reporting data security incidents, the allocation of risk, a method for dispute resolution, and details on how eHealth Exchange is governed. Each eHealth Exchange participant knows what the requirements are and that every other participant is required to comply with the same requirements. Failure to comply will result in penalties including suspension of data exchange privileges or, in extreme cases, expulsion from eHealth Exchange. Knowing that common rules exist and must be followed is a key component of any trust community. In the case of eHealth Exchange, it has created a foundation for governance of the multiparty network of very diverse stakeholders.

While a section by section analysis of the DURSA is beyond the scope of this book, some of the key provisions of the DURSA are:

- *Permitted Purposes*: Use of eHealth Exchange is limited to specific permitted purposes. Participants may not request information for reasons that fall outside the scope of these enumerated permitted purposes.
- *Permitted Users*: Every Participant is responsible for deciding which individuals within its organization or network are allowed to access eHealth Exchange. Each Participant must have a process to authenticate its users and to monitor their use of eHealth Exchange.
- *Minimum Level of Participation*: This requires that any eHealth Exchange participant that submits a request related to treatment is required to respond to requests from other participants when the permitted purpose of those requests is also treatment.
- *Autonomy Principle*: Participants in eHealth Exchange are diverse and include health plans, IDNs, HIEs, federal government agencies, and other governmental organizations. It is important to respect the business rules that these participants have in place.
- *Notification of Security Incidents*: Participants are required to notify the eHealth Exchange Coordinating Committee within 1 hour of

[3] The current version of the DURSA is available online at http://sequoiaproject.org/ehealth-exchange/onboarding/dursa/

determining that a security incident may have occurred involving the transmission of information using eHealth Exchange. A participant must submit a detailed report which includes specific information set out in the DURSA within 24 hours of the suspected incident. This is an extremely aggressive notification standard that meets the strictest federal requirements.

- *Allocation of Risk*: Governmental agencies cannot agree to indemnify nongovernmental parties, so the DURSA does not include traditional indemnification provisions by design. However, participants do agree to be responsible for their own actions, when using eHealth Exchange, that cause damage or injury to another participant. In this way, risk is allocated to the party that is most able to control it.
- *Data Privacy*: The DURSA establishes the requirements of HIPAA as a contractual standard even if a participant is not otherwise subject to HIPAA as a covered entity or a business associate.
- *Mandatory "Flow Downs"*: Participants are required to flow down to every organization or individual in their network the DURSA requirements related to Security Incident notification and other critical provisions. This assures that everyone using eHealth Exchange is following the same set of rules.

Having a common set of rules that are known by all participants and are mandatory for participation in eHealth Exchange helped to create a trust framework that is both durable and flexible. However, there must be oversight of the community so that participants know the requirements are being followed and there are consequences for not following them. eHealth Exchange is not a legal entity, so traditional governance models, like board of directors, were not available to it. Additionally, there was no federal legislation that granted authority to a governance body over eHealth Exchange. Careful thought was given to determining the key characteristics of an effective governance model for data exchange. The following key principles of governance were developed by NeHC[4] under contract to ONC.

- *Distributed Governance*: Governance should not be solely vested in any single organization or group. The complexity of the governance functions and the diversity of core competencies required to execute these functions make it very clear that effective governance will require the active participation of multiple organizations, individuals and groups, including consumers. Governance of the "network of networks" is and will continue to be inherently complex and requires a diverse range of competencies and perspectives, thus making it very clear that effective governance requires active participation by and distribution among public and private organizations.
- *Representative Governance*: One of the hallmarks of eHealth Exchange is its diversity in terms of those who participate in the exchange of health information. The ONC Strategic Plan affirms that this diversity is purposeful and should be encouraged. The governance model should be designed to balance the collective needs of eHealth Exchange with the unique needs of individual stakeholders, thus promoting stakeholders' continued use of and participation in eHealth Exchange. Many stakeholders including, but not limited to governmental stakeholders, are subject to specific legal requirements that govern their participation in eHealth Exchange.

[4] The National eHealth Collaborative (NeHC) was a public–private partnership established through an ONC grant. NeHC's efforts focused on enabling secure and interoperable health information exchange through education and stakeholder engagement. NeHC merged with The HIMSS Foundation in Dec. 2013.

Any governance structures should take these requirements into consideration.

- *Transparency and Openness*: The foremost basis for establishing trust is engaging in governance activities that are transparent and open to stakeholders. The degree, type, and mechanism for openness and transparency will vary in accordance with the specific functions or activities.
- *Responsive*: Governance exists for the benefit of the governed. This concept has many implications and challenges for governance but among the most significant is that the governance process be responsive to the needs and concerns of both governmental and nongovernmental stakeholders. This responsiveness includes giving timely attention to governing issues and remaining flexible enough to accommodate multiple demands on the governing body.
- *Accountability*: Those charged with eHealth Exchange governance occupy a position of public trust. eHealth Exchange is a vital component of the national infrastructure as part of both the health care system and the electronic HIE infrastructure. Individuals and organizations who participate in the governance process must recognize that they, as well as the actual governing authority(ies), are accountable to the stakeholders, and the public more broadly, in the discharge of their duties. To the extent that multiple groups are involved in governance, their individual interests may at times be in conflict with the interests of eHealth Exchange. There will need to be processes to address such conflicts.

Using the principles of governance, the eHealth Exchange decided that the best approach to governance of the network of networks was a self-governance model that was driven by the eHealth Exchange participants themselves. The result is a Coordinating Committee composed of representatives of the participants. eHealth Exchange was not created by a legislative or regulatory action, and is not a corporation. Therefore, the legal basis for the Coordinating Committee had to be created from whole cloth. The DURSA created the Coordinating Committee by agreement of all signatories and identifies the scope of the Coordinating Committee's authority. Each eHealth Exchange participant, by signing the DURSA, agrees contractually to submit to the authority of the Coordinating Committee to oversee eHealth Exchange. The authority of the Coordinating Committee is specifically set out in the DURSA as below. While broad, it is not unlimited. Following the principle of distributed governance, each eHealth Exchange participant is responsible for governing itself and those who exchange information via eHealth Exchange using that participant's digital credentials.

SECTION 4.03 GRANT OF AUTHORITY

The participants hereby grant to the Coordinating Committee the right to provide oversight, facilitation, and support for the participants who transact message content with other participants by conducting activities including, but not limited to, the following:

- Determining whether to admit a new participant;
- Maintaining a definitive list of all transaction patterns supported by each of the participants;
- Developing and amending Operating Policies and Procedures in accordance with Section 11 of this agreement;
- Receiving reports of breaches and acting upon such reports in accordance with Section 14.03 of this agreement (Breach Notification);
- Suspending or terminating participants in accordance with Section 19 of this agreement (Suspension and Termination);
- Resolving disputes between participants in accordance with Section 21 of this agreement (Dispute Resolution);

- Managing the amendment of this agreement in accordance with Section 23.02 of this Agreement;
- Evaluating, prioritizing, and adopting new Performance and Service Specification, changes to existing Performance and Service Specifications and the artifacts required by the validation plan in accordance with Section 10 of this agreement;
- Maintaining a process for managing versions of the Performance and Service Specifications, including migration planning;
- Evaluating requests for the introduction of Emergent Specifications into the production environment used by the participant to Transact Message Content;
- Coordinating with ONC to help ensure the interoperability of the Performance and Service Specifications with other HIE initiatives including, but not limited to, providing input into the broader ONC specifications activities and ONC Standards and Interoperability Framework initiatives; and
- Fulfilling all other responsibilities delegated by the participants to the Coordinating Committee as set forth in this agreement.

The composition of the Coordinating Committee is a critical issue. The governance principles developed as part of creating eHealth Exchange require that a governing body be representative in order to be effective. The eHealth Exchange has evolved since it was formed in 2007 and the composition of the Coordinating Committee has evolved as well in order to remain representative of the stakeholders. Initially, the Coordinating Committee was composed of representatives from the first governmental and nongovernmental signatories to the DURSA (the "charter Participants"). This approach was taken to assure that the Coordinating Committee reflected the input of those with the most at stake in the success of eHealth Exchange.

This was a transitional model, however, and the DURSA required this approach to sunset after a period of years in favor of a more pure representative model in which nongovernmental participants elected a specific number of Coordinating Committee members and each federal agency that participated in eHealth Exchange appointed individuals. Over time, the role of various federal agencies changed such that it seemed more prudent to have the federal agencies, as a group, select up to five individuals to serve on the Coordinating Committee as voting members which is the current model. This approach assures that the perspective of the federal agencies involved in eHealth Exchange is retained with the Coordinating Committee, which is critical, while not imposing an undue burden on each agency to designate a representative. The remaining nine voting members of the Coordinating Committee are selected by the nonfederal participants. There is also an *ex officio* seat (nonvoting) reserved for ONC to assure that the Coordinating Committee and ONC continue to communicate effectively.

This Coordinating Committee governance model has proven to be effective in leading eHealth Exchange through its initial years as major policy issues were debated and resolved. The business and legal environment for HIE has changed dramatically since eHealth Exchange was created in 2007 and the Coordinating Committee has been responsible for keeping eHealth Exchange current and relevant in a rapidly changing landscape. This has been very challenging and yet, because the Coordinating Committee was built on solid governance principles, it has been able to adapt and remain effective. Governance must be flexible and responsive to be effective and we expect the Coordinating Committee will continue to evolve as the environment changes.

EMERGING TRENDS

The emerging governance structure will likely follow emerging HIE business models. For example, if health care organizations continue to join nationwide level HIE initiatives, then governance will likely be driven by nationwide level organizations. Another possible emerging model is a collaboration of regional HIOs through organizations like the Strategic Health Information Exchange Collaborative (SHIEC). A third possible model is a governance structure directed by or heavily influenced by the federal government. The U.S. Department of Health and Human Services has published information notices regarding governance and has indicated it will continue to promote "rules of the road" related to governance.

SUMMARY

Governance is an essential requirement of HIE. Yet governance is a voluntary activity, which must be embraced by all stakeholders. Stakeholder engagement is vital as an HIO seeks to gain consensus regarding data access and data use policies. A governing body representative of the diversity in an HIE establishes data sharing agreements to enforce the policies and practices. Governance defines what data will be shared, how it will be shared, to whom it will be shared, and when it will be shared. An effective governance framework engenders trust, scales to accommodate additional stakeholders and approved use cases, and adapts to market and regulatory changes.

As HIOs mature, they encounter numerous governance hurdles. Successful HIOs will persuade participants to place HIE needs above the needs of their individual organizations. As nationwide data sharing networks emerge and expand, HIOs will be faced with a new set of challenges to operate within a nationwide governance framework.

QUESTIONS FOR DISCUSSION

1. As detailed in the Governing Body section, a group of primary care physicians and specialists request approval to access a care summary from the exchange without a patient registration transaction, which is the approved use case. Why do you think the governing body denied the request? Should it have been approved?
2. An established regional HIO is considering joining the eHealth Exchange at the request of a nationwide health care organization (eg, Walgreens) operating in its market. However, the policies and data sharing agreements of the regional HIO conflict with the policies and DURSA supported by the eHealth Exchange. The HIO does not want to change its policies and data sharing agreements, but it wants to share data with the nationwide health care organization. What recommendation would you make to the parties involved?

References

[1] Office of the National Coordinator for Health Information Technology Health Information Exchange Governance. Washington, DC: U.S. Department of Health and Human Services; 2015. [cited August 20, 2015]; Available from: <http://www.healthit.gov/policy-researchers-implementers/health-information-exchange-governance>.

[2] Allen C, Des Jardins TR, Heider A, Lyman KA, McWilliams L, Rein AL, et al. Data governance and data sharing agreements for community-wide health information exchange: lessons from the beacon communities. EGEMS (Washington, DC) 2014;2(1):1057. http://dx.doi.org/10.13063/2327-9214.1057.

[3] Security and Privacy. 45 CFR 160.103; 45 CFR 164.502, 164.504(e).

[4] Protection of Human Subjects. 45 CFR Part 46.

[5] eHealth Exchange. Data Use and Reciprocal Agreement; 2015 [cited August 20, 2015]; Available from: <http://healthewayinc.org/images/Content/Documents/Application-Package/2011.03.05-restatement-i-of-the-dursa-final.pdf>.

[6] Middleton B., Fleming M., Wiegand T., Merritt D., Bakalar R., Georgiou A., et al. Best Practices for Community Health Information Exchange. Center for Community Health Leadership; [cited August 20, 2015]; Available from: <https://healthit.ahrq.gov/sites/default/files/docs/library/CCHL_BPG.pdf>.

[7] Dimitropoulos L.L., Loft J. Health information privacy and security collaboration. Rockville, MD: Agency for Healthcare Research and Quality; May 2014 [cited August 20, 2015]; Available from: <https://healthit.ahrq.gov/ahrq-funded-projects/privacy-and-security-project>.

CHAPTER

5

Managing the Business of Health Information Exchange: Toward Sustainability

John P. Kansky

Indiana Health Information Exchange, Indianapolis, IN

OUTLINE

LEARNING OBJECTIVES

At the end of the chapter, the reader should be able to:

- Define sustainability and explain how it is applied to health information exchange (HIE).
- Explain how sustainability differs for the three forms of HIE: Private HIE, Government-facilitated HIE, and Community-based HIE.
- Describe, in financial terms, the ways in which an unsustainable HIE business can move to a sustainable financial position.
- Describe the importance of the alignment of mission, organizational structure, and business model and examples of how misalignment can undermine an HIE's sustainability.
- Identify and understand challenges to HIE sustainability resulting from factors outside the HIE itself.

INTRODUCTION

Much has been written, presented, and debated about the sustainability of health information exchange (HIE). In fact, the health-care industry seems to have a mild obsession with the question of how to sustain HIE. Whether for-profit or not-for-profit, organizations that are created to perform HIE (the verb) are businesses (HIE, the noun). The obsession with the sustainability of HIE can be attributed, in part, to the fact that most HIEs were founded in the last 10 years; and, as with many young businesses, they are operating on temporary funding sources and generating more expense than revenue. Anyone running a business that is losing money is going to be obsessed with how to get to the point their business is making money (and therefore sustainable). Because so few HIEs are making money today, sustainability is a national obsession.

At the base of the debate is usually the question of whether HIEs *can* be run sustainably. This is the wrong question. HIEs can certainly be run sustainably. Therefore a much better set of questions—explored in this chapter—are related to *how* to operate a sustainable HIE.

SUSTAINABILITY FOR THE THREE FORMS OF HIE ARE DIFFERENT

An exploration of sustainability in the context of HIE must begin with a working definition. The following is the author's definition of sustainability based on experience in the field of health information technology and, specifically, the work of growing and managing a large HIE:

> Sustainability: The ability to continuously operate a company or organization that fulfills a defined mission while remaining financially viable. In the context of HIE this means delivering HIE services in some useful way without going broke—indefinitely.

So, sustainability in this context refers to *financial* sustainability. For an HIE business to meet the above definition, it must be performing HIE (the verb) in some useful way (HIE services) and generating enough money to keep operating. As covered in chapter "What is Health Information Exchange?", there are three forms of HIEs: *Private HIE*, *Government-facilitated HIE*, and *Community-based HIE*. The sustainability of each type can be quite different, and each situation is explained briefly below. However, when people in the health-care industry debate or question HIE sustainability, they are focusing on a specific challenge—the challenge of creating value through health information exchange and monetizing this value (ie, getting someone to pay) with enough success to financially sustain the HIE organization. This chapter is dedicated to an exploration of that sustainability challenge. As you will see, this specific challenge of sustainability is most typically characteristic of free-standing, community-based HIE businesses that are not part of a larger company or government.

The sustainability of private, proprietary HIEs is at the will of the central organization that operates and controls the HIE. That organization created the HIE to serve some business purpose and as long as the HIE is perceived to be fulfilling that purpose, the central organization will sustain its operation—financially and otherwise. For example, if a large hospital system decided to create a private HIE to share information across its enterprise and with selected business partners, it creates and sustains that HIE "function" with revenue generated through patient care. If the hospital system ever decided the private HIE was no longer providing value in excess of the cost of its operation, the hospital system would simply stop operating the HIE. This scenario is not a very interesting or controversial sustainability challenge, so it will not be further explored in this chapter.

The sustainability of HIEs operated by state governments are often similar to that of private HIEs. The source of funding of the HIE is identified or created by the state government. This could be from state tax revenues, through a levy (eg, a fee charged on all health insurance claims filed in the state), or simply covered within the budget of the agency in which it operates (often the public health department or Medicaid agency). If the state perceives value in continuing to operate the HIE, it will continue to identify and provide the funds to do so. However, in some states with government-run HIEs, state leaders believe that the HIE should be able to provide value to stakeholders, independent of the state, and that the value of HIE should be monetized to cover the cost of its operation. Therefore, the state expects the leaders of the HIE to figure out how to operate sustainably without relying upon government funds. This sustainability challenge is similar or identical to the challenge faced by free-standing, community-based HIE businesses; and, therefore, this is the focus of the remainder of this chapter.

While the name "community HIE" might sound quaint or parochial, in fact some of the largest and most robust HIEs in the country are of this form. A community-based HIE is typically a free-standing, not-for-profit business whose mission and purpose is to improve the quality, safety, and efficiency of health and/or health care through HIE. The organization fulfills that mission by providing HIE services to customers in the health-care supply chain (eg, to hospitals, health insurance companies, physician groups, etc.). These services produce value for the customers and, in exchange, the customers are willing to pay fees to the HIE—as long as the fees charged by the HIE are less than the customer's perceived value of the service. If the HIE's cost of operating a given service is at or below the fees customers are willing to pay, the service is sustainable. If not, it is not. Community HIEs that operate sustainably create a profile of sustainable services (ie, more than one or two) which together generate enough revenue to exceed the total cost of operating the HIE. Simple, right?

The explanation above is an accurate description of the basis of sustainable HIE, but it glosses over details and nuance that we will now explore. Much of what comes next is more about business than HIE.

BUSINESS 101 FOR HEALTH INFORMATION EXCHANGES

HIEs, dry cleaners, oil refineries, and health clubs are all businesses and all have certain basic characteristics in common. Whether for-profit or not-for-profit, to be sustainable they all must produce revenue in excess of expenses. They all have fixed and variable costs as well as overhead. At the beginning of the chapter, we asserted simply that if an HIE delivers a profile of sustainable services, and if the total revenue from all services exceeds the cost of operating the HIE, then it is sustainable. While true, it is important to explore a few key business and microeconomic concepts embedded in that simple explanation.

Key Business Definitions:

- Total revenue—The sum of all income produced and earned by the HIE—presumably from fees charged to customers through the delivery of services.
- Total expense—The sum of all costs of operating the HIE including all fixed and variable costs.
- Variable costs—The costs that grow as the provision of services grows. New customers or growing transaction volumes cause variable costs to rise. Typical variable costs for an HIE include data storage and any vendor fees that vary with volume. (If we operated a hot dog cart, buying more hot dogs would be a variable cost.)
- Fixed costs—The costs that the HIE incurs regardless of transaction volumes or the addition of new customers. Typical fixed costs for an HIE include rent, insurance, depreciation, and salaries. (If we operated a hot dog cart, the rental of the cart would be a fixed cost.) Some fixed costs can be directly attributed to the cost of delivering services while the rest are sometimes referred to as overhead.
- Overhead—The portion of fixed costs that an HIE incurs that are not directly related to the delivery of its products or services, but rather, support the overall business operations. Overhead[1] includes rent, selling and marketing costs, and management salaries.
- Gross margin—The amount of revenue each service generates in excess of its own costs.
- Excess revenues (over expenses)—As the name suggests, when the HIE's total revenue is greater than its total expenses, it generates *excess revenue over expenses*. In for-profit businesses, this is called *profit* or *net income*.

HYPOTHETICAL CASE STUDY TO ILLUSTRATE SUSTAINABILITY

So, for a given HIE to be sustainable, total revenue must be greater than total expenses over the long term. Let us explore that more deeply through the example of a hypothetical HIE we will call *HyHIE* (Table 5.1).

In the simple example above, HyHIE is sustainable and can add $200k a year to its "rainy-day and reinvestment fund." However, what if circumstances were subtly different? What if HyHIE had 7% fewer customers? Or one fewer services? Or had to charge 8% lower prices? Or had an increase of 9% in fixed costs? In all these scenarios, HyHIE is no longer sustainable.

There are many community-based HIEs today that are not currently operating sustainably (ie, their total expenses exceed their total revenues), but they have some temporary

[1] To be clear, some fixed costs are part of overhead and some are not. For example, rent and management salaries are not considered directly related to the delivery of its products or services—and therefore overhead. The salary of a database administrator or helpdesk associate would not be overhead as their effort is directly part of service delivery. This nuance is relevant to good accounting, but not important to the concepts of HIE sustainability in this chapter.

TABLE 5.1 Facts Describing the Hypothetical Case Study HyHIE

HyHIE's portfolio of sustainable services	Service 1 (S1), Service 2 (S2), Service 3 (S3), and Service 4 (S4)	• Each service generates $1 million per year in revenue • Each service costs $700k to deliver (but only $200k of the cost of each service is variable cost) • Therefore, each service generates a "gross margin" of $1M – $700k = $300k
Total revenue	= S1 revenue + S2 revenue + S3 revenue + S4 revenue	= $4M/year
HyHIE's fixed costs	For example rent, insurance, and salaries	= $3M/year (this would include the $2M fixed cost component of S1, S2, S3, and S4 plus other costs like rent)
HyHIE's variable costs	For example ... the variable cost component of delivering S1, S2, S3, and S4	= $200k + $200k + $200k + $200k = $800k/year
Total expense	= Fixed costs + Variable costs	= $3.8M/year
Excess revenue over expense	= Total revenue – Total expense	= $4M – $3.8 = $200k/year

source(s) of funding on which they rely to operate. What we learn from the HyHIE example is that moving an HIE business from an unsustainable to a sustainable financial position means some combination of the following:

- Increasing revenue by:
  - adding more customers
  - adding more services
- Increasing the gross margin per service (raising prices or reducing service delivery costs)
- Reducing overhead costs.

INCREASING HIE REVENUE

HIEs can increase their revenue in three ways[2]: by adding customers, by adding services, or by increasing service prices to their customers. A closer examination of each reveals some important microeconomic and business principles that are important to HIEs. As price increases are directly related to gross margin, a means of increasing revenue that will be discussed as part of increasing the gross margin per service.

Increasing Revenue by Adding Customers

As the HIE sells services that yield revenue it uses to cover its cost of operations, each additional customer provides a little more revenue. And as we are assuming we cannot offer services that cost more to deliver than they generate in revenue, we know that some of the revenue from each additional customer helps us cover our fixed costs and gets us closer to sustainability. Let us suppose we have a service we offer to hospitals. If only half the hospitals in our market currently buy the service, we can add more customers simply by convincing more hospitals of the value of participating in the service. Alternatively, the same service could be used by independent labs or imaging centers. We could therefore add customers by selling the service to them.

[2] HIEs often have temporary sources of revenue, such as one-time government grants. These temporary sources, while they are revenue, are almost always specifically intended to financially support the HIE while it build itself into a truly sustainable organization.

But what if we operate in one specific healthcare market and all (or nearly all) the potential customers already buy the service? Can we expand into a new market (eg, a nearby city that has some referral traffic with our market)? If we continue extrapolating this a bit, it allows us to see how an important microeconomic principle applies to HIE sustainability. As we see that each additional customer makes it easier to be sustainable, doesn't having more potential customers also make sustainability easier? If we sell services to hospitals, it is easier to sell services to more hospitals if there are 100 hospitals in our market than if there are 10. So it is easier to sustain an HIE business in a large market than in a small one. This leads to a question that cannot be answered precisely here (we leave it to the economists). The question is "What is the optimal size market for sustainable health information exchange?" Given that most community HIEs operate in markets smaller than an entire state (or in small states[3]), experience tells us the answer is *bigger*.

TABLE 5.2 Sources of New HIE Service Ideas

Sources of New HIE Service Ideas	Explanation/Examples
The service portfolios of other successful HIEs	If another HIE is successfully sustaining, for example, an electronic results delivery service, your HIE may be able to offer a similar or identical service
Business challenges (pain points) brought to the HIE by customers (or potential customers)	A customer, knowing the data and capabilities of the HIE, may present a business problem to the HIE. For example, they might ask if the HIE can improve a specific population health management initiative by providing additional data
Self-generated service concepts (through formal or informal idea generation)	Whether through formal product development ideation or concepts that come up opportunistically, members of the HIE's product management team will occasionally recognize new opportunities to create value for customers.
Opportunities created by federal or state regulations	Government regulations, such as meaningful use, create opportunities for HIEs to produce valuable services for customers

Increasing Revenue by Adding Services

Community-based HIEs that operate sustainably create a profile of sustainable services which together generate enough revenue to exceed the total cost of operating the HIE. More specifically, financial sustainability is achieved when the portfolio of services is generating enough gross margin to cover the HIE's overhead costs. As we know that each sustainable HIE service provides additional revenue and gross margin, each new service helps get the HIE closer to sustainability. Therefore, successful HIE businesses keep adding services that (1) advance their mission and purpose and (2) generate additional revenue and gross margin.

But how does one identify HIE services that are sustainable? By no means specific to HIE, there is an entire field of study around the identification, development, and management of products and services known as product management.[4] In general, HIE services, like services in any industry or market, produce value for customers by making something in their world better or easier. A good service enables the customer to do something useful that they either cannot do on their own or cannot do as efficiently or effectively on their own. In practice, there are four main sources of new service ideas or concepts as summarized in Table 5.2.

[3] For example, the state of Delaware includes about a dozen hospitals.

[4] Readers can learn more about best practices in the identification and development of services—not specifically HIE services—by researching Product Management and New Product Development.

Regardless of the source, identifying the concept for a HIE's next potential sustainable service is the easy part. Concepts must be vetted for technical, economic, and legal/cultural feasibility; prioritized; developed; launched; marketed; and managed. To yield one sustainable service offering, HIEs should expect to pursue three to five service concepts. Abandoning concepts that prove to be unfruitful at the earliest possible stage of development is healthy as it keeps product development costs to a minimum. One adage of entrepreneurship and innovation also applies to product development—*fail early, fail often*. That is to say, do not be afraid to pursue new ideas but also do not be afraid to *pull the plug* if an idea does not work out.

As an HIE seeks to grow its profile of sustainable services, the importance of the HIE's mission and the economic realities of sustainability must be considered simultaneously and balanced. It helps to think of potential HIE services in two groups illustrated in Fig. 5.1.

There are many services that an HIE could deliver that are consistent with its mission (the left side of the Venn diagram in Fig. 5.1). Some of these services will have ready customers who are willing to pay for value they perceive, but some services will not. Consider an example of a service that could improve the quality of health care. An HIE could combine and analyze large and complex health-care data sets from multiple payors and provider organizations and identify specific gaps in best practice clinical care for specific patient populations. These identified gaps could be communicated to health-care providers who are treating these patients—even in real time as the patients present in different settings across the health-care system. However, it could be difficult to identify the customer segment(s) who would be willing to cover the significant cost of such a service given its complexity and the volume of data needed to provide it at scale.

Alternatively, there are services an HIE could deliver that have ready, paying customers (the right side of the Venn diagram in Fig. 5.1). Some of these services will be consistent with a given HIEs mission, but some services will not. For example, an HIE might have access to data that a for-profit marketing research firm would value to support product planning for its customers. However, most community-based HIEs would view this use of the data as outside their mission.

Therefore, services on which a sustainable HIE can be based are at the intersection of these two groups (the overlapping portion of the

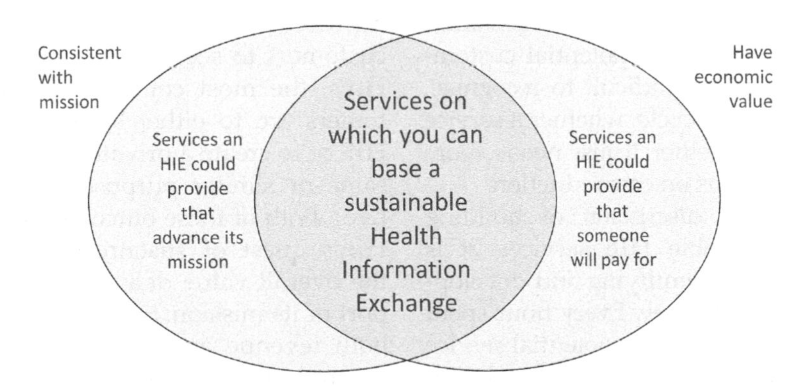

FIGURE 5.1 There are services that a health information exchange could theoretically provide for which there is no apparent business model. There are also services that have business models that are outside the mission of a typical HIE.

Venn diagram in Fig. 5.1). An HIE service portfolio should be composed of services that are both consistent with the mission of the organization and have intrinsic economic value to existing or new customers.

Imbedded in the above explanation is the concept of an unsustainable HIE service. An unsustainable service may serve the mission of the HIE and be technically achievable and viable in every other way, but not generate enough revenue to cover the cost of providing the service. Raise the price and customers would not buy it. Lower the price and the HIE is selling at a loss. Unsustainable. Reasons a given service might be unsustainable are as follows:

- Produces too little value (not a good service—abandon it)
- Produces good value but costs too much to deliver.

For the case in which a service produces value but costs too much, an unsustainable service could be turned into a sustainable service by sufficiently reducing the cost of delivering the service. For example, if the service is too costly because the HIE is delivering it in a cost-inefficient way, it could be rendered sustainable by finding a way to deliver it more efficiently. Alternatively, the service may be too expensive to deliver only because the scale of the customer base is too small. That service could be rendered sustainable by selling it to more customers and/or broadening the market of potential customers. In practice, it can be difficult to recognize, especially early in its life cycle, whether a service is unsustainable or whether it just needs more sales effort or more focus on cost reduction.

Before leaving the discussion of building a portfolio of sustainable HIE services, it is important to note that identifying and developing HIE services costs money. Every hour spent investigating the feasibility of a potential service offering, designing it, developing it, and selling it is 100% cost and 0% revenue until the first customer signs a contract and begins paying. And many more customers must be signed and implemented before the service is making a positive contribution to the organization's bottom line. The money to fund the development typically comes from one of two sources: excess revenue generated by other services or (more commonly) one time sources of funding (eg, a grant). Grants, while increasingly scarce, can be excellent sources of funding for the development of sustainable services as long as there is a disciplined and clearly understood goal that what the grant funds *will result in a sustainable service*. HIEs cannot be operationally sustained on grant funds, which are inherently temporary.

INCREASING THE GROSS MARGIN PER SERVICE

Increasing gross margin means making slightly more *profit* from a service you already offer and deliver to customers. For a given service, an HIE can increase a service's gross margin in two ways: raise prices or reduce the cost of delivering the service.

Setting Prices

Of these two choices, it is tempting to assume that raising prices is easier, but a customer's perspective would be different. In microeconomic terms, raising prices forces customers to seek alternatives. For community HIEs, the most common alternatives for customers are to either stop participating in the HIE or to create a private HIE that can serve the same or similar purpose (from their perspective). Both of these outcomes are harmful to the HIE's quest of sustainability and undermine the overall value delivered by the HIE in support of its mission. Setting prices that maximize both revenue and customer participation is a theoretical goal, and there is no practical way of knowing if you have ever achieved it. As it is important to the mission and value proposition of an HIE to have as much participation from health-care stakeholders in the markets they serve, any price that is greater than the HIEs total cost of delivering the service that does not drive customers away is a financial victory.

Setting prices is much easier in theory than it is in practice. Establishing a price and explaining that price to potential customers is straightforward, in theory, if an HIE knows two numbers: (1) the total cost (including overhead[5]) of delivering the service to that customer; and (2) the total economic benefit of the service that the customer will receive from the service.

Any price that is above the first number but below the second means that both the HIE and the customer come out ahead. The problem is that in reality, an HIE is not likely to precisely know what it will cost to implement and deliver a service to a specific customer and even more unsure of the economic benefit to the customer.

What typically happens in the real world is that the HIE pleads its case for how its service will provide value, economic or otherwise, and the skeptical customer asks for empirical evidence. While there are a few research studies that support the economic value of HIE (more are needed; see chapters: The Evidence Base for Health Information Exchange and Measuring the Value of Health Information Exchange), these studies inevitably do not fit the specific circumstances and therefore are not helpful in convincing skeptical potential HIE participants. In the end, some organizations are convinced of the value and participate while others do not. Increasingly HIE is becoming an assumed part of the health-care supply chain, and markets are moving toward strengthening HIEs in terms of function and value as opposed to deciding whether or not to participate.

Reducing the Cost of Service Delivery

Remember that financial sustainability is reached when the gross margin from all services exceeds the organization's overhead. If price is held steady and the costs associated with the delivery of services are reduced, the gross margin from that service increases. Given how difficult it can be to raise prices, reducing the cost of service delivery is extremely helpful.

Accountants refer to an organization's total cost of service (or product) delivery as *cost of goods sold* or *COGS*. For an HIE, COGS is chiefly made up of the costs associated with the people needed to deliver the HIE's services and a whole bunch of things related to data, computers, and software. Sometimes the people are employees and sometimes they are contractors. Sometimes the computers and software belong to the HIE and sometimes they are licensed or delivered as a service (eg, cloud computing or software as a service). In either case, lowering COGS is about figuring out how to deliver the service with the lowest cost combination of people and computing. This might mean outsourcing your data center operation, or it might mean insourcing your data center operation. It might mean reducing your workforce by X people to lower payroll expenses, or it might mean hiring X people to perform a function at a lower cost than a third party was charging.

In most cases, the per-customer cost of delivering a service will drop as the customer base grows. Therefore growing the scale of your HIE helps to reduce costs and increase margin. Thus lowering service delivery cost might be achieved by merging with a neighboring HIE, for example. Significant HIE consolidation is

[5]Accountants have methods of attributing the organization's overhead fairly to its various revenue generating services. You must include a fair amount of overhead in the total cost of a service to know its gross margin at a given price.

happening as evidenced by recent mergers in New York, Michigan, and Texas.[6]

Yet there is no magical formula. Reducing service delivery costs in the pursuit of sustainability is about deeply understanding your costs and working hard at exploring alternatives approaches, negotiating hard with suppliers, and sometimes making difficult business decisions.

REDUCING OVERHEAD COSTS OF AN HIE BUSINESS

HIEs tend to be high fixed-cost businesses, like an oil refinery or a steel mill as opposed to a high variable cost business such as a consulting firm. Some fixed costs can be directly attributed to the cost of delivering HIE services, like leasing a data center, while the rest, generally speaking, are overhead. As the biggest financial challenge to sustainability for a given HIE is to generate enough gross margin from services to cover its overhead, overhead is viewed as a necessary evil. Minimizing overhead is an important mantra for the leadership of any HIE or any other high fixed-cost business.

Minimizing overhead is characterized by having a small leadership team, fair but not overly generous compensation levels, adequate but not extravagant office space, and prudent insurance coverage. The author once worked for a company that issued business cards to employees in five different colors and had an open bar at company parties; it was not an HIE, and that company soon went bankrupt.

While managing for minimal overhead might seem as simple as being fiscally conservative, there are conundrums. For example, consider sales expenses. Costs associated with sales are overhead. But stop selling, and your HIE will not grow. If an HIE's strategy to reach sustainability hinges on increasing the number of customers, and therefore the scale of the HIE, doubling the size of the sales force may well be the key to sustainability. This, however, will double the sales component of overhead. Once again, there is no magic formula.

Earlier we discussed increasing revenue by adding customers. While technically not reducing overhead, it is worth noting that as an HIE's customer base grows, overhead costs are *diluted*. That is to say that if the HIE's scale increases and overhead stays the same, the overhead per customer is reduced. Anheuser-Busch InBev produces more beer than your local microbrewery but both businesses are sustainable. However, take note that their prices per pint are not the same. Anheuser-Busch has much lower overhead per pint and therefore can charge much lower prices. The smaller the scale of the company, the higher the prices it must charge to cover overhead. Customers are price sensitive because they have alternatives, which is usually to not participate in the HIE.

PLANNING FOR SUSTAINABILITY

No different than any other businesses, HIEs should have and follow a plan for their business which spells out their goals and strategies for achieving them.[7] When setting goals and strategies, the mission of the organization and how best to achieve it should be the first concern. For an HIE that is not currently generating revenue over expenses, sustainability

[6] Since December 2013 at least three significant HIE mergers have been announced: Healthix and Brooklyn Health Information Exchange in New York, Michigan Health Connect and the Great Lakes HIE in Michigan, and the exchanges in Dallas and San Antonio in Texas.

[7] Readers can learn more about best practices in planning for any business by researching Strategic Planning.

should be a close second. Just like the restaurateur who has opened a new location, obsessing over sustainability is absolutely appropriate until profitability is achieved. However, sustainability need not be a permanent preoccupation. While your HIE is moving toward sustainability (ie, losing money), it is important to make decisions about every aspect of the HIE business with long-term sustainability in mind. However, once the HIE is sustainable, prudent management and fiscal discipline should enable the leadership team to focus on new ways of delivering value to customers and innovative means of achieving the mission. Sustainability, at that point, should be an ongoing reward for good, careful management.

Start With Sustainability in Mind

For a cross-country driving trip to be successful and efficient, one needs a plan for the route, places to stay along the way, and enough money to cover the expenses of the journey. But even with all these things, choosing the wrong vehicle or not packing the right accouterments can doom the journey before it begins. So it is with HIEs. Certain key characteristics of the organization, if not well-chosen and correctly aligned, can make long-term sustainability difficult or impossible to achieve. These include mission, organizational structure (including corporate governance), and business model.

Mission

The mission of the HIE, as with any company, should be the bedrock of planning and decision-making. An HIE's mission statement might say that the organization exists to "enable the highest quality health care" or "raise the health status of citizens." The mission statement might say "in central Indiana" or "in the Midwest." It might say "support patient engagement" or "advance health IT research." In each case, following the mission will lead the organization in different directions. For example, a difference as subtle as "enable the highest quality health care" versus "raise the health status of citizens" can make a big difference. Focusing on health *care* suggests finding ways to help health-care providers, whereas raising the health status of citizens suggests promoting or advancing public health, disease prevention, nutrition, and exercise.

Organizational Structure

The term organizational structure, in this context, refers to whether an HIE is for-profit or not-for-profit, how its board governs it, who makes up the board, and how the bylaws of the corporation are written. While there is no one right organizational structure, a sustainable HIE is more likely to result if careful consideration is given to these most basic aspects of organizational design. For example, if the mission of the organization is heavily focused on research, a board of business leaders from for-profit businesses may be a misalignment. If the organization is for-profit, a board made up of academicians or government leaders could lead to problems.

As HIEs face business challenges related to sustainability, the individuals in leadership roles and on the board of the organization will make the most important decisions. Imagine explaining to your board that the best strategy to attain sustainability is to increase the margin of services by raising prices if the board is made up of leaders from your customer organizations. The structure of the HIE should match the long-term strategy and purpose of the organization, and the governing board of the HIE must understand and support that alignment. Be prepared to make difficult changes when those changes are necessary to remove barriers and move toward sustainability.

Business Model

In the most general terms, an HIE's business model is a cohesive idea about how the organization will do something useful (ie, produce value) and how the organization will generate revenue so it can do so sustainably. More specifically, the business model answers questions like:

- What kind of services the HIE will deliver?
- To what types of organizations will those services will be delivered?
- What is the value proposition of the services to those organizations?
- How will the HIE generate revenue to cover its cost?

These decisions must be in line with the organization's mission, and the leadership and board of the HIE must understand and believe in the business model. For a given HIE, many possible versions of a business model could ultimately be successful, but there are many potential pitfalls. Getting the details right is important. The answer to a question as simple as "who pays the HIE" can sink an otherwise sound service concept.

As we saw in the HyHIE case study, loss of revenue from one service can render an HIE unsustainable. An example will help. Suppose the business model of the HIE is based on services that give hospital-based clinicians better information. A part of the value proposition of these services is that the additional information will prevent unnecessary procedures, thereby improving the quality of the care delivered to the patient (eg, faster care with less trauma, less radiation) while reducing the cost of care. Does the HIE business model presume that it will charge the hospital based on the improvement in quality, or does it plan to charge the payor (eg, insurance carrier) based on the reduction in cost? There is no "right answer."

If the leadership and board understand and believe in the business model, they will act in concert to find an answer that leads to sustainability. Together, they can make the necessary decisions around the HIE's business model and help gain support for it among health care and business stakeholders in the market. This alignment and understanding is necessary for a successful and sustainable HIE business.

CHALLENGES TO SUSTAINABILITY

As we have explored in this chapter, there are many financial aspects of an HIE business that must be artfully managed to achieve sustainability. But outside the HIE, in the wider ecosystem of health care and governmental policy, there are other challenges to sustainable HIE that go beyond managerial accounting. While not an exhaustive list, Table 5.3 provides some examples of the challenges facing HIEs.

SUMMARY

HIE on any real scale has existed less than 20 years. During that period, the advancement of technology and standards and the government's involvement in HIT policy-making has been dramatic. The pace of change in the American health-care system has been equally dramatic. In that context, HIE businesses have emerged and their growth and evolution has accelerated. The national obsession with HIE sustainability is an understandable byproduct of those environmental circumstances. HIE businesses *can* be run sustainably. There is ample opportunity in our fragmented and inefficient health-care system to create value—especially when technology and information are your tools. Any business that can create value can figure out the combination of mission, organizational, structure, business model, services, and disciplined financial management that are required to succeed.

TABLE 5.3 Examples of Challenges to HIE Sustainability

Challenge	Explanation
The country does not know how to do HIE yet	HIE is in its early stages of maturity. Look at several HIEs and observe the many differences in even the most basic aspects of their approaches. Look further at how many new standards and new government regulations have been created in the last 5 years. The country is still figuring out what approaches and business models will be the most effective and efficient
Alternative to HIE is the status quo	Because health-care providers and public health officials have been operating for decades in the absence of HIE, the natural tendency is to continue with the status quo. HIE leaders must not only have a compelling value proposition; they must also be able to communicate an understanding of that value to others. HIE can be a difficult concept to understand and explain, so many organizations are not participating [1]
Lack of economic evidence	Skeptical or confused decision-makers want evidence of the economic value of HIE. Studies demonstrating which HIE services deliver value (and which do not) are too few. See chapter "The Evidence Base for Health Information Exchange" for an assessment of the current evidence on HIE
Adoption requires change	HIEs cannot produce value unless the customers of the HIE adopt and use their services. Just as health-care providers are having to adapt their workflows to reap the benefits of EHRs, adoption of HIE services sometimes requires adaptation. Many HIE services fail to produce improvements in health and health care only because they are not used and adopted by health workers.
Challenging and Confusing Government Direction	Since 2010, the federal government has begun trying to use policy to advance and promote HIE. The resulting regulations have elevated the level of activity and interest in HIE; but also created significant confusion and, in some cases, have forced prescriptive standards and actions that stifle innovation [2]

QUESTIONS FOR DISCUSSION

1. Using concepts in this chapter, what arguments would you make to support the basic tenet that HIE businesses *can* be run sustainably?
2. What examples of sustainable HIE services are you aware of? Do you understand the business model behind these services?
3. For any HIE service that you are aware of, discuss ways an HIE could try to increase the gross margin from that service.
4. For any existing HIE you are aware of, discuss ways that HIE could try to increase its revenue.
5. What ideas do you have for HIE services that you feel could produce value and be sustainable?
6. What is needed in terms of government policy to make sustainable HIE a natural and indispensable element of delivering health care and maintaining health in our country?
7. What can the leaders of individual HIEs do to make HIE a natural and indispensable element of delivering health care and maintaining health in their market?

References

[1] Dixon BE, Miller T, Overhage JM. Barriers to achieving the last mile in health information exchange. J Healthc Inf Manag 2013;27(4):55–60.

[2] Basch P, McClellan M, Botts C, Katikaneni P. High value health IT: policy reforms for better care and lower costs. Washington: The Brookings Institution; 2015. March [cited August 11, 2015]. Available from: http://www.brookings.edu/~/media/research/files/papers/2015/03/16-health-it-policy-brief/16-high-value-health-it-policy-reforms-mcclellan.pdf.

CHAPTER

6

Privacy, Security, and Confidentiality: Toward Trust

Eric Thieme

Faegre Baker Daniels, Indianapolis, IN

OUTLINE

LEARNING OBJECTIVES

At the end of this chapter, the reader should be able to:

- Define trust, privacy, confidentiality, and security.
- Define an HIPAA covered entity and business associate.
- Understand how HIPAA interacts with state laws.
- Define protected health information (PHI).

- Understand permissible uses and disclosures of PHI under the HIPAA Privacy Rule.
- Understand the required and addressable security controls under the HIPAA Security Rule.
- Understand what is a breach of unsecured PHI under the HIPAA Breach Notification Rule.
- Understand three primary contracting models for HIE participation.

INTRODUCTION

Trust is having confidence in how another party will behave in a given situation.[1] If you have a high degree of confidence in how another party will behave in a given situation, then you have a high degree of trust in that other party. If the behavior of another party is unknown in a given situation, then the degree of trust in that party is low.

Laws, rules, regulation, and contracts exist to foster trust. They define how particular parities should behave in given situations. In a contract, one party might promise to do A in situation Z and B in situation X. The contract establishes expected behaviors in given situations and acts as a mechanism to enforce behaviors or apply penalties if a party does not behave as required by the contract. As parties behave according to the contract over time, more and more trust is established.

Laws, administrative rules, and regulations work in much the same way. A law might say if Z occurs, then all regulated parties must do A. The law or regulation will carry with it enforcement penalties to which regulated parties will be subject if they do not comply with the law. As parties comply with the law or regulation over time, more and more trust is established across the society.

These concepts of trust, built over time through contract, laws, and regulations, are paramount in developing a successful health information exchange (HIE). Health-care providers and health plans are trusted by their patients and members to safeguard health information. In order for these entities to share health information, a sufficient fabric of trust must be created by the HIE through contracts and practices, as well as laws and regulations at both state and federal levels. Compliance with HIE contracts as well as applicable laws and regulations is demonstrated through strong HIE governance (as described in chapter: Engaging and Sustaining Stakeholders: Toward Governance), which breads further trust. As HIE participants work together over time, they develop a higher degree of certainty in how each other will act in a given situation, which translates into a higher degree of trust.

The concepts of privacy, security, and confidentiality are established through contracts, laws, and regulations. They represent situations in which parties must develop a high degree of certainty around how other parties will act (ie, trust) in order for an HIE initiative to be successful. It is the combination of contracts, laws, and regulations that define expected behaviors around privacy, security, and confidentiality that establish the trust necessary for a successful HIE.

[1] This chapter will define several terms, such as trust, privacy, confidentiality, and security. The definitions are the author's description of what these terms mean in the context of health information exchange, rather than definitions from third party sources. Different parties may have different definitions; the ones provided in this chapter are used in the context of health information exchange.

Privacy

Privacy is the freedom to choose what information is shared or not shared with other parties. For example, privacy is an individual's right to not disclose information about themselves to others, such as not disclosing an individual's genetic predisposition to cancer on an employment application. Legislatures may choose to enact laws that prohibit the compelled disclosure of information in order to protect an individual's privacy.

Confidentiality

Confidentiality is the obligation to keep secret information with which one is entrusted. For example, confidentially obligations are imposed under the Health Insurance Portability and Accountability Act (HIPAA) by prohibiting covered entity health-care providers from disclosing protected health information (PHI) to the media without a patient's authorization. Confidentiality obligations are often mislabeled as privacy obligations. For example, the HIPAA Privacy Rule would be more appropriately labeled as the Confidentiality Rule as it imposes obligations upon covered entities not to make certain disclosures of information (ie, to maintain confidentiality).

Security

Security is the combination of administrative, technical, and physical safeguards that ensure confidentiality and promote privacy. Security is comprised of the safeguards that prevent inappropriate uses and disclosures of information. For example, strong passwords, encryption, and door locks all represent security safeguards that exist to keep information in the right hands.

This chapter will explore the contractual and legal mechanisms that exist to promote privacy, confidentiality, and security in order to foster trust among HIE participants.

FEDERAL AND STATE LAWS PERTAINING TO HIE

The "rules of the road" for HIE are defined by a combination of laws and regulations at both state and federal levels as well as contracts among HIE participants. Federal and state laws establish a baseline, and then HIE participants may create additional rules through contracts among HIE participants. Contracts among HIE participants cannot override or conflict with federal or state laws and regulations, but they may provide for obligations above and beyond federal or state laws and regulations.

The interaction between state and federal law in the HIE space can be complex and confusing. Generally, federal laws preempt state laws when the two are in conflict. In many cases, Congress will "occupy the field" and create laws or regulations that preempt all state laws and regulations. For example, Congress regulates medical devices through a scheme that preempts all state laws and regulations. In other cases, Congress will establish a national minimum in an area and allow states to enact more stringent laws or regulations. This is the case with HIPAA and regulation of uses and disclosures of health information. When in conflict, HIPAA preempts state laws except to the extent state law is more stringent than HIPAA [1]. For example, HIPAA allows health-care providers to disclose PHI for treatment purposes without patient consent or authorization [2]. This creates a federal "floor." States are free to enact laws that require health-care providers to obtain patient consent before disclosing PHI for treatment purposes because imposing a consent requirement is more stringent than the HIPAA federal floor. Therefore, an HIE initiative must analyze its state laws to determine if they are more stringent than HIPAA. If they are, then the HIE and its participants must comply with the more stringent state law requirements, keeping in mind that if a state law is silent on an issue, then the federal floor of HIPAA must be followed.

Sensitive Data

Many states have enacted laws that are more stringent than HIPAA with respect to several categories of "sensitive data." Data considered sensitive under state laws are often mental and behavioral health data, communicable disease data, genetic information, and sexually transmitted disease data. State laws will generally impose more stringent patient consent requirements on the disclosure of these types of data. HIPAA and federal law generally do not provide additional protections or consent requirements upon communicable or sexually transmitted diseases. HIPAA and federal law do provide specific protections for psychotherapy notes (under HIPAA) [3] and drug and alcohol addiction treatment data (under 42 CFR Part II). These types of data require specific patient consent each time they are disclosed. It is important for any HIE initiative to research state and federal laws relating to sensitive data and determine how such data will be handled by the HIE. Many HIEs take the approach of prohibiting their participants from sending HIPAA psychotherapy notes and Part II drug and alcohol addiction treatment information. They will also take the same approach with respect to state-regulated sensitive data. This way the HIE never handles data that have special consent requirements attached to it. Rather than outright prohibiting such types of data, some HIEs require that their participants specifically represent and warrant that consent for disclosure has been obtained for any data that are shared with the HIE. This allows sensitive data types to be shared via the HIE, but imposes additional administrative burdens upon HIE participants.

HIPAA and the HITECH Act

The primary federal laws applicable to HIE initiatives is the Health Insurance Portability and Accountability Act of 1996 (HIPAA) and the Health Information Technology for Economic and Clinical Health Act (HITECH Act). HIPAA was passed in 1996 and allowed for the Department of Health and Human Services (HHS) to issue privacy and security regulations. HHS implemented these regulations in what are known as the Privacy Rule (finalized in December of 2000) and the Security Rule (finalized in February of 2003). In 2009, as part of the American Recovery and Reinvestment Act (ARRA or the Stimulus Package), the HITECH Act was passed and, among other things, made a number of changes to HIPAA, which were implemented through regulations issued by HHS (most of which were finalized in Jan. 2013, some of which are still forthcoming). These two laws (HIPAA and HITECH) and their implementing regulations (the Privacy Rule and the Security Rule) create the federal floor of laws and regulations that impact HIE's use and disclosure of PHI.

What is Regulated?

HIPAA, by virtue of the Privacy Rule, the Security Rule, and the HITECH Act, applies to "covered entities" and their "business associates." A *covered entity* is (1) a health-care provider that engages in certain electronic transactions (essentially any health-care provider that accepts insurance of any kind will engage in covered electronic transactions), (2) a health plan, or (3) a health-care clearinghouse (an entity that converts health information into standard formats required by HIPAA) [4].

A *business associate* is a person or entity (other than a member of a covered entity's workforce) that creates, receives, maintains, or transmits PHI for or on behalf of a covered entity; essentially a person or entity that performs services for a covered entity that involve PHI [4]. Examples of business associates include billing companies, practice management companies, hosted EHR vendors, and lawyers. Under the HITECH Act, a health information organization (or an HIE) is specifically named as a business associate [4].

HIPAA requires that all covered entities have contracts with their business associates (called business associate agreements or BAAs) [5]. BAAs must contain a number of specific provisions regarding confidentiality and security [6]. Before the HITECH Act, business associates were not directly subject to HIPAA, they were merely obligated to comply with the terms of their BAAs with covered entities. This left the federal government in a difficult position when a business associate suffered a breach of PHI. The federal government had no direct recourse against the business associate; it was left to the covered entity to pursue contractual remedies against the business associate under its BAA. To avoid this lack of recourse, the HITECH Act provided that business associates must now comply with all aspects of the Security Rule and virtually all of the aspects of the Privacy Rule [7]. This means that the federal government now has a direct cause of action against a business associate in the event of a breach [8].

Having established that covered entities and business associates are the entities regulated by HIPAA, the next question is: What type of information is subject to HIPAA? HIPAA regulates *protected health information*, which is individually identifiable health information transmitted or maintained in any form or medium (excluding certain education records and student medical records) [4]. *Individually identifiable health information* is health information, including demographic information, created or received by a covered entity that relates to the past, present, or future physical or mental health or condition of an individual that identifies the individual or could reasonably be used to identify the individual [9].

The Privacy Rule lists 18 specific identifiers that, when paired with some type of health information, result in PHI. Those identifiers are as follows:

1. Names
2. All geographic subdivisions smaller than a state, including street address, city, county, precinct, zip code, and their equivalent geocodes, except for the initial three digits of a zip code if certain population requirements are met
3. All elements of dates (except year) for dates directly related to an individual, including birth date, admission date, discharge date, date of death; and all ages over 89 and all elements of dates (including year) indicative of such age, except that such ages and elements may be aggregated into a single category of age 90 or older
4. Telephone numbers
5. Fax numbers
6. Electronic mail addresses
7. Social security numbers
8. Medical record numbers
9. Health plan beneficiary numbers
10. Account numbers
11. Certificate/license numbers
12. Vehicle identifiers and serial numbers, including license plate numbers
13. Device identifiers and serial numbers
14. Web Universal Resource Locators (URLs)
15. Internet Protocol (IP) address numbers
16. Biometric identifiers, including finger and voice prints
17. Full face photographic images and any comparable images
18. Any other unique identifying number, characteristic, or code, except for certain coding systems that allow for reidentification of data [10].

These identifiers are broad and show that HHS takes an expansive view in determining what might reasonably be used to identify an individual. Many individuals hold the false belief that if they simply remove a name they have deidentified PHI. The truth is that only once these 18 identifiers are removed from PHI, will the PHI be considered "deidentified" under HIPAA and no longer subject to regulation under HIPAA? [11–13]. Covered entities (and their business associates with permission from their covered entity) may deidentify PHI and use deidentified information for any purpose [14]. This is an important term to consider in any covered entity–business associate relationship: Will the covered entity permit the business associate to deidentify PHI and use the deidentified information for other purposes? Many vendors seek to deidentify information and monetize it through sales or licensing arrangements. Some HIEs could benefit and increase their sustainability if they are permitted to deidentify PHI and use the deidentified data for other purposes. Deidentification can raise privacy concerns as individuals may feel that a third party should not profit from the use of their deidentified data. Deidentified data can also be used for many public goods by researchers looking to promote public health or analyze the efficacy of different treatments. The issue of deidentification is an important one to discuss with HIE stakeholders and reach agreement upon how the issue will be addressed by an HIE.

The Privacy Rule and the Security Rule

Knowing who (covered entities and business associates) and what (PHI) is regulated by HIPAA, the next question is: What is required under HIPAA? The Privacy Rule establishes permissible uses and disclosures of PHI and the Security Rule establishes a set of required and addressable security controls.

The Privacy Rule

Under the Privacy Rule, covered entities and business associates may only use or disclose PHI if the Privacy Rule permits the particular use or disclosure or if the person who is the subject of the PHI authorizes the use or disclosure [15]. It is important to note the distinction between "use" and "disclosure." A use of PHI is the sharing, employment, application, utilization, examination, or analysis of such information *within an entity* that maintains such information [4]. A disclosure of PHI is the release, transfer, provision of, access to, or divulging in any other manner of information *outside the entity* holding the information [4].

Under the Privacy Rule, the following are the primary uses and disclosures of PHI that are permitted without a patient's authorization:

- To the individual to whom the PHI relates
- For treatment, payment, or health-care operations
- For public health activities
- As required by law
- For certain research activities where a privacy board or an institutional review board has waived the authorization requirement [16].

Except in the case of treatment, the Privacy Rule requires that covered entities and business associates make reasonable efforts to limit uses and disclosures of PHI to the minimum amount necessary to accomplish the intended use or disclosure [17].

For the purposes of an HIE, most uses and disclosures will be for treatment, health-care operations, or public health activities. Just because the Privacy Rule permits a particular use or disclosures does not mean that a business associate (or an HIE) may automatically make such use or disclosure; the business associate (or an HIE) must obtain permission from its covered entity(ies) to make a particular use or disclosure [18]. It is critical that an HIE establish the types of uses and disclosures that will be made of data shared with the HIE and obtain appropriate permissions for such uses and disclosures in its agreement (including a BAA) with the HIE participants.

HIE use cases for treatment purposes are fairly straightforward and self-explanatory. For example, providing data at the point of care or delivering a clinical lab result is a treatment disclosure [19].

Public health use cases encompass, for example, delivering immunization reports to public health authorities or providing data for public health syndromic surveillance [19].

Health-care operations use cases that are emerging as the next frontier of HIE use cases. Health-care operations includes, among other things, conducting quality assessment and improvement activities, including outcomes evaluation and development of clinical guidelines, provided that the obtaining of generalizable knowledge is not the primary purpose of any studies resulting from such activities; patient safety activities; population-based activities relating to improving health or reducing health-care costs, protocol development, case management and care coordination, contacting of health-care providers and patients with information about treatment alternatives; and related functions that do not include treatment [19]. These uses and disclosures, sometimes called "secondary use," are some of the higher value services that an HIE can offer. As these are permitted under the privacy rule without patient authorization [20], it is important for an HIE to secure permission from its covered entity participants for the HIE to make these uses of PHI if these services are part of the HIE's plans.

An important change that the HITECH Act made to the Privacy Rule is in the area of requests by patients for their information not to be shared in certain circumstances. The Privacy Rule provides that patients may request that covered entities not to make certain uses or disclosures of their information [21]. The Privacy Rule goes on to state that covered entities are not obligated to grant such requests except in one situation [22]. That situation is when a patient pays out-of-pocket in full for health care and requests that their health-care provider not share information relating to such health care with the patient's health plan [23]. In this situation the provider must honor the request and refrain from sharing the information with the patient's health plan [23]. This can create unique challenges for HIEs that share data with health plans, as many do and as more and more will to increase their sustainability. HIEs must have in place a mechanism for their health-care provider participants to either; (1) not send information that is subject to a restriction request or (2) notify the HIE that certain data are subject to a restriction request so that the HIE can take steps to ensure that the data are not shared with the patient's health plan. This right is rarely exercised by patients, but it is nonetheless something for which HIEs must be prepared if they are going to share data with health plans.

The Privacy Rule establishes the situations in which covered entities and business associates may use and disclose PHI. The Privacy Rule is sometimes used as an excuse for providers and health plans to not share data with each other. The truth is that the Privacy Rule is designed to allow sharing of health data among health-care providers and health plans in the interest of patient treatment, improving quality, and population health management. If an entity is declining to share data because "HIPAA does not allow it," it is important to do a deep analysis to determine what provision of HIPAA does not allow the particular data sharing. The truth is that if the sharing would enhance patient care or public health, then it is probably allowed under HIPAA. HIPAA does a good job of protecting confidentiality by limiting uses and disclosures to covered entities and business associates and then ensuring confidentiality by imposing security control requirements upon covered entities and business associates under the Security Rule.

The Security Rule

The Privacy Rule establishes permissible uses and disclosures of PHI. The Security Rule is equally as important in establishing the baseline security controls that are required or addressable by covered entities and business associates [24]. The Security Rule establishes a number of general requirements that apply to all covered entities and business associates and then describes a number of implementation specifications that are either "required" or "addressable" by covered entities and business associates [24]. This framework provides a great deal of flexibility and allows covered entities and business associates to consider their size, complexity, capabilities, technical infrastructure, cost and probability and criticality of potential risks when implementing security controls [25]. If a particular control is required (shown as (R) in Table 6.1), then it must be implemented by a covered entity or business associate [26]. If a particular control is addressable (shown as (A) in Table 6.1), then the covered entity or business associate must assess whether each control is a reasonable and appropriate safeguard

TABLE 6.1 HIPAA Security Rule Controls

Administrative Procedures [28]	Physical Safeguards [29]	Technical Security Measures [30]
Security management process—Policies and procedures to prevent, detect, contain and correct security violations, including: • Risk assessment (R) • Reduce risk to an appropriate level (R) • Workforce sanctions (R) • Review system activities (R)	*Facility access controls*—Policies and procedures to limit physical access to PHI, including: • Contingency operations plans (A) • Facility security plan (A) • Access control and validation procedures (A) • Maintenance records (A)	*Access control*—Policies and procedures to allow PHI access only to those persons or programs that have been granted access rights, including: • Unique user identification (R) • Emergency access (R) • Automatic logoff (A) • Encryption (A)
Security responsibility—Identify a security official (R)	*Workstation use*—Policies and procedures that specify functions and physical attributes of workstations and the surrounding areas (R)	*Audit controls*—Hardware, software or mechanisms that record and examine activity in systems (R)
Work force security—Limit PHI access to appropriate members of the workforce, including: • Authorization and supervision of employees (A) • Clearance of workforce members (A) • Procedures for terminating access to PHI as necessary (A)	*Workstation security*—Physical safeguards for all workstations that access PHI (R)	*Integrity*—Policies and procedures to protect PHI from improper alteration or destruction, including: • Mechanism to authenticate PHI to ensure it has not been altered or destroyed (A)
Information access management—Access to PHI is limited as required by the Security Rule, including: • Isolating health-care clearinghouse functions (R) • Access authorization policies (A) • Access modification policies (A)	*Device and media control*—Policies and procedures that govern the receipt and removal of hardware and media that contain PHI, including: • Disposal of media (R) • Media reuse (R) • Accountability for movement (A) • Data backup and storage (A)	*Person or entity authentication*—Procedures to verify that a person or entity seeking access to PHI is the one claimed (R)

(*Continued*)

TABLE 6.1 *Continued*

Administrative Procedures [28]	Physical Safeguards [29]	Technical Security Measures [30]
Security awareness and training—A security and awareness training program for all workforce members, including: • Security reminders (A) • Protection from malicious software (A) • Log-in monitoring (A) • Password management (A)		*Transmission security*—Technical security measures to guard against unauthorized access to PHI while in transit, including: • Integrity controls (A) • Encryption (A)
Security incident procedures—Policies and procedures to address security incidents through response and reporting (R)		
Contingency plan—Policies and procedures for responding to emergencies and system failures, including: • Data backup (R) • Disaster recovery plan (R) • Emergency operation plan (R) • Testing and revision of plans (A) • Application and data criticality analysis (A)		
Evaluation—Perform periodic technical and nontechnical evaluations of security controls (R)		
Business associates—Covered entities and business associates must obtain written BAAs from their business associates and subcontractors, respectively (R)		

in its environment, when analyzed with reference to the likely contribution to protecting PHI and either implement the control or document its decision to not implement the control [27]. The controls are divided into three categories: Administrative, Physical, and Technical, as shown and described in Table 6.1.

Breach Notification Rule

The HITECH Act established a national requirement for individuals to be notified in the event of a breach of their PHI [31]. The HITECH breach notification rule requires that a covered entity notifies an individual of a breach of the individual's "unsecured" PHI [32]. Unsecured PHI is PHI that has not been encrypted or destroyed in accordance with guidelines issued by the Secretary of HHS [10]. This concept of "unsecured" PHI illustrates the value and importance of encrypting PHI (ie, a breach of encrypted PHI is not a "breach" for purposes of the breach notification rule). Even though encryption is only an "addressable" control under the Security Rule [33], the "safe harbor" that encryption provides under the breach notification rule is increasingly making encryption a de facto requirement. An HIE needs to seriously consider encryption of data both while it is at rest (eg, when stored) and in transit (eg, when being transferred via email or file transfer protocol). Many covered entities will require their business associates to utilize encryption to take advantage of the breach notification rule's encryption safe harbor.

Under the breach notification rule, in the event of a breach of unsecured PHI, covered entities must notify individuals and business associates must notify covered entities after performing a risk assessment [32,34]. An impermissible acquisition, access, use, or disclosure of unsecured PHI is presumed to be a breach under the rule unless the covered entity or business associate demonstrates that there is a low probability that the PHI has been compromised based upon a risk assessment of at least the following factors:

- the nature and extent of the PHI involved, including the types of identifiers and the likelihood of reidentification;
- the unauthorized person who used the PHI or to whom the disclosure was made;
- whether the PHI was actually acquired or viewed; and
- the extent to which the risk to the PHI has been mitigated [10].

The notice to individuals (or from a business associate to a covered entity) must include, to the extent possible:

- a brief description of what happened, including the date of the breach and the date of the discovery of the breach, if known
- a description of the types of unsecured PHI that were involved in the breach (such as whether full name, social security number, date of birth, home address, account number, diagnosis, disability code, or other types of information were involved)
- any steps individuals should take to protect themselves from potential harm resulting from the breach
- a brief description of what the covered entity involved is doing to investigate the breach, to mitigate harm to individuals, and to protect against any further breaches and
- contact procedures for individuals to ask questions or learn additional information, including a toll-free telephone number, an email address, website, or postal address [35].

Additionally the media must be notified of a breach that affects more than 500 individuals and HHS must be notified of all breaches (immediately if the breach is over 500 individuals and annually for breaches that affect less than 500 individuals) [36,37].

As all HIEs are business associates, they must be sure to have plans and procedures in place to notify their covered entities in the event of a breach. HIE participation agreements or their BAAs should address roles and responsibilities in the event of a breach. For example, who will bear the costs associated with notification? Additionally, many BAAs will require that a business associate notify a covered entity of any impermissible use or disclosure of PHI, regardless of whether a risk assessment demonstrates that there is a low probability that the PHI has been compromised [38]. This may result in situations where a business associate notifies a covered entity of an impermissible use or disclosure, but the covered entity elects to not notify individuals based upon the covered entity's risk assessment.

HIPAA Enforcement

Before the HITECH Act, HIPAA had a reputation for being a "paper tiger" due to its lack of enforcement and relatively low fines and penalties when enforced. The HITECH Act greatly increased the penalties for HIPAA violations (from $100 to $50,000 up to a $1.5

Million cap), which can include jail time [39]. Additionally the HITECH Act empowered State Attorneys General to bring HIPAA enforcement actions [40]. Further, HITECH calls for the sharing of HIPAA violation penalties with individuals harmed by violations (although regulations implementing this provision have not yet been issued) [41]. Lastly, the HITECH Act requires that HHS conduct HIPAA audits of covered entitles and business associates [42]. The combination of these enforcement enhancements under the HITECH Act gives HIPAA the enforcement strength that has been lacking and has made HIPAA compliance a much higher priority at covered entities and business associates.

CONTRACTS

Federal and state laws establish the baseline rules of the road for HIE. When HIE participants come together to form an HIE initiative, they are likely to want to agree upon additional rules that will govern their relationship and foster trust among participants. As a threshold issue, there are different contracting structures that may be used in an HIE. Generally, they can be divided into three categories as shown in Table 6.2.

HIE contracting has evolved a great deal in recent years. The trend is toward multiparty agreements; however, many two-party HIE participation agreement and point-to-point agreement frameworks still exist. Each model has pros and cons and various reasons why it is used.

Point-to-Point Agreements

Party-to-party or point-to-point agreements tend to be used when the number of HIE participants is low and the parties involved do not wish to create a sophisticated HIE governance structure. Sometimes point-to-point agreements are referred to as data use agreements or DUAs, especially in the government context. Point to point agreement frameworks can be found in small communities where there are, for example, only two hospitals that have decided to share data with each other in certain circumstances. The two parties will enter

TABLE 6.2 HIE Contracting Structures

Structure	Characteristics
Party-to-party or point-to-point agreements	• Direct agreements between individual parties exchanging data with each other • No HIE entity involved • Example: Jurisdiction by jurisdiction agreements with the CDC for biosurveillance
Two-party HIE participation agreements	• Individual agreement between an HIE entity and a participant • HIE participants do not have direct contractual privity with each other • Involvement of an HIE entity • Example: HIE X has 27 "one-off" or individualized agreements with the 27 entities that participate in its HIE
Multiparty agreement	• A common set of terms and conditions to which an HIE entity and all participants agree • The HIE and all participants are in direct contractual privity with each other • Involvement of an HIE entity • Example: The DURSA governing the eHealth Exchange or the INPC Terms and Conditions used in Indiana

into direct agreements with each other that will define the circumstances under which data will be exchanged. There is no HIE entity to mediate the exchange; the two entities share data directly with each other. Eventually, a third party may come a long that wants to exchange data. Under the point-to-point model, the third party would sign an agreement with both the existing parties and data sharing would occur. The obvious downside to this model is that it does not scale up. If a fourth and fifth party came along in this example, they would need to each contract with the first three parties as well as each other. Once this type of growth occurs, the parties probably need to look at a different model that allows for broader participation and the possible creation of an HIE entity to mediate the exchange.

Two-Party Agreements

The two-party HIE participation agreement model comes into play when an HIE entity exists and it needs to contract with HIE participants to facilitate exchange. Under this model, the HIE signs an agreement with each HIE participant. The HIE will want the multiple agreements it signs to be as similar as possible, but in all likelihood there will be variation in the agreements it signs. The HIE participants only have a contractual relationship, or privity, with the HIE entity. They do not have contractual relationships with each other. This model has been used by numerous HIE entities across the country. The challenge to this model is that variation among the agreements the HIE signs can create challenges for the HIE entity in administering its exchange. If the HIE has different obligations to different HIE participants, the administrative costs of running the HIE will increase. Further, if the HIE wishes to make changes to its agreement, for example, to allow for a new data use, the HIE must go to each HIE participant and ask for a contractual amendment. This creates additional administrative overhead and could lead to "hold out" problems if some of the HIE participants are not willing to agree to the amendment. Further, because the HIE participants do not have direct contractual privity with each other, they will not have contractual rights against each other in the event of a breach. For example, if an employee at HIE participant A wrongly discloses PHI that was obtained through the HIE from HIE participant B, HIE participant B may have breach notification obligations, but does not have contractual recourse against the bad actor at HIE participant A. HIE participant B would only have a contractual right against the HIE entity (who then in turn would have a contractual right against HIE participant A), which could be problematic as the HIE entity might lack sufficient capital or insurance coverage to make HIE participant B whole.

Multiparty Agreements

The multiparty agreement model is the most sophisticated model of the three and has many advantages; however, it can be challenging to implement, as all HIE participants and the HIE entity must agree to the same terms. This requires a significant amount of negotiations and consensus building across participants. Sometimes so much so that HIE initiatives that seek to implement this model fail to get past the contract negotiation phase. If consensus around a common set of terms and conditions can be reached, then the HIE will have a lower contractual administration burden as all HIE participant have the same rights and obligations. Further, contractual amendment mechanisms can be built into the agreement that allow amendments and new data uses without having to obtain signatures from each HIE participant. Under the Data Use and Reciprocal Support Agreement (DURSA) used by the eHealth Exchange [43] and the INPC Terms and Conditions used by the Indiana

Health Information Exchange, amendments and new data uses can be proposed to designated committees that have the contractual authority to approve amendments and new data uses. Once approved by the designated committee, the amendment or new data use can go into effect. Lastly, under this model, all HIE participants and the HIE entity have direct contractual privity with each other, which allows for direct contractual actions in the event of a contractual breach. Also, by way of example, the INPC Terms and Conditions provides for cross-indemnification by all HIE participants; meaning that each participant can look directly to other participants for indemnification in the event that one participant causes harm to another.

Regardless of the contracting model implemented by an HIE, contracts among or with HIE participants serve as a mechanism to create and build trust by defining how particular parties will behave in given situations. A through contract will address as many situations as possible so that HIE participants will trust in how each other will act in those situations, which breads more and more trust over time.

SUMMARY

Trust among HIE participants is paramount to any HIE initiative. The initiative will never get off the ground and actually engage in data sharing if the participants do not trust each other. Trust is confidence in knowing what another party will do in a given situation. Laws, regulations, and contracts are mechanisms that dictate how parties will behave in given situations and therefore are trust enablers. The HIPAA Privacy and Security Rules, as enhanced by the HITECH Act, serve as the primary pieces of federal regulation that govern privacy, security and confidentiality in the health-care space, therefore they are the primary regulations that establish how health-care entities, such as HIE participants, will act in given situations. They establish permitted uses and disclosures of PHI and set forth the baseline security controls that health-care entities must put in place. State laws, particularly in the area of sensitive data, can be enacted to add additional requirements on the use and disclosure of health information, particularly in the area of patient consent, and must be addressed by any HIE initiative. Finally, contractual arrangements among IHIE entities and their participants can establish additional rules for how parties will behave in given situations. Different contracting models lead to different levels of trust and sophistication in HIE arrangements. An HIE initiative that understands the federal and state legal landscape and implements a contracting structure that address critical legal issues will bread trust among its participants and enable a higher level of exchange.

QUESTIONS FOR DISCUSSION

1. How is "trust" defined in the context of HIE?
2. Explain the difference between "privacy" and "confidentiality.".
3. What are the primary federal laws the regulate privacy and security in the health-care space?
4. What uses and disclosures of protected information are permitted under HIPAA without patient consent or authorization?
5. May states enact legislation that is more stringent than HIPAA?
6. Is encryption a required or addressable control under the HIPAA Security Rule?
7. What benefits does encryption provide under the Breach Notification Rule?
8. What are the three categories of security controls under the HIPAA Security Rule?
9. What type of contracting structure are most HIE initiatives trending towards?

References

[1] General rule and exceptions, 45 C.F.R. 160.203(b); 2002.
[2] Uses and disclosures of protected health information: general rules, 45 C.F.R. 164.502(a)(1)(ii); 2013.
[3] Uses and disclosures for which an authorization is required, 45 C.F.R. 164.508(a)(2); 2013.
[4] Definitions, 45 C.F.R. 160.103; 2013.
[5] Uses and disclosures of protected health information: general rules, 45 C.F.R. 164.502(e)(2); 2013.
[6] Uses and disclosures: organizational requirements, 45 C.F.R. 164.504(e)(2); 2013.
[7] Security standards: general rules, 45 C.F.R. 164.306; 2013.
[8] Definitions. 45 C.F.R, 160.402; 2013.
[9] Definitions. 45 C.F.R, 150.103; 2013.
[10] Other requirements relating to uses and disclosures of protected health information, 45 C.F.R. 164.514(b); 2013.
[11] Uses and disclosures of protected health information: General rules, 45 C.F.R. 164.502(d)(2); 2013.
[12] Other requirements relating to uses and disclosures of protected health information, 45 C.F.R. 164.514(a); 2013.
[13] Other requirements relating to uses and disclosures of protected health information, 45 C.F.R. 164-514(b); 2013.
[14] Uses and disclosures of protected health information: general rules, 45 C.F.R. 164.502(d); 2013.
[15] Uses and disclosures of protected health information: general rules, 45 C.F.R. 164.502(a); 2013.
[16] Uses and disclosures of protected health information: general rules, 45 C.F.R. 164.502(a)(1); 2013.
[17] Uses and disclosures of protected health information: general rules, 45 C.F.R. 164.502(b); 2013.
[18] Uses and disclosures of protected health information: general rules, 45 C.F.R. 164.502(a)(3); 2013.
[19] Definitions, 45 C.F.R 164.501; 2013.
[20] Uses and disclosures to carry out treatment, payment, or health care operations, 45 C.F.R. 165.506(c); 2013.
[21] Rights to request privacy protection for protected health information, 45 C.F.R. 164.522(a)(1)(i); 2013.
[22] Rights to request privacy protection for protected health information, 45 C.F.R. 164.522(a)(1)(ii); 2013.
[23] Rights to request privacy protection for protected health information, 45 C.F.R 164.522(a)(1)(vi); 2013.
[24] Security standards for the protection of electronic protected health information, 45 C.F.R. 164, Subpart C; 2003.
[25] Security standards: general rules, 45 C.F.R 164.306(b); 2013.
[26] Security standards: general rules, 45 C.F.R 164.306(d)(2); 2013.
[27] Security standards: general rules, 45 C.F.R. 164.306(d)(3); 2013.
[28] Administrative safeguards, 45 C.F.R. 164.308; 2013.
[29] Physical safeguards, 45 C.F.R. 164.310; 2013.
[30] Technical safeguards, 45 C.F.R. 164.312; 2013.
[31] Notification in the case of breach of unsecured protected health information, 45 C.F.R. 164, Subpart D; 2009.
[32] Notification to individuals, 45 C.F.R 164.404; 2013.
[33] Technical safeguards, 45 C.F.R. 164.312(e); 2013.
[34] Notification by a business associate, 45 C.F.R. 164.410; 2013.
[35] Notification to individuals, 45 C.F.R. 164.404(c); 2013.
[36] Notification to the media, 45 C.F.R. 164.406; 2013.
[37] Notification to the Secretary, 45 C.F.R 164.408; 2013.
[38] Uses and disclosures: organizational requirements, 45 C.F.R. 164.504(e)(2)(ii)(c); 2013.
[39] Amount of a civil money penalty, 45 C.F.R. 160.404; 2013.
[40] Improved Enforcement, Section 13410(e) of the HITECH Act.
[41] Improved Enforcement, Section 13410(c)(3) of the HITECH Act.
[42] Audits, Section 13411 of the HITECH Act.
[43] The Data Use and Reciprocal Support Agreement (DURSA) is available at http://sequoiaproject.org/wp-content/uploads/2015/03/restatement_i_of_the_dursa_9.30.14_final.pdf.

PART III

TECHNICAL ASPECTS OF MANAGING HEALTH INFORMATION EXCHANGE

CHAPTER

7

The Evolving Health Information Infrastructure

David Broyles[1], Brian E. Dixon[2], Ryan Crichton[3], Paul Biondich[4] and Shaun J. Grannis[4]

[1]Indiana University Richard M. Fairbanks School of Public Health, Indianapolis, IN [2]Indiana University Richard M. Fairbanks School of Public Health; and the Center for Biomedical Informatics, Regenstrief Institute, Inc., Indianapolis, IN [3]Jembi Health Systems, Cape Town [4]Indiana University, School of Medicine; and the Center for Biomedical Informatics, Regenstrief Institute, Inc., Indianapolis, IN

OUTLINE

LEARNING OBJECTIVES

By the end of the chapter, the reader should be able to:

- Define the concept of a health information infrastructure.
- List and describe three key technical aspects of a health information infrastructure.
- Explain the concept of architecture from an information science perspective and how it is used in strategic planning for a health information infrastructure.
- Explain the role of transactions in health information exchange (HIE).
- List and describe the three types of interoperability important to HIE.
- Describe the role and core functions of an interoperability layer (IL) in supporting HIE.
- List and describe the components of an IL.

INTRODUCTION

This is the first chapter in the section of the book that covers the technical aspects of HIE. In this chapter, we define and describe the key concept of a health information infrastructure or the ecosystem in which HIE occurs. Information infrastructures are enabled by technical architectures, so we define a model HIE architecture and the core technical aspect of the model that facilitates HIE—the IL. Additional details on interoperability and the standards that support the syntactic form of interoperability can be found in the chapter "Syntactic Interoperability and the Role of Standards." Semantic interoperability and standards are covered in the chapter "Standardizing Health Care Data Across an Enterprise."

THE HEALTH INFORMATION INFRASTRUCTURE

The health information infrastructure for a nation, state, or community is an ecosystem composed of the people, processes, procedures, tools, facilities, and technologies which supports the capture, storage, management, exchange, and creation of data and information to support individual patient care and population health. While individual organizations such as hospitals possess discrete people (eg, health care workers), processes (eg, medication administration protocols, referral patterns), and information systems (eg, electronic health records (EHRs), remote monitoring, laboratory information systems), communities are composed of a larger set of technologies, organizations, and people that create a health information infrastructure [1]. Thus, an information infrastructure is a sort of network of networks, and HIE is the method by which data and information are shared among the organizations, people, and technologies that comprise the defined ecosystem.

The Health Information Infrastructure is an Ultra Large-Scale System

As described by the Institute of Medicine in its report on the digital infrastructure for supporting the learning health system [2], a health information infrastructure is similar to the concept of an ultra large-scale (ULS) system as defined in computer science. A ULS system is a set of characteristics that tend to arise as a result of the scale of the system (in this case the complex and fragmented organization as well as delivery of health care) rather than a prescriptive set of required technical components. Previous work on the ULS concept [3] has identified the following key characteristics of ULS systems:

- *Decentralization*: The scale of ULS systems means that they will necessarily be decentralized in a variety of ways—decentralized data, development, evolution, and operational control.
- *Inherently conflicting, unknowable, and diverse requirements:* ULS systems will be developed and used by a wide variety of stakeholders with unavoidably different, conflicting, complex, and changing needs.
- *Continuous evolution and deployment:* There will be an increasing need to integrate new capabilities into a ULS system while it is operating. New and different capabilities will be deployed and unused capabilities will be dropped; the system will be evolving not in phases but continuously.
- *Heterogeneous, inconsistent, and changing elements:* A ULS system will not be constructed from uniform parts: there will be some misfits, especially as the system is extended and repaired.
- *Erosion of the people/system boundary:* People will not just be users of a ULS system; they will be elements of the system, affecting its overall emergent behavior.
- *Normal failures:* Software and hardware failures will be the norm rather than the exception.
- *New paradigms for acquisition and policy:* The acquisition of a ULS system will be simultaneous with the operation of the system and require new methods for control.

SUPPORTING THE HEALTH INFORMATION INFRASTRUCTURE

To organize and support an integrated health information infrastructure, where the various actors in the ecosystem can effectively exchange data and information, HIE networks must facilitate three important technical aspects of an infrastructure (the organizational, political, and legal aspects will be considered in later chapters): an *architecture* that defines how everything "fits together" and provides a common understanding for creating and managing the components of the infrastructure; methods for *transactions* between information systems or the exchange of data and information; and methods for *interoperability* or the ability for receiving information systems to do something with the data or information exchanged. The specific information systems and applications used in HIE are defined and managed by individual hospitals, physician offices, health systems, public health agencies, and payors. These include systems such as laboratory information systems, radiology information systems, emergency department information systems, etc. Where an HIE infrastructure can provide the most value is in defining the big picture and providing pathways that enable data exchange.

Architecture

In computer science, the term *software architecture* refers to the high-level design of a system, the methods by which components are created, and the documentation of the system structures. In other words, the *architecture* of an information infrastructure defines how its various parts "fit together." Fig. 7.1 is an example of an architecture from the US Nationwide Health Information Network (now referred to as the eHealth Exchange). The image succinctly identifies the various components of the network, including infrastructure components, available services to members of the network as well as the use cases for information exchange implemented to date. The architectural depiction comes from a much larger document [4], which provides guidance to system engineers and developers on the tools and methods they should use when creating, maintaining, and

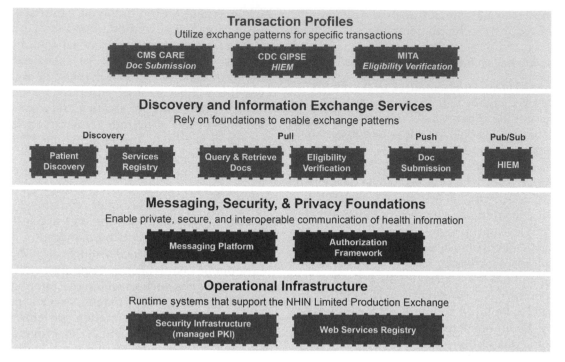

FIGURE 7.1 Architectural components of the US Nationwide Health Information Network (NHIN). *Adapted from Ref. [4].*

implementing components of the system. An architecture for HIE is derived from consensus discussions among the stakeholders involved in the network (eg, health systems, public health authorities, and pharmacies) who agree upon the components for exchange as well as the methods by which data and information will be exchanged.

When stakeholders agree upon an architecture, most often they agree to use one of several types of architectural patterns or styles. An *architectural pattern* is a general reusable approach to a commonly occurring problem in software architecture within a given context like HIE. An *architectural style* is a reusable set of design decisions and constraints that are applied to an architecture to induce chosen desirable qualities [5]. While computer scientists disagree on the exact differences between the two idioms, they both provide a common language or vocabulary with which to describe classes of systems [6]. Commonly used architectural patterns and styles include:

- Client/Server—Distributed systems that involve a separate client and server system, and a connecting network. The simplest form of client/server system involves a server application that is accessed directly by multiple clients, referred to as a two-tier architectural style. Historically, the client/server style indicated a desktop application that communicated with a database server containing much of the business logic or with a dedicated file server. This style is recommended when implementing business processes that will be used by people throughout an organization.

- Component-Based Architecture—Decomposes the system into reusable functional or logical components that expose well-defined communication interfaces. Essentially the system is composed of prefabricated components that perform specific functions. A set of components function together as an application server. Aspects of a user interface are typically implemented as components. Other common types of components are those that are resource intensive, not frequently accessed, and must be activated using the just-in-time approach (common in distributed component scenarios); and queued components executed asynchronously using message queuing.
- Service-Oriented Architecture (SOA)—Application functionality is provided as a set of services that are loosely coupled because they use standards-based interfaces that can be invoked, published, and discovered. Services in SOA are focused on providing a schema and message-based interaction with an application through interfaces that are application scoped as opposed to components. SOA approaches are common for Software as a Service as well as cloud-based applications. The SOA style is recommended for message-based communication between segments of the application in a platform-independent way, when you want to take advantage of federated services such as authentication or when you want to expose services that are discoverable through directories. Because services are independent and focus on a performing a narrow task, maintenance is easier when compared to other styles.

Whereas client/server types are common for health information systems operating within a clinic, hospital, or health system, HIE applications typically use component-based or SOA types. Furthermore, SOA dictates that services operate in distributed environments and focus on document-centric communication [7], making this type very suitable for HIE since health information infrastructures share many aspects of a ULS system. More recent HIE initiatives have favored SOA approaches in their design and development, including the eHealth Exchange [8,9].

Transactions

A health information transaction can be defined as the exchange of electronic health information between two extraneous entities for a specific purpose [10]. HIEs are designed to promote a variety of health information transactions. An example of a common transaction is the delivery of laboratory test results to the physician that ordered the test [10]. The transaction occurs between the information system at the laboratory and the EHR system in the clinic or health system. Laboratory reports can also be sent from the lab information system to other health system stakeholders such as a public health agency [11]. Thus transactions support routine business processes among health care system stakeholders. Other examples include sending medication orders to the pharmacy, retrieving a report from a specialty physician, and registering a new patient who visits the clinic for the first time.

In Table 7.1, we summarize common classes of transactions that can occur within a health system. While individual transaction types (eg, medication order, lab result delivery) are designed around a specific process in health care, these transaction classes represent a broader set of transactions that can occur. There is a Save/Update Records class that represents the variety of transactions in which data or information about a patient is "pushed" or delivered from one system to another for either storage in the EHR or display to a clinician. Another class referred to as Requests/Queries represents transactions in which one

TABLE 7.1 Transaction Classes Commonly Handled by Health Information Infrastructures

Transaction Class	Description
Save/Update Records	Information regarding a patient encounter can be saved to the individual's electronic health record
	Demographic information about a patient can be updated in the client registry
	A new patient is registered in the health system for the first time
Requests/Queries	A list of a patient's previous encounters restricted to a specific time frame can be retrieved
	Client information can be obtained by providing the client ID number
	Information about a specific health care facility can be retrieved if the point of service application calling the system provides the facility ID number
	A point of service system can request a list of a clients that match specific criteria outlined in the parameters of the query
	A point of service application can request a list of health care facilities that match specific criteria outlined in the parameters of the query
Alerts	The system can relay alert messages regarding patient care to physicians and other providers
	Public health authorities can be alerted to a new report of a disease like Ebola; they may be closely monitoring in a state or nation

information systems asks or requests information from the EHR or another information system about a patient or population (eg, all patients with diabetes, veterans). A third class, Alerts, represents transactions in which a business rule is triggered by data in the system and a user is alerted about an emerging state (eg, new blood pressure reading is high, diagnosis of a highly contagious disease).

Interoperability

Successful transactions between disparate information systems require multiple layers of interoperability including foundational, syntactic, and semantic [12,13]. Foundational interoperability refers to the technical infrastructure necessary to share information between systems [13]. Syntactic interoperability requires that messages sent between two information systems must be transmitted in a format that is recognized by both systems [14]. Semantic interoperability refers to the ability of one system to correctly decipher and process the information received from another information system without prior consultation [15].

Foundational Interoperability

Disparate health information systems that wish to exchange information must adhere to a series of standardized communication protocols. Initially, the heterogeneous systems must be linked together to form a communication network. Many exchanges use Transmission Control Protocol/Internet (TCP/IP) connections to fulfill this requirement [12]. Information exchange also requires an application protocol such as the Hypertext Transfer Protocol (HTTP) [12,16]. Web services such as SOAP (Simple Object Access Protocol) or Representational State Transfer (REST) that define how and where to send the messages are also critical to structured information exchange [12]. Although foundational interoperability is necessary for data exchange, these requirements can be fulfilled relatively easily in relation to syntactic and semantic interoperability concerns.

Syntactic Interoperability

Successful communication between systems also requires messages to be transmitted using a structure and syntax that is ascertainable to both systems [13]. Formats such as Extensible Markup Language (XML) are frequently used to satisfy this demand [12,14]. Enabling successful communication becomes increasingly complex as more heterogeneous systems with their own unique formatting are involved in the information exchange [12]. For this reason, HIEs have typically adopted messaging standards such as Health Level Seven (HL7) version 2 or 3 [12,17–19]. In the chapter "Syntactic Interoperability and the Role of Standards," the book provides a more detailed discussion on syntactic interoperability, including HL7, and the process for developing and selecting technical standards.

Semantic Interoperability

The ability to successfully receive a message does not assure that the system receiving the message will be able to interpret and complete a request. If an external system attempting to communicate with the HIE system uses terminology or coding that is incompatible with the internal standards of the HIE, then the data must be translated into standardized format before it can be interpreted. Additionally, the response must be translated back into the language used by the external system. In many HIE structures, this can be a time-consuming and expensive process [20–22]. In the chapter "Standardizing Health Care Data Across an Enterprise," the book more fully discusses syntactic interoperability as well as methods and tool for managing terminologies.

OPEN HIE—A MODEL HEALTH INFORMATION INFRASTRUCTURE

Interoperability between multiple disparate health systems presents a particularly complex challenge for HIEs to overcome [21,23,24]. The interoperability of health information systems is a prominent issue in the United States due to the fragmented makeup of the health information infrastructure [25]. Although maintaining many disassociated information systems empowers the United States to meet a diverse variety of local health care needs, this degree of flexibility also has some drawbacks [25]. The majority of these health information systems were designed and structured to meet the unique needs of the implementing health care organization [26]. Planning for interoperability with external systems is generally a low priority in the development process [27]. Although standards for health data exist, many health care providers still identify clinical observations using locally specific terminology that is not harmonious with external systems [21]. As a result, health data is often collected in an inconsistent manner from one organization to another [28]. This often prevents the information systems of the separate organizations from corresponding with each other successfully without a uniform method of standardizing the data [28]. The lack of standardization that results from this approach makes it difficult to assemble the information from these fragmented local databases into a strong national system [25].

The OpenHIE model is designed to promote the sharing of health information in countries with a diverse array of health information systems through a middle-out approach to national HIE [25]. The middle-out strategy adapts to the varying needs and capabilities of the heterogeneous entities involved in the HIE [25]. The OpenHIE model facilitates interoperability by combining existing applications through relatively simple and inexpensive interfaces rather than implementing new systems or major redevelopment efforts [29]. This enables the OpenHIE solution to avoid some of the financial and technical barriers experienced by many conventional HIE solutions [25,30]. As a result, OpenHIE can be implemented more quickly than other solutions and with few disruptions to any existing operational health information systems that will be participating in the HIE [17].

In order for numerous heterogeneous health information systems to communicate successfully, the architecture of an HIE must offer flexible processes and technology that are capable of accommodating the constantly changing demands associated with health information. The OpenHIE model addresses this challenge through a component-based architecture. The component-based design enables multiple services to work together to provide a secure mechanism for sharing health care information while maintaining the flexibility of the system. This allows OpenHIE to meet the needs specific to the country where it is being implemented. As a result, OpenHIE has the potential to make the health care industry of an implementing nation more efficacious and boost the quality of service by enabling accurate and timely access to critical patient information [11,30–32].

The OpenHIE architecture is depicted in Fig. 7.2. Each component supports well-described core health data management functions and interoperates with other components to ensure that health information from various point of service applications is rationalized to support person-centric and population-based health care needs. Reference implementations of each of the components exist to validate and highlight the functionality enabled within the architecture and also are designed to support real-world needs. Different compositions of

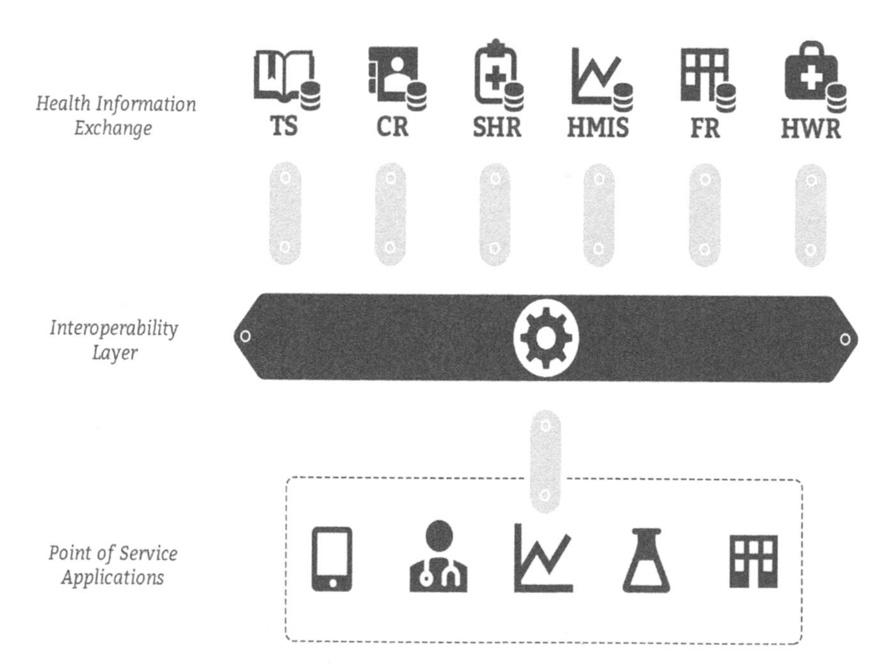

FIGURE 7.2 The OpenHIE model with architectural components.

these components can be used within a given environment to support myriad workflows.

The components of the OpenHIE architecture depicted in Fig. 7.2 include:

- *IL* serves as the core method for connecting the components of the HIE with point of service applications. Detailed description of the IL is provided in the remainder of this chapter.
- *Terminology Service (TS)* that manages local as well as reference terminologies, collections of unique concepts that describe diagnoses, treatments, and outcomes. Detailed description of the TS is provided in the chapter "Standardizing Health Care Data Across an Enterprise."
- *Shared Health Record (SHR)* that serves as a repository of person-centric records detailing visits, diagnoses, treatments, laboratory results, and other observations documented during care delivery or by public health authorities. Detailed description of the SHR is provided in the chapter "Shared Longitudinal Health Records for Clinical and Population Health."
- *Health Management Information System (HMIS)* that stores and redistributes population level information normalized through the HIE. Detailed description of the HMIS is provided in the chapter "Shared Longitudinal Health Records for Clinical and Population Health."
- *Client Registry (CR)* that manages the unique identities of people receiving health services or who live in a community. Detailed description of the CR is provided in the chapter "Client Registries: Identifying and Linking Patients."
- *Facility Registry (FR)* that manages unique health facilities located within a community, state or nation. Detailed description of the FR is provided in the chapter "Facility Registries: Metadata for Where Care Is Delivered."
- *Health Worker Registry (HWR)* that manages unique health workers at all levels of the health system, including doctors, nurses, pharmacists, social workers, and community health workers. Detailed description of the HWR is provided in the chapter "Health Worker Registries: Managing the Health Care Workforce."
- *Point of Service Applications* are health information systems external to the HIE that have a need to interface with the HIE components. Mobile applications, laboratory information systems, and monitoring devices likely have a need to store data in the HIE and/or retrieve data from the HIE. These applications interact with the HIE components via the IL.

Interoperability Layer

In the OpenHIE model, the foundation of the flexible architecture is the *interoperability layer* or *IL* [27]. The IL is a middleware system that enables easier interoperability between disparate information systems by bringing all of the infrastructure services and external applications together [33]. The OpenHIE structure includes both systems that request services and systems that provide those services. Service requestors are the external point of service applications such as a pharmacy information system or laboratory information system that are making requests of the internal OpenHIE components [27,34]. Service providers are the systems that accommodate these requests [27]. The service providers in the OpenHIE infrastructure consist of the domain services represented in Fig. 7.2 including the CR, provider registry, FR, SHR, and the TS. The job of the IL is to facilitate the transaction between the service requestor and the service provider.

The IL receives transaction requests from external client systems, conducts the correspondence between the internal components of the HIE, and possesses functions that can facilitate manageable interoperability between systems [35]. The IL serves several core functions that facilitate HIE for OpenHIE.

1. The IL simplifies the security for the HIE by providing a single point of access for all external systems that are attempting to communicate with the components of the HIE such as the CR, the provider registry, the FR, or the SHR.
2. The IL keeps a record of all of the transactions that take place in the OpenHIE.
3. The IL is responsible for routing messages to the appropriate service provider within the infrastructure.

In addition to the core functions provided by the IL, it also offers mediation functionality. If a point of service application sends a request in a format that is not recognizable to the service provider, the IL assists the transaction by furnishing an adapter that transforms the message into a format accepted by the internal components of the HIE. Similarly, the adapters will transform the data back into a format expected by the point of service application that initiated the transaction. When necessary, the IL orchestrates complicated transactions to remove that complexity from the consumer systems.

Structure of the IL

The IL was designed to address the problem of interoperability between health care systems through an architectural framework that incorporates the use of web services and progressive middleware [36]. The OpenHIE IL is composed of two components including the core component and the orchestrators and adapter services component. This architectural approach is based on the Enterprise Service Bus (ESB) model. An ESB is a middleware system that integrates messaging, web services, transformation, and routing to coordinate transactions among discordant applications [16,36]. These advanced middleware systems can be leveraged to overcome interoperability constraints between heterogeneous health information systems [16,33,37]. ESBs can accept transaction requests and then perform mediation tasks to fulfill the transaction [16,27]. Additionally, the individual mechanisms of the ESB can operate independently of one another which allows them to continue to function in the event that one component fails [27,38]. Fig. 7.3 illustrates the components of the IL and the role they serve in the OpenHIE infrastructure. The components are described in greater detail below.

Core Component

The core component of the IL serves as the entry point into the HIE. It functions as a web service proxy and executes some supplementary tasks on the incoming requests to eliminate the need for other domain services to furnish them. It provides security for the HIE, logs transactions, identifies and displays errors that occur between services, and routes the incoming requests to the proper services. This requires an authentication and authorization service, a log service, and an audit service. When the IL receives confirmation from all of these services that the applicable information has been collected and saved, it passes the message to the router so that it can be sent to the appropriate service.

Providing a single point of entry for all incoming messages serves to streamline the transaction process [39]. The IL can accommodate requests from a diverse range of systems through exposing an external application programming interface (API) [18,40]. The external API is publicly accessible to systems with the proper privileges and handles all transactions with point of service applications such as laboratory or pharmacy information systems. Requests from these external systems can be collected through an application protocol such as HTTP and then translated into a

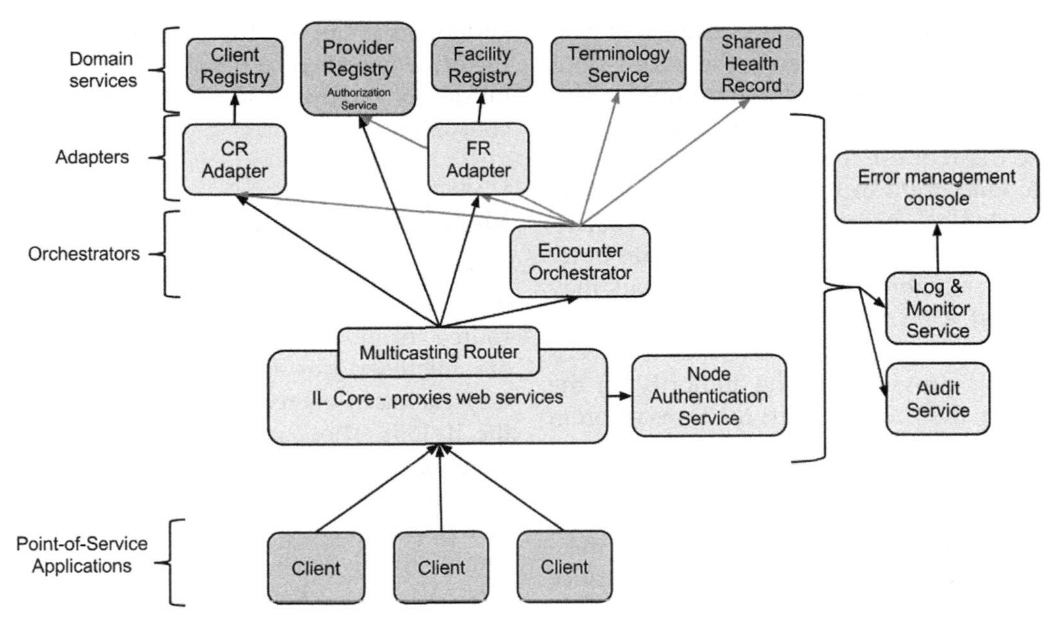

FIGURE 7.3 Architecture of the OpenHIE model illustrating the detailed components of the interoperability layer.

configuration that is recognizable to all components of the IL [27]. The use of an API enables OpenHIE services to be called in real time by external point of service systems [41]. The point of service systems calling the IL can provide the necessary parameters for the system designated by the API and then allow the IL to facilitate an automated response [41]. This approach is advantageous over conventional systems that often relied on asynchronous approaches to interoperability [40,41].

Security

The core component of the IL also manages security for the entire HIE. Using the IL as the sole point of entry into the HIE mitigates potential security barriers to information exchange because the requesting systems can submit a message without ascertaining the location and security demands of the system that is providing the service [27]. The node authentication service depicted in Fig. 7.3 ensures that only authorized systems can interact with the components of the OpenHIE. Transactions that are received by the IL are acquired over a secured HTTPs connection through the external API [41]. The IL uses the Audit Trail and Node Authentication (ATNA) profile from Integrating the Healthcare Enterprise (IHE) to authenticate transactions (see chapter: Syntactic Interoperability and the Role of Standards, for more on IHE). The ATNA profile relies on Mutual Transport Layer Security to ensure that transactions only take place when the digital certificate of a point-of-service application is trusted by the IL and the digital certificate of the IL is trusted by the point-of-service application.

The point of service applications that are calling the IL are responsible for authenticating users. For example, a provider may want to call the HIE to obtain a list of a patient's encounters within the last year. Once the provider has entered the correct password, they can submit a transaction request to the IL. This transaction request includes a provider ID number. When the IL receives an authenticated request, it calls the provider registry to verify the permissions associated with the provider ID number. This step verifies that the provider has the authority to make the request. This is important because some mobile point of service applications may be restricted to requesting data from specific services within the infrastructure, while other more robust point of service applications may have unrestricted access to all of the services provided in the infrastructure. Once it is verified that the provider has the authority for the transaction, the IL will record the transaction in the SHR and notify the provider or other point of service application that the transaction was successful. If the provider does not have the authority for the transaction, an exception message would be returned to their point of service application. The results would be written to the audit log of the IL.

Monitoring/Logging

Another function of the core component of the IL is to log and monitor the transactions that occur. The log and monitor and audit services portrayed in Fig. 7.3 provide an audit trail for each transaction by storing every message as well as the crucial characteristics of the message including the sender's identity, details about the information that was received, the time and date the message was received, and the response to the message. This enables auditing when necessary and provides insight into the movement of messages through HIE.

The logging mechanism of the IL also improves system performance and error management within the OpenHIE infrastructure. Areas within the system that may be experiencing restrictions to the flow of information or inefficiencies can be identified more easily. All failed transactions are logged and can be grouped by the underlying source of the error. System administrators can use this information to correct recurring issues more efficiently [27]. Transactions that failed due to an internal system error can be rerun once the root cause of the error has been rectified without placing the burden of having to resubmit a request on the consumer.

Mediation Component

The IL also offers a mediation component that executes the transactions that are routed from the core component. Mediators are microservices that carry out supplementary exercises on requests that are received by the IL [33]. These mediation microservices are disassociated components of the IL that each provides a distinct function. The two types of mediators that incorporated into the architecture of the IL include adapters and orchestrators. Adapters change the incoming requests into an acceptable format when necessary, while orchestrators enable a business process to be carried out.

Adapters

Adapters allow the IL to transform incoming transactions into a format that the HIE recognizes [27]. Transformation ensures that the transaction will have syntactic interoperability. For example, a message that arrives in HL7 version 3 format may need to be converted into HL7 version 2 format in order to be recognized by the system because HL7 version 3 uses XML data objects to identify values while HL7 version 2 uses delimiters to separate values [19]. Adapters are also responsible for facilitating semantic interoperability for the transaction by translating the codes from the messages into the standardized language used by the IL. This requires a call to the terminology server that maps the standards used by the IL to the vocabulary used by the various participating systems [27]. Each of the internal OpenHIE components such as the CR or FR has a designated adapter as characterized in Fig. 7.3 to perform these services [35].

Orchestrators

The orchestration microservice enables the timely completion of transactions that require multiple tasks to be executed. The orchestrator may need to call numerous components of the HIE in order to assemble a valid response to the point of service application that initiated the transaction. For example, the completion of a request may require the verification of multiple identifiers that may be stored in separate registries within the HIE infrastructure such as the provider registry, FR, and CR. The illustration in Fig. 7.3 exemplifies how the encounter orchestrator may delegate tasks throughout the OpenHIE during a transaction.

These mediation services are summoned only when there is a requirement to translate or orchestrate a transaction. The core component will communicate directly with the domain service for transactions that do not require an adapter or orchestrator. The mediation services also log the messages that they dispatch to the domain services. The mediation components that are available in the IL are generally unique to the needs of the country that is implementing OpenHIE. Developing orchestrators and adapters as independent services within the architecture adds flexibility to the system because these subcomponents can be added or removed as needs change [35]. An alternative approach is to combine orchestration and adaptation services into a single component, referred to as an interface engine which is described in more detail in the chapter "Syntactic Interoperability and the Role of Standards".

BENEFITS OF THE OPENHIE IL

Collectively, the OpenHIE IL provides a solution to overcome many of the prominent barriers that can inhibit health information sharing. The ability to restrict access to a single entry point simplifies security, monitoring, and error management for the entire HIE infrastructure. The ability of the IL to process requests without the use of a specific message format is critical because no individual standards can exhaustively meet the demands of all prevailing and forthcoming information systems [28]. The flexibility of the IL structure enables OpenHIE to adapt as clinical guidelines, technology, and the needs of the stakeholders evolve over time [29]. Services can be added or changed as needed, and the loose component-based architecture can be leveraged to accommodate fluctuations in transaction volumes.

SUMMARY

The technical attributes of a health information infrastructure are paramount to the effectiveness of large-scale information exchange efforts. HIEs must have a well-developed architecture, mechanisms for transmitting data from one system to another, and processes to provide interoperability between disparate information systems. In this chapter, we have discussed the core technical components of a robust health information infrastructure and described one model for achieving HIE within a community, state, or nation. While OpenHIE offers advantages, it is not the only way to achieve HIE. Regardless of the architecture selected, stakeholders who want to engage in HIE must make design decisions about the layers of interoperability or else the various disparate information systems that exist within a given health care ecosystem will not be able to exchange data or information.

In the rest of this section of this book, we describe other important technical components of a health information infrastructure that can facilitate HIE. In the chapter "Syntactic Interoperability and the Role of Standards," we discuss syntactic interoperability and available technical standards that support HIE between information systems. Then in the chapter "Standardizing Health Care Data Across an

Enterprise," we describe semantic interoperability and available internationally recognized data standards for consistent representation of data and information across information systems. In the chapter "Shared Longitudinal Health Records for Clinical and Population Health," we discuss the role of an SHR that enables longitudinal examinations of individual patients as well as populations. Linking patient records from disparate facilities and health information systems requires a client or patient registry, which we discuss in the chapter "Client Registries: Identifying and Linking Patients." Then in the chapter "Facility Registries: Metadata for Where Care Is Delivered," we describe facility registries which uniquely identify the places where patients receive care in a health system. Finally, we discuss health worker registries in the chapter "Health Worker Registries: Managing the Health Care Workforce" that uniquely identify the various individuals who provide care in a community or health system, including physicians, nurses, medical assistants, etc. When used together, these various components of a health information infrastructure not only facilitate HIE between information systems but they enable providers, community, and public health organizations to answer questions about who receives care where in the community by whom as well as the outcomes of that care. This is ultimately the goal of HIE—to facilitate better quality, more efficient care that leads to improved health for individuals and populations.

Acknowledgments

The authors thank the OpenHIE Community of Practice for sharing its collective knowledge and wisdom for use in the book, not only in this chapter but also in this entire technical section.

QUESTIONS FOR DISCUSSION

1. What characteristics of the health system support the argument that a health information infrastructure can be classified as an Ultra Large-Scale System?
2. Compare and contrast the HIE architectural styles and patterns. Which approach might be the most effective on a national scale?
3. Which type of interoperability is most important to architectural design of an HIE?
4. Why is a flexible HIE architecture so important in a country like the United States with multiple heterogeneous health information systems?
5. What function provided by the interoperability layer is the most important to HIE endeavors? Why?

References

[1] Dixon B, Grannis S. Public health informatics infrastructure Magnuson JA, Fu JPC, editors. Public health informatics and information systems. London: Springer; 2014. p. 69–88.

[2] Institute of Medicine Digital infrastructure for the learning health system: the foundation for continuous improvement in health and health care: Workshop series summary. Washington DC: The National Academies Press; 2011.

[3] Feiler P, Sullivan K, Wallnau K, Gabriel R, Goodenough J, Linger R, et al. Ultra-large-scale systems: the software challenge of the future. Pittsburg: Software Engineering Institute, Carnegie Mellon University; 2006. Available from: <http://resources.sei.cmu.edu/library/asset-view.cfm?assetID=30519>.

[4] Nationwide Health Information Network Nationwide health information network (NHIN) exchange: architecture overview. Washington, DC: Department of Health and Human Services, U.S.; 2010. (updated April 21, 2010; cited June 16, 2015); Available from: <http://www.himss.org/files/HIMSSorg/content/files/Line%2013%20-%20NHIN_Architecture_Overview_Draft_20100421.pdf>.

[5] Taylor RN, Redmiles DF, van der Hoek A. Architectural styles. Irvine, CA: Institute for Software Research, University of California, Irvine [cited June 10, 2015]; Available from: <http://isr.uci.edu/architecture/styles.html>.

[6] Microsoft Corporation Architectural patterns and styles. Microsoft application architecture guide, 2nd ed. Redmond, WA: Microsoft Corporation; 2009.

[7] Koskela M, Rahikainen M, Wan T. Software development methods: SOA vs. CBD, OO and AOP. Available

from: <http://citeseerx.ist.psu.edu/viewdoc/summary?doi=10.1.1.111.9582>.

[8] Hosseini M, Ahmadi M, Dixon BE. A service oriented architecture approach to achieve interoperability between immunization information systems in Iran. AMIA Annu Symp Proc 2014;2014:1797–805. Epub January 1, 2014.

[9] Simonaitis L, Dixon BE, Belsito A, Miller T, Overhage JM. Building a production-ready infrastructure to enhance medication management: early lessons from the nationwide health information network. AMIA Annu Symp Proc 2009;2009:609–13. Epub January 1, 2009.

[10] Centers for Medicare and Medicaid Services. Transaction & code sets standards. 2014 [cited May 17, 2015]; Available from: <https://www.cms.gov/Regulations-and-Guidance/HIPAA-Administrative-Simplification/TransactionCodeSetsStands/index.html?redirect=/TransactionCodeSetsStands/02_TransactionsandCodeSetsRegulations.asp>.

[11] Dixon BE, McGowan JJ, Grannis SJ. Electronic laboratory data quality and the value of a health information exchange to support public health reporting processes. AMIA Annu Symp Proc 2011;2011:322–30. Epub December 24, 2011.

[12] Gliklich RE, Dreyer NA, Leavy MB. Registries for evaluating patient outcomes: a user's guide [Internet], 3rd ed. Rockville, MD: Agency for Healthcare Research and Quality; 2014.

[13] Healthcare Information and Management Systems Society. What is Interoperability? 2013 [cited February 12, 2015]; Available from: <http://www.himss.org/library/interoperability-standards/what-is-interoperability>.

[14] Vergara-Niedermayr C, Wang F, Pan T, Kurc T, Saltz J. Semantically interoperable XML data. Int J Semant Comput 2013;7(3):237–55. Epub October 10, 2014.

[15] Dolin RH, Alschuler L. Approaching semantic interoperability in Health Level Seven. J Am Med Inform Assoc 2011;18(1):99–103. Epub November 26, 2010.

[16] Andry F, Wan L. Health information exchange network interoperability through IHE transactions orchestration. International Conference on Health Informatics. Vilamoura, Portugal: 2012.

[17] Barbarito F, Pinciroli F, Mason J, Marceglia S, Mazzola L, Bonacina S. Implementing standards for the interoperability among healthcare providers in the public regionalized Healthcare Information System of the Lombardy Region. J Biomed Inform 2012;45(4):736–45. Epub January 31, 2012.

[18] Lee M, Heo E, Lim H, Lee JY, Weon S, Chae H, et al. Developing a common health information exchange platform to implement a nationwide health information network in South Korea. Healthc Inform Res 2015;21(1):21–9. Epub February 24, 2015.

[19] Viangteeravat T, Anyanwu MN, Nagisetty VR, Kuscu E, Sakauye ME, Wu D. Clinical data integration of distributed data sources using Health Level Seven (HL7) v3-RIM mapping. J Clin Bioinformatics 2011;1:32. Epub November 23, 2011.

[20] Lin MC, Vreeman DJ, McDonald CJ, Huff SM. A characterization of local LOINC mapping for laboratory tests in three large institutions. Methods Inf Med 2011;50(2):105–14. Epub August 21, 2010.

[21] Dixon BE, Vreeman DJ, Grannis SJ. The long road to semantic interoperability in support of public health: experiences from two states. J Biomed Inform 2014;49:3–8. Epub April 1, 2014.

[22] Baorto DM, Cimino JJ, Parvin CA, Kahn MG. Combining laboratory data sets from multiple institutions using the logical observation identifier names and codes (LOINC). Int J Med Inform 1998;51(1):29–37. Epub September 28, 1998.

[23] Vest JR, Gamm LD. Health information exchange: persistent challenges and new strategies. J Am Med Inform Assoc 2010;17(3):288–94. Epub May 6, 2010.

[24] Kuperman GJ. Health-information exchange: why are we doing it, and what are we doing? J Am Med Inform Assoc 2011;18(5):678–82. Epub June 17, 2011.

[25] Coiera E. Building a National Health IT System from the middle out. J Am Med Inform Assoc 2009;16(3):271–3. Epub May 2, 2009.

[26] Berges I, Bermudez J, Illarramendi A. Toward semantic interoperability of electronic health records. IEEE Trans Inf Technol Biomed 2012;16(3):424–31. Epub January 6, 2012.

[27] Crichton R, Moodley D, Pillay A, Gakuba R, Seebregts C. An architecture and reference implementation of an open health information mediator: enabling interoperability in the rwandan health information exchange Weber J, Perseil I, editors. Foundations of health information engineering and systems. Berlin Heidelberg: Springer; 2013. p. 87–104.

[28] Gold MR, McLaughlin CG, Devers KJ, Berenson RA, Bovbjerg RR. Obtaining providers' 'buy-in' and establishing effective means of information exchange will be critical to HITECH's success. Health Aff (Project Hope) 2012;31(3):514–26. Epub 2012/03/07.

[29] Arzt NH. Service-oriented architecture in public health. J Healthc Inf Manag 2010;24(2):45–52.

[30] Adler-Milstein J, Bates DW, Jha AK. Operational health information exchanges show substantial growth, but long-term funding remains a concern. Health Aff (Project Hope) 2013;32(8):1486–92. Epub July 11, 2013.

[31] Dixon BE, Zafar A, Overhage JM. A framework for evaluating the costs, effort, and value of nationwide health information exchange. J Am Med Inform Assoc 2010;17(3):295–301. Epub May 6, 2010.

[32] Vest JR. Health information exchange: national and international approaches. Adv Health Care Manage 2012;12:3–24. Epub August 17, 2012.

[33] Crichton R. The open health information mediator: an architecture for enabling interoperability in low to middle income countries. Master of Science Thesis. Durban, South Africa: University of KwaZulu-Natal; 2015. Available from: <http://www.cair.za.net/research/outputs/open-health-information-mediator-architecture-enabling-interoperability-low-middle>.

[34] Liu S, Zhou B, Xie G, Mei J, Liu H, Liu C, et al. Beyond regional health information exchange in China: a practical and industrial-strength approach. AMIA Annu Symp Proc 2011;2011:824–33. Epub December 24, 2011.

[35] El Azami I, Cherkaoui Malki MO, Tahon C. Integrating hospital information systems in healthcare institutions: a mediation architecture. J Med Syst 2012;36(5):3123–34. Epub Novemver 17, 2011.

[36] Koufi V, Malamateniou F, Vassilacopoulos G. A big data-driven model for the optimization of healthcare processes. Stud Health Technol Inform 2015;210:697–701. Epub May 21, 2015.

[37] Ryan A, Eklund P. The health service bus: an architecture and case study in achieving interoperability in healthcare. Stud Health Technol Inform 2010;160 (Pt 2):922–6. Epub September 16, 2010.

[38] Van Den Bossche B, Van Hoecke S, Danneels C, Decruyenaere J, Dhoedt B, De Turck F. Design of a JAIN SLEE/ESB-based platform for routing medical data in the ICU. Comput Methods Programs Biomed 2008;91(3):265–77. Epub July 5, 2008.

[39] Khan WA, Khattak AM, Hussain M, Amin MB, Afzal M, Nugent C, et al. An adaptive semantic based mediation system for data interoperability among Health Information Systems. J Med Syst 2014;38(8):28. Epub June 27, 2014.

[40] Blobel B, Holena M. Comparing middleware concepts for advanced healthcare system architectures. Int J Med Inform 1997;46(2):69–85. Epub October 7, 1997.

[41] Healthcare Information and Management Systems Society. Integrating the HIE into the EHR workflow. 2011. Available from: <http://files.himss.org/2011-08-08-IntegratingtheHIEintotheEHRWorkflow.pdf>.

CHAPTER

8

Syntactic Interoperability and the Role of Standards

Masoud Hosseini[1,2] *and Brian E. Dixon*[2,3,4]

[1]Department of BioHealth Informatics, Indiana University, School of Informatics and Computing, Indianapolis, IN [2]Center for Biomedical Informatics, Regenstrief Institute, Inc., Indianapolis, IN [3]Indiana University, Richard M. Fairbanks School of Public Health, Indianapolis, IN [4]Department of Veterans Affairs, Center for Health Information and Communication, Veterans Health Administration, Health Services Research and Development Service CIN 13-416, Richard L. Roudebush VA Medical Center, Indianapolis, IN

OUTLINE

LEARNING OBJECTIVES

By the end of this chapter you will be able to:

- List and describe the different levels of interoperability and the role of each in health information exchange (HIE).
- Describe the principles of messaging and its role in HIE.
- Categorize messaging standards and distinguish their application in health care.
- Describe the process for developing standards in health care.
- Identify and describe available resources and services for organizations seeking to implement standards.

INTRODUCTION

In the previous chapter, we defined interoperability and described how an interoperability layer facilitates data exchange between core health information exchange (HIE) services and the many health information system (HIS) applications that may have a need to send or receive data and information. At the heart of interoperability is messaging, or the process by which data and information are exchanged between two computer systems. In this chapter, we more fully describe the concept of syntactic interoperability and the standards that support messaging between HIS including HIE services. We further describe the development and maintenance of standards, a process important to creating and sustaining interoperability in the health-care ecosystem. In chapter "Standardizing Health Care Data Across an Enterprise", we extend our discussion to include semantic interoperability and standards.

SYNTACTIC INTEROPERABILITY

Successful transactions between disparate information systems require multiple layers of interoperability as described in the previous chapter [1,2]. Whereas technical interoperability provides a foundation for successfully transmitting messages from system A to system B; syntactic interoperability provides a structure and syntax that enables the message to be ascertainable by both systems [2].

Let's return to the example of mailing a letter from chapter "What Is Health Information Exchange". The technical interoperability afforded by the postal service allows us to drop any kind of letter in the mail and have it delivered to our destination, provided of course that it contains a valid address and correct amount of postage. However, the technical infrastructure of the postal service is agnostic about the kind of letter we mail. Syntactic interoperability, on the other hand, cares about and therefore provides structure and syntax for the envelope as well as the contents.

Let's say we wish to send out cover letters and resumes because we are searching for a new job. The kind of envelope and type of information inside the envelope in this scenario are unique and vary from when we wish to send love letters, postcards while on vacation, or payments for our new car. Syntactic interoperability allows us to explicitly define the type of envelope and its contents for messages that will contain information about a person seeking a job.

In computer science, the structure of a message is defined as the *schema*. For example, the schema of HL7 (Health Level 7) v3 messages is based on the Extensible Markup Language (XML). Unlike programming languages, such as Java or C#, which give instructions to the computer to perform an action, markup languages are structural methods for annotating text. Text can be converted into a markup language structure by labeling specific "chunks" or sections of data using *tags* that are defined in the given markup language. XML is a markup language for generating messages that adhere to a predefined structure consisting of specific sections designed to contain specific types of information. For example, one can define an XML *schema* that labels (or marks up) the following data in a document: patient first name, patient last name, date of birth, gender, and diagnosis.

Thinking about the letters we send when job hunting, a schema for the message would define two sections: cover letter and resume. The schema for the cover letter section would further define specific "parts" such as where the addressee information should be, where we should put the salutation, and where we should put our interest in the specific job to which we are applying. The schema for the resume section would define specific subsections and the types of information to go in those subsections, including education level, employment history, and specialized skills. In fact, when we use a software application such as Microsoft Word to create our cover letter and resume, we likely used a *template* which provided us a structure in which we added our own specific information. Likewise in HIE, we use schemas and templates to create and interpret messages that are sent and received by HIS.

Schemas and templates constrain the vast array of possible message types and information that could potentially be put into any given message. Being compliant with constraints leads to robust and standard messages the facilitate interoperability. Fig. 8.1 presents a section of HL7 v3 message that defines the guardian or caretaker for a patient. There are specific *tags*, enclosed in < >, for each type of information (eg, id, name, etc.) in the section. There is also a structure to the section as indicated by the indentation as well as the color coding inside the tags. We can infer from this section that John Doe is the guardian and his telephone number is 555-555-5001. Complete messages in health care are much more complex, but they are constructed using these basic "building blocks."

```
<guardian>
    <id extension="1234" root="2.16.840.1.123456.7.5"/>
    <guardianPerson>
        <id extension="1234" root="2.16.840.1.123456.35.6"/>
        <name>
            <given>Doe</given>
            <family>John</family>
        </name>
        <telecom value="tel:555-555-5001" use="HP"/>
        <birthTime value="200808820102314.243+0200" />
    </guardianPerson>
</guardian>
```

FIGURE 8.1 An example section from an XML-based message representing guardian information for a fictitious patient.

HEALTH INFORMATION MESSAGING STANDARDS

Syntactic interoperability is achieved through the use of standards. Standards in health IT are broadly organized in four categories [3]:

- Vocabulary/code sets/terminology (semantic interoperability)
- Structure and Content (syntactic interoperability)
- Transport (foundational interoperability)
- Services (syntactic interoperability).

Effective messaging in health care requires two categories of syntactic standards: one which governs the construction of the message (Structure and Content) and one that facilitates the envelope in which the message is placed (Services). Fortunately there are maturing, robust standards to achieve syntactic interoperability. In this section, we describe existing syntactic standards and their general purpose and use. Detailed, in-depth coverage of syntactic standards is outside the scope of this book, but is offered through a text by Benson [4], a monograph by Corepoint Health [5], and a variety of training courses offered by HL7 International [6].

Structure and Content Standards

Health Level Seven—HL7

Health Level Seven (HL7) is the leading and most widely recognized syntactic standard in health IT. The "level 7" in its name refers to the application layer of the OSI (Open Systems Interconnection) model, a conceptual model that characterizes and standardizes interactions within a computer system regardless of its underlying technology. The seventh layer of the OSI model describes application-layer functions that typically includes synchronizing communication between computer systems.

HL7 is an event trigger model in which the sending application transmits a message after a trigger is fired. The main cause for a trigger is a health-care event, such as the registration of a patient at a primary care clinic, discharge of a patient from an acute care hospital, or completion of a laboratory test for the presence of a disease. Receiving systems can then act upon the message, inferring the action that occurred based on the message type and responding to that action. For example, an A01 message indicates the registration of a patient. A computer system that receives an A01 message could respond by querying the HIE network for recent information on the patient available at other institutions for presentation to a clinician prior to the clinical encounter. The receipt of an ORU message for a laboratory result in which a test for the presence of *Methicillin-resistant Staphylococcus aureus* could cause a different computer system to examine the value of the result and alert a clinician to review the result or an infection preventionist to initiate an isolation protocol.

The first version of the HL7 standard was published in 1987, yet there have been many revisions to the standard since its debut. Version 2 (v2) of the HL7 standard is widely adopted and used by HIS in the United States. Yet there are a variety of v2 versions, including v2.3, v2.5.1, and v2.6. Successive, incremental improvements to v2 resulted in clearer, more detailed and documented versions that sought to expand the standard to additional clinical domains while also supporting better normalization. Because of this, the v2 standard is backward compatible, enabling applications to correctly receive and appropriately handle different versions in the v2 family.

Version 2 messages are human readable, non-XML messages, and the data are encoded in segments, fields, and components using a variety of delimiters. Fig. 8.2 presents a sample Admission, Discharge, Transfer (ADT) v2.3 message, which is one of the most common messages in use today. Segments are presented in red (gray in the print version) and the fields

```
MSH|^~\&|GoodEMR|Location1|LIS|Location1|201502042115||ADT^A01|ADT000
01|P|2.3|
EVN|A01|201502042115||
PID|||MRN12345^5^M11||DOE^JOHN^A||19800711|M||C|1 MERIDIAN
STREET^^INDIANAPOLIS^IN^46280|
NK1|1|GOODMAN^CINDY^J|WIFE||||||NK^NEXT OF KIN
PV1|1|I|200^11^01||||006666^GOOD^BARBARA^J.|||SUR||||ADM|A0|
```

FIGURE 8.2 A sample HL7 v2.3 Admission Discharge Transfer (ADT) message.

are separated by pipe (|) delimiter. There are other delimiters, such as the carrot (^), used for separating components within fields.

Although v2 incrementally improved over time, many in the health IT world felt it only normalized 80% of a given interface between two systems [5]. This meant that an additional 20% was customized when, for example, an interface was established between a hospital's laboratory information system and that hospital's electronic health record (EHR) system. The customization was necessary because many aspects of v2 were inherently designed to be flexible, allowing several "design choices" to be made when implemented. In addition to being flexible, critics charged that v2:

- lacked a consistent data model, meaning that the display or storage of data by a clinical information system directly impacts what portions of the HL7 standard it could successfully support;
- lacked clear, well-defined application and user roles, allowing vendors to choose which set of HL7 messages would be supported for a given set of clinical functions; and
- focused too much on US settings, meaning that international users felt the standard did not support HIE in a variety of contexts.

Because of these criticisms, the HL7 community created Version 3 (v3) of HL7 standard. The community first released v3 in 2005. Unlike v2, the HL7 v3 standard represents a suite of specifications explicitly designed around the HL7 Reference Information Model (RIM). The RIM provides a comprehensive, consistent data model that contains a combination of storyboards, classes, data types, use cases, as well as different triggers and events that together create an information framework needed for generating HL7 messages. The v3 standard provides a single source that allows health IT vendors to work with the full set of messages, data types, and terminologies in the RIM needed to build a complete implementation. Furthermore, the RIM and v3 standard were designed with globalization in mind, supporting implementation of HIE around the world. The following are the benefits of v3 as provided on the HL7 International website [7]:

- Focuses on semantic interoperability by specifying that information be presented in a complete clinical context that assures that the sending and receiving systems share the meaning (semantics) of the information being exchanged.
- Provides consistent representation of data laterally across the various HL7 domains of interest and longitudinally over time as new requirements arise and new fields of clinical endeavor are addressed.
- Designed for universal application so that the standards can have the broadest possible global impact and yet be adapted to meet local and regional requirements.

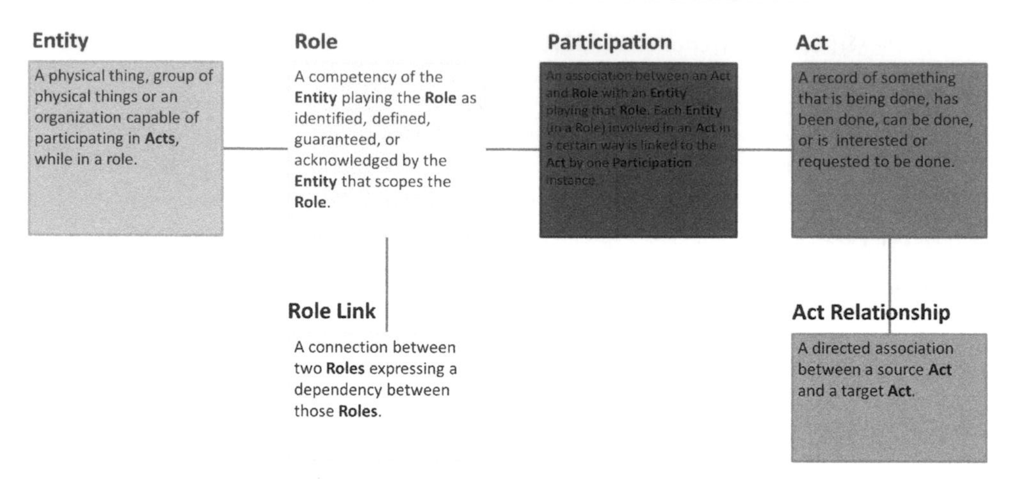

FIGURE 8.3 The HL7 Reference Information Model (RIM) core classes and the relationships between them.

The HL7 RIM includes three core classes (Entity, Role, and Act) that are linked together by three association classes (Participation, Act Relationship, and Role Link) as represented in Fig. 8.3. Every event in HL7 is an *Act*, which is analogous to verb in the English language. Each *Entity*, such as a person, can play different *Roles* such as "patient" or "provider." For an Act to occur, an Entity with a specific Role must *Participate* in some action. Acts relate to each other through *Act Relation* classes and Roles can connect to each other through the *Role Link*.

Fig. 8.4 represents how the RIM supports modeling the performance of a knee replacement surgery. As you see in Fig. 8.4, John Doe, Dr Nelson, Dr Smith, and Good Hospital are different entities (green (light gray in the print version) rectangles) that have different roles (yellow (white in the print version) rectangles) in knee replacement surgery procedure (red (gray in the print version) rectangle). For example, John Doe has patient role and Dr Nelson is a physician. However, same roles might have different participations (blue (dark gray in the print version) rectangle) in a single act. For example, Dr Nelson and Dr Smith both have physician role; however, Dr Nelson participates as a surgeon and Dr Smith participates as an Anesthesiologist in this surgery. Also, there is a lighter red (medium gray in the print version) rectangle in the picture that represents the Act Relationship class and connects two different acts to each other. In Fig. 8.4, John Doe had a knee observation before his surgery and the Act Relationship class connects those two Acts because the information in that observation is pertinent to the knee surgery.

Digital Imaging and Communications in Medicine (DICOM)

DICOM (Digital Imaging and Communications in Medicine) is the most widely adopted standard in the world for the exchange and management of medical images. Since introducing DICOM in 1993, providers have been able to use fully digital images with high resolution instead of physical X-ray films. Using DICOM, images generated by different types of medical imaging devices (eg, X-ray, CT, MRI, ultrasound) can be integrated into picture archiving and communication systems (PACS) and they can be exchanged in HIE networks [8]. The DICOM standard not only encodes the image but also a set of metadata and attributes

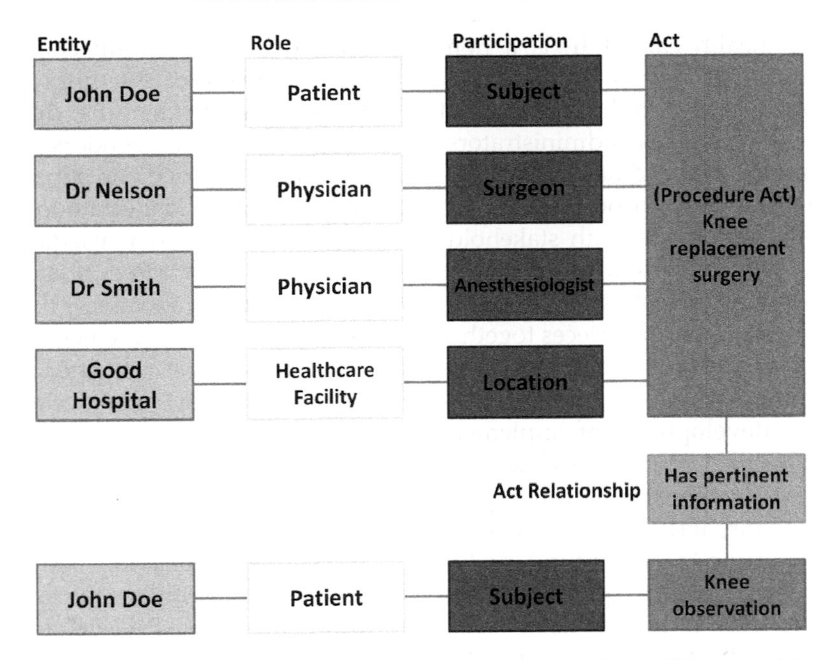

FIGURE 8.4 Example scenario using HL7 modeling for a participation involving different entities and their roles in a knee replacement surgery act.

that describe the image and can be used by other applications in health-care delivery.

National Council for Prescription Drug Programs (NCPDP)

The National Council for Prescription Drug Programs (NCPDP) standardizes electronic exchange of data for prescribing, dispensing, monitoring, managing, and paying for medications and pharmacy services. Currently there are 26 different standards developed by NCPDP; yet only three of them are endorsed for implementation (Telecommunication, SCRIPT, and Manufacturer Rebate). The NCPDP telecommunication standard provides a structure to electronically submit third-party drug claims as well as perform eligibility verification and prior authorization. SCRIPT supports transmitting prescription information electronically in support of fulfilling new prescriptions, prescription refill requests, relaying medication history, and transactions for long-term care.

Standards for HIE Services

A valid, well-constructed message is a major step towards HIE, yet it is only one component of syntactic interoperability. To successfully exchange information, one also needs syntactic standards for the envelope and transactions that will move valid messages from Hospital A to Hospital B. In this section of the chapter, we review existing, mature efforts that support HIE implementers' efforts to establish interoperable exchange of information. While some may not consider these initiatives to be true technical standards, they provide guidance and support for standardizing transactions, in many ways helping to provide the extra 20% effort needed to achieve interoperability.

Integrating the Health-Care Enterprise (IHE)

Integrating the Health-care Enterprise (IHE) works to support efficient and secure interoperability in health care. IHE is a nonprofit organization that brings together key stakeholders, including health-care subject matter experts (eg, clinicians, administrators) and health IT vendors, to coordinate interoperability activities. However, IHE does not develop standards. Instead, IHE works with stakeholders to implement already developed standards through a common, standards-based framework (called the IT Infrastructure) that pieces together various standards across the entire OSI model.

Upon its common framework, IHE facilitates collaborative development of implementation guidelines it calls "IHE Profiles" across a range of use cases in health care as well as public health. For example, IHE has developed an RFD (Retrieve Form for Data Capture) profile that uses available standards to query a remote server for a form (eg, a public health case reporting form), display the form to a user for completion, and then return a completed form to some other HIS. The IT infrastructure and profiles from IHE are used by more than 160 vendors globally. In fact, IHE has strong adoption outside the United States.

There are four major services provided by IHE to address interoperability issues in health care globally:

1. *Problem Identification*: Many clinical and IT experts gather together and identify different use cases and scenarios in health care that require HIE. These experts focus on certain domains and extract the needs for interoperability as well as clinical workflow.
2. *Profile Specification*: After identifying the gaps and challenges in health information interoperability, the experts focus on identifying established standards for communication among systems in these use cases to develop HIE Profiles. HIE profiles describe, in detail, how to use different messaging, terminology, and technical standards to enable HIS to communicate. Vendors in health IT use these profiles to address interoperability challenges in critical areas in health-care settings.
3. *Connectathon Testing*: After developing systems using IHE profiles, vendors participate in a carefully planned and supervised event called the IHE Connectathon to test their application and exchange data with other vendors' products to evaluate the level of interoperability and assess the maturity and accuracy of their implementation.
4. *Integration Statements*: After testing their systems at the IHE Connectathon, vendors publish IHE Integration Statements to state that their product is tested based on IHE guidelines and they are compliant with IHE Profiles. Integration Statements demonstrate that a given application supports IHE profiles and facilitates the process of product acquisition in health-care facilities.

It is challenging for vendors to develop applications that are interoperable with different systems. IHE profiles and Connectathon events enable vendor to test similar implementation of standards with their products.

eHealth Exchange

The eHealth Exchange formerly known as the Nationwide Health Information Network (NwHIN) is the foundation for national health interoperability in the United States. Unlike IHE, the eHealth Exchange is itself an HIE network. The network consists of state and regional HIE networks as well as federal agencies such as the Social Security Administration and Department of Veterans Affairs.

The eHealth Exchange functions as a federated network in which health information is maintained at the source and queried when it is needed. Supporting its transactions is a framework of technical standards carefully selected and supported by the eHealth Exchange. Thus the eHealth Exchange provides HIE services for its members rather than technical infrastructure or data.

The eHealth Exchange was first developed by the Office of the National Coordinator for Health Information Technology (ONC) but is now managed by a nonprofit organization called the Sequoia Project. The Sequoia Project also manages Carequality, a public–private collaborative building consensus among health IT data exchange programs to develop a common interoperability framework, enabling seamless exchange among HIE networks.

Standards & Interoperability (S&I) Framework

The Standards & Interoperability (S&I) Framework, established by ONC, provides a collaborative environment in the United States among public and private sectors to develop tools, services, and guidelines to facilitate interoperability in health care. Like IHE, the S&I Framework brings clinical subject matter experts and health IT professionals together to focus on a singular challenge in health care for which a robust "profile" can be developed. Through a well-defined process, a group of stakeholders can define a narrow use case, identify available standards, and create implementation guidance that enables adoption of the standards. However, unlike IHE, the S&I Framework also asks its teams to then take the next steps of creating a reference implementation of the profile, then facilitate pilot projects that test the use case in a few communities, and then develop HIS certification and testing criteria to support scaling HIE across the nation.

To date the S&I Framework has completed work on several projects, including Transitions of Care, Health eDecisions (clinical decision support), and Provider Directories for the Direct Project. At the time of writing, the S&I Framework had active projects focused on Structured Data Capture, Data Provenance, and Public Health Laboratory Results. Information on the S&I Framework as well as the various products it has created to date can be found on its website: http://www.siframework.org/.

DEVELOPING STANDARDS FOR HEALTH CARE

The development and maintenance of technical standards are overseen by Standards Development Organizations (SDOs), which can be private or public organizations. The American Society for Testing and Materials (ASTM) and HL7 are two important SDOs in the United States that develop standards for clinical and administrative information. There are also SDO accreditation organizations, such as the American National Standards Institute (ANSI), which oversees SDOs in the United States and coordinates standards development with international SDOs so that American products can be used worldwide.

In this section, we will describe how healthcare standards are developed and what the processes are that SDOs go through to develop a new standard or improve an existing one. We further discuss the different methods of stand ards development.

Standards Development in Health Care

Standards can develop through "bottom-up," "top-down," or both approaches. Standards that achieve market penetration through organic (bottom up) adoption by industry are said to be de facto or market-driven standards. At the opposite end of the spectrum, standards endorsed or required for use by government authorities are said to be de jure "according to the law" standards. Most standards in health care tend to be de facto. However, some de jure methods have been quite effective, such as the Meaningful Use regulations in the United States which provides incentives to hospitals and providers who use certified EHR technology. The EHR certification process requires use of designated standards [9]. There is evidence that this approach is working. A recent ONC report to Congress [10] noted that more than six in ten hospitals electronically exchanged patients' health data with providers outside their organization, an increase of more than 50% since 2008.

Once the need for a standard is recognized, SDOs such as HL7 recruit and assemble a collaborative team which is called technical committee or working group comprised of experts in the area of interest and individuals that will be influenced by the standard. Working group members meet to discuss and develop a draft standard. The draft standard is distributed among all members of the SDO to be voted upon, usually through Web-based portal that allows for the balloting of standards. During the balloting period, members can comment on the draft standard and revisions can be made.

The first version of a standard might be referred to as an *Informative Standard*, because it informs the community about an HIE challenge and proposes a solution. The next version of the standard is typically considered to be a *Draft Standard for Trial Use*, meaning that it has been defined to a point that would allow a group of vendors or providers to pilot test its use. After some period of time, during which various implementers have had the chance to trial the standard and feedback has been collected from the implementers, a standard can be revised and approved as a *Normative Standard*. The title Normative suggests a final, consensus-based designation that the standard is ready for widespread adoption.

Even after a standard becomes normative, it can be further refined or updated. Future versions might be developed due to many reasons such as requirement changes, gaps in the current standard, or expanding the scope of the standard. Version 2 of the HL7 standard, for example, has been considered normative since the 1990s. Yet this standard continues to be updated.

Other Methods of Standard Development

Ad hoc is another classification of standards developed by group of people or organizations interested in a specific use case. Their informal agreement on a solution for a specific challenge is considered to be an *Ad hoc* standard. DICOM is a very popular *Ad hoc* standard for exchanging medical images. DICOM is the result of collaborative work between the American College of Radiology (ACR) and the National Electrical Manufacturers Association (NEMA).

RESOURCES FOR IMPLEMENTERS

Implementers of HIE not only need mature technical standards but also guidance and tools to support implementation for a given use case. While efforts like IHE and the Sequoia Project can support normalization of cross-enterprise and HIE transactions, there are additional resources available. The first is an implementation guide (IG), a document that outlines constraints on top of standards and profiles for a very specific use case in clinical or population health. The second is an interface engine, a technology designed to implement standards, profiles, and IGs. Together these resources can be used by implementers to take mature standards and implement them in a community, state, or nation.

Implementation Guides

Technical standards provide a foundation upon which a specific HIE implementation rests. While necessary, standards alone are not sufficient to achieve interoperability as they are inherently accommodating across a range of use cases. Therefore, for a given use case, standards must be constrained and guidance must be provided to implementers, which is the purpose of an *IG*.

IGs are often published by SDOs as well as affinity groups such as ministries of health, professional societies, and industry groups. In example, the IG for Syndromic Surveillance in the United States is published by the Centers for Disease Control and Prevention [11], whereas the IG for electronically reporting laboratory results is published by HL7. The IGs are usually focused on a narrow use case, such as the electronic ordering of a laboratory test or the electronic reporting of a patient's death. A list of several IGs available from HL7 is available on its website [12].

Unlike profiles, IGs do not focus on transactions but message structure and content. The IGs outline what information is required for a given use case, even where it might be generally considered to be optional by the base standard. For example, a field for a patient's race may be required in many US public health use cases, but it may be optional in many global contexts since some countries do not allow the capture of racial information in EHR systems. For use cases involving HL7 v2, the IGs typically specify the message types to be used. For HL7 v3 based use cases, the IGs specify the templates and sections that are to be included in addition to specifying the data elements within sections.

To implement many of the OpenHIE services described in this book, it is recommended that readers consult the IGs available at www.ohie.org. Just like the HL7 and CDC IGs, the IGs by OpenHIE provide guidance on implementing a specific set of standards and processes that will create interoperability for a given use case.

Interface Engines

Implementers need a method by which to interface, or connect, various health IT systems using standards and IGs. An *interface engine* is a mediator technology that supports standard-based implementation of HIE. The engine is software that "listens" for messages on a channel (eg, think pipeline or roadway), and they can also send messages through a channel to other systems. By using interface engines, it allows implementers to avoid programming a significant amount of information about HL7 standards, guidance from the IG and other details into the source system (eg, an EHR system). Instead the interface engine mediates traffic or messages between the EHR and outside systems.

The interface engine is typically programmed to receive certain types of messages, then do something when messages arrive. For example, when ELR (electronic laboratory reporting) messages arrive, the interface engine could be instructed to pass the message along to the EHR for storage in the patient's medical record. It might also be programmed to forward a copy of the message to the public health department if the result pertained to a disease required to be reported to health authorities (eg, sexually transmitted infection). This second option might require the interface engine to open the message and inspect its contents. Therefore interface engines are versatile software allowing both simple communication of messages from one system to the next as well as more complex tasks such as interpreting a message and taking an action based on the contents.

Interface engines can also be programmed to translate messages as they pass through. For example, an interface engine might convert HL7 v2 messages to v3 messages, or vice versa. Other use cases might require transforming an incoming message to a nonstandard version that can be incorporated into a proprietary or legacy system. The potential number of configurations and uses of interface engines are endless given their flexibility and design to support the full spectrum of messages available in the health-care domain. Furthermore, as mentioned in chapter "The Evolving Health Information Infrastructure," interface engines provide mediation services that combine orchestration and adapter functions. Therefore an important design choice in HIEs is whether to implement distinct adapters and orchestrators or use an interface engine.

There are several commercial interface engines available in the marketplace, including:

- Mirth Connect
  - Costa Mesa, CA, USA
  - https://www.mirth.com/

- Corepoint Health Integration Engine
  - Frisco, TX, USA
  - http://www.corepointhealth.com/
- InterSystems Ensemble
  - Cambridge, MA, USA
  - http://www.intersystems.com/
- Siemens OPENLink
  - Malvern, PA, USA
  - http://usa.healthcare.siemens.com/
- Summit Healthcare Express Connect
  - Braintree, MA, USA
  - http://www.summit-healthcare.com/
- Orion Health Rhapsody Integration Engine
  - Boston, MA, USA
  - https://orionhealth.com/
- Infor Cloverleaf Integration Suite
  - New York, NY, USA
  - http://www.infor.com/

EMERGING TRENDS

In this section, we discuss several emerging trends in the realm of syntactic standards. First, we examine emerging standards that are up-and-coming and therefore likely to impact the future of HIE. Second, we describe an emerging effort to better support HIE implementers identify and select the standards they will use. Third, we describe the standards proposed for supporting Stage 3 of the Meaningful Use program. While the final rule for Stage 3 is not available at the time of writing the book, we introduce and describe standards that are likely to support HIE use cases that will expand in the future. Finally, we explain the report recently delivered to Congress about Health Information Blocking.

Emerging Technical Standards

HL7 FHIR (Fast Healthcare Interoperability Resources) is an emerging innovative standard for exchange of information. As we explained in previous sections, HL7 members developed a very comprehensive standard in version 3 and addressed many of the gaps in HL7 v2, however, because of its complexity still now majority of health-care organizations and HIEs utilize v2 messages instead v3. FHIR standard first introduced in 2011 to overcome the complexity of the RIM standard and hide all of those complexities from developers' sight. FHIR is designed to be compatible with previous versions of HL7 standard (v2 and v3) to enable legacy systems to function in HIE. Since FHIR is much simpler to be implemented and uses straightforward RESTful technology, it is very promising standard for future of HIE.

2015 Interoperability Standards Advisory

At the beginning of 2015, the ONC published an open draft of an Interoperability Standards Advisory [3] designed to identify the best available interoperability standards and implementation specification for industry use. These standards and associated implementation specifications are grouped into four categories mentioned in "Health Information Messaging Standards" section:

- Vocabulary/code sets/terminology (semantic interoperability)
- Structure and Content (syntactic interoperability)
- Transport (foundational interoperability)
- Services (syntactic interoperability).

Overall, the advisory provides a list of available, mature standards, and implementation specifications that can be used for operational HIE in the United States. Such formal lists can prompt dialogue among industry stakeholders when more than one standard is available. They can also provide a starting place for HIE initiatives within a country. Other nations may choose to do something similar.

Standards for Meaningful Use Stage 3

The Notice of Proposed Rulemaking (NPRM) for Meaningful Use Stage 3 was released in Mar. 2015 by the US Centers for Medicare & Medicaid Services (CMS). The rule, which is likely to be finalized near the time of publication, builds upon prior rules in Stage 1 and Stage 2 of the CMS EHR Incentive Programs within the United States. The Stage 3 proposed rule specifies criteria for the Meaningful Use program in 2015–17 that eligible providers and hospitals must meet in order to qualify for incentive payments.

According to CMS, Stage 3 aims to expand interoperability of health data and sharing among providers. The proposed criteria in the NPRM are presented in eight-key objective areas, one of which is HIE. For the HIE objective, CMS proposes three measures as follows:

1. Providers should submit electronic Transmission of Care (TOC) and referrals for more than 50% of patients treated.
2. Providers should receive electronic records for more than 40% of patients transitioned or referred to them.
3. Providers should perform medication, allergy, and problem list reconciliation for 80% of transfer and referral patients.

In addition to the measures in the defined HIE objective area, CMS also proposes several new criteria for eligible hospitals and providers, including:

1. Patients must be able to access data through a portal, personal health record (PHR), or application programming interface (API) to view, download, or transmit their information with 24 hours of its availability.
2. EHR systems must incorporate patient generated data, such as data from a home monitoring device or mobile application.
3. EHR systems should have the capability to transmit physician-based reports of communicable disease cases to public health authorities.

These proposed criteria all require standardized, structured exchange of data between EHR systems and HIS in operation within other provider organizations, public health departments, or patient-controlled technologies. When the final rules are published, they will likely include some or all of these criteria. The final rules, therefore, will continue to drive adoption of HIE and the standards that support exchange of data between various information systems.

Information Blocking

In Apr. 2015, shortly after the release of the NPRM, the ONC delivered a report to the US Congress explaining that some health-care providers and IT developers are engaging in "information blocking" which limits health information sharing or HIE. According to ONC "information blocking occurs when persons or entities knowingly and unreasonably interfere with the exchange or use of electronic health information."

Sharing health information is a major focus health IT policy in the United States, and information blocking interferes with this national goal. The report provides some guidelines for identifying information blocking in the health-care domain and describes steps to prevent it. The report also describes steps already taken or proposed actions by ONC to address information blocking. Unfortunately the report highlights that action by ONC will not be enough as many types of information blocking are beyond the reach of current federal law. The report is likely to stimulate dialogue and potential action by the federal government to amend or create laws that aim to curb information blocking, paving the way for greater HIE and interoperability.

SUMMARY

Technical standards provide a foundation for interoperability in HIE. While necessary, standards are not sufficient for achieving the goal of seamless HIE among health-care stakeholders. Additional effort is necessary to integrate complex HIS, which requires collaboration among providers, vendors, and other stakeholders. Integration profiles and IGs, created by multi-stakeholder groups, are required to fully connect systems in support of interoperability. Work continues to evolve standards, refine IGs, and support implementation of standards in many countries. While the road ahead is long, the end result will be more efficient health systems that support better outcomes for both patients and populations.

QUESTIONS FOR DISCUSSION

1. If XML is designed to be an *extensible* markup tool, why does the health-care industry need a clinical document architecture?
2. What alternatives to the HL7 Reference Implementation Model (RIM) exist and how do they compare in scope to the RIM?
3. What is the process by which an individual or organization can get involved in developing standards with HL7 or integration profiles with IHE?
4. What are the similarities and differences between the international IHE group and the S&I Framework initiative in the United States?
5. Why do we need implementation guides? Shouldn't technical standards be sufficient for achieving interoperability?

References

[1] Gliklich RE, Dreyer NA, Leavy MB. Registries for evaluating patient outcomes: a user's guide [Internet], 3rd ed. Rockville, MD: Agency for Healthcare Research and Quality; 2014.
[2] Healthcare Information and Management Systems Society. What is interoperability? 2013 [cited February 12, 2015]. Available from: <http://www.himss.org/library/interoperability-standards/what-is-interoperability>.
[3] Office of the National Coordinator for Health Information Technology. 2015 Interoperability Standards Advisory. Washington, DC: U.S. Department of Health and Human Services; 2015 [cited July 2, 2015]. Available from: <http://www.healthit.gov/sites/default/files/2015interoperabilitystandardsadvisory01232015final_for_public_comment.pdf>.
[4] Benson T., 2nd ed. Principles of health interoperability HL7 and SNOMED, xxv Dordrecht: Springer; 2012. 316 pp.
[5] The HL7 evolution. Corepoint Health; 2010 [cited July 3, 2015]. Available from: <http://corepointhealth.com/sites/default/files/whitepapers/hl7-v2-v3-evolution.pdf>.
[6] Health Level 7 International. Training; 2015 [cited July 2, 2015]. Available from: <http://www.hl7.org/implement/training.cfm?ref=nav>.
[7] Health Level 7 International. HL7 Version 3 Product Suite [cited July 3, 2015]. Available from: <http://www.hl7.org/implement/standards/product_brief.cfm?product_id=186>.
[8] The DICOM Standard 2015b. NEMA; 2015 [cited July 3, 2015]. Available from: <http://medical.nema.org/standard.html>.
[9] Dolin RH, Alschuler L. Approaching semantic interoperability in Health Level Seven. J Am Med Inform Assoc 2011;18(1):99–103. Epub November 26, 2010.
[10] Office of the National Coordinator for Health Information Technology Report to Congress: Update on the adoption of health information technology and related efforts to facilitate the electronic use and exchange of health information. Washington, DC: Department of Health and Human Services; 2013.
[11] Centers for Disease Control and Prevention Phin messaging guide for syndromic surveillance: emergency department, urgent care, inpatient and ambulatory care settings. Atlanta, GA: Centers for Disease Control and Prevention; 2015. Available from: <http://www.syndromic.org/storage/documents/PHIN_Release_1.9/PHIN_Messaging_Guide_for_Syndromic_Surveillance_2_0_20150303.docx>.
[12] Health Level 7. Implementation Guides; 2015 [cited July 5, 2015]. Available from: <http://www.hl7.org/implement/standards/product_section.cfm?section=5>.

CHAPTER

9

Standardizing Health-Care Data Across an Enterprise

Jennifer M. Alyea[1], Brian E. Dixon[1,2], Jack Bowie[3] and Andrew S. Kanter[4]

[1]Indiana University Richard M. Fairbanks School of Public Health, Indianapolis, IN [2]Center for Biomedical Informatics, Regenstrief Institute, Inc., Indianapolis, IN [3]Apelon, Inc., Hartford, CT [4]Department of Biomedical Informatics, Columbia University, New York, NY; and Intelligent Medical Objects, Inc., Northbrook, IL

OUTLINE

LEARNING OBJECTIVES

By the end of this chapter, the reader should be able to:

- Describe the utility of standard reference terminologies in health information exchange.
- Identify factors to consider when selecting context-appropriate terminology standards.
- Describe the process of mapping between terminologies, as well as identify types of tools available to assist in mapping.
- Explain why a Terminology Service is important in health information exchange, and describe the process for its implementation.

INTRODUCTION

As described throughout the book, health information exchange (HIE) involves the integration, aggregation, and communication of health data from a variety of distinct sources. As data are exchanged, it becomes a challenge to maintain their original meaning or semantics. Thus, for HIE to achieve semantic interoperability, data must be standardized, or normalized, to ensure the receiving system can correctly interpret and use the data it received. This involves clear communication within messages of both the data and an information model with which the data are to be interpreted.

The chapter "Standardizing and Exchanging Messages" discussed the importance of standardizing messages and information models. In this chapter, we describe the process of and challenges inherent in standardizing data within HIE messages. We will examine the concept of a terminology and explain how one terminology can be translated or "mapped" to another. The chapter will further describe the need and use of reference (standard) terminologies to create semantic interoperability. Finally, we discuss the purpose and implementation of a Terminology Service, which is a set of technical components (eg, hardware, software) designed to facilitate data standardization and achieve semantic interoperability.

ROLE OF TERMINOLOGIES IN HEALTH CARE

A *terminology* is the body of terms used with a particular technical application in a subject of study, theory, or profession. Terminologies vary in their purposes, scopes, and structures. This is especially true in health care where there is a high degree of specialization. Although there exists a nearly universal terminology for human anatomy that is taught to a variety of health professions, there is a wide array of specialized terminologies used in health-care settings. Nursing, for example, has three major terminologies: NANDA International (NANDA-I), the Nursing Interventions Classification (NIC), and the Nursing Outcomes Classification (NOC). The nursing terminologies provide sets of terms to describe nursing judgments, treatments, and nursing-sensitive patient outcomes.

Terminologies in health-care support the documentation of observations, treatments, and outcomes that clinicians put in the patient chart—which is increasingly performed using electronic health record (EHR) systems. Although there exist a fair number of "major" or standard terminologies like the NIC and NOC, there are many more terminologies developed for specific purposes. A *local terminology* is one that is created for a specific purpose by a single organization, such as a laboratory, hospital, clinic, or pharmacy. For example, a local terminology may be used by the laboratory supporting a large health system to provide "user friendly" terms to physicians who order the tests.

Although useful to providers in a particular health system, a local terminology may be difficult to interpret by providers in another health system. For example, Health System A might refer to a glycated hemoglobin (HbA1c) test as "Glycohemoglobin," whereas Health System B may refer to a similar test as "Hemoglobin A1c." Although a human clinician can use his or her clinical knowledge and expertise to reason that the two tests likely mean the same thing, computers cannot perform such reasoning in isolation. Therefore, to ensure that meaning or semantics are transferred along with the test results during HIE, health information systems should use a reference terminology. A *reference terminology* is a formal, canonical terminology developed and maintained by a national or international standards development organization (SDO). A reference terminology is often referred to as a *standard*, *terminology standard*, or *standard terminology*. SDOs and the development of standards is described in the chapter "Standardizing and Exchanging Messages".

Terminologies consist of *terms* which are also referred to as concepts. A term can represent a clinical observation (eg, weight, blood pressure, response to a question asked of a patient), a laboratory result, or a clinical diagnosis. Most terms, especially those in standard terminologies, are represented by both a code and a description. The code is often a unique, numeric identifier that abstractly represents the concept. A description can be a shorthand name or descriptor that is human-readable. For example, a code 12345 might have a description of "Hemoglobin A1c." Some standard terminologies often have multiple axes or dimensions for each term to more precisely define them.

STANDARD TERMINOLOGIES IN HEALTH CARE

The use of reference terminologies is the foundation for facilitating semantic interoperability—maintaining data's original meaning during HIE. Standardized reference terminologies accomplish this by providing a structured, comparable technical language that enables the data to have meaning outside of the originating system. As a result, comparability of data can allow for accurate and consistent measurement, aggregation, analysis, and reporting of information. Terminology standards also allow data reusability, allowing standardized terms to be stored as a single concept and used multiple ways in a variety of applications [1]. Examples of standard terminologies in health care are presented in Table 9.1. Although additional

TABLE 9.1 Commonly Used Standard Terminologies in Health Care

Terminology	Full Name	Responsible Organization
CPT	Current Procedural Terminology	American Medical Association (http://www.ama-assn.org)
ICD	International Classification of Diseases	World Health Organization (http://www.who.int)
LOINC	Logical Observation Identifiers, Names and Codes	Regenstrief Institute (http://www.loinc.org)
RxNorm	RxNorm	US National Library of Medicine (http://nlm.nih.gov/research/umls/rxnorm/)
SNOMED CT	Systematized Nomenclature of Medicine—Clinical Terms	International Health Terminology Standards Development Organisation (http://www.ihtsdo.org)

reference terminologies exist, we have included those most commonly used in HIE transactions within the United States. For a more comprehensive description of the predominant terminology standards, the reader is referred to the work of Giannangelo [2].

SELECTION OF STANDARD TERMINOLOGIES FOR HIE

Given there are a variety of standard terminologies, HIE leaders must determine which terminology standard(s) should be selected. The process of selecting terminology standard(s) for a given HIE service or context of use requires consideration of several factors [3], including:

- underlying health needs and priorities of the health system;
- overall goals and objectives of the HIE or specific HIE service;
- the types or categories of data to be exchanged among a network of systems; and
- the workflow which will generate the data to be exchanged or in which data will be queried.

The goals and objectives for a given HIE service or use case (context of use) are the primary driver for which terminology standard(s) are to be selected. For example, the goal for an HIE or an initial service may be to improve childhood vaccination rates in a low-income population. A simplified HIE use case may be to report the proportion of children who have received all required vaccinations by age 5 at a given point-in-time within every low-income neighborhood in a geographic area in order to prioritize targeted interventions. This use case requires a standard terminology that can adequately capture the case definition and has good coverage of the intervention being tracked (injectables and vaccines). Given these requirements, a good candidate terminology to consider would be NDC (National Drug Code) maintained by the US Food and Drug Administration (FDA). The NDC includes all drugs manufactured, prepared, propagated, compounded, or processed for commercial distribution, including injectables and vaccines. If this use case were outside the United States, then a different standard terminology might be more appropriate. Moreover, in some cases it will be necessary to select more than one standard vocabulary to achieve the goals of an HIE use case.

The entire NDC catalogue includes much more breadth than what is necessary for the vaccination use case. Therefore, the HIE might consider selecting a *value set*, a subset of terms drawn from a standard vocabulary, instead of the entire NDC. Numerous value sets have been predefined by various authorities, including the US Centers for Disease Control and Prevention (CDC) and the US National Library of Medicine (NLM). The CDC maintains a set of value sets used for a series of public health HIE use-cases [4], and the NLM maintains values sets for clinical quality measures [5].

Although useful in many scenarios, a value set can also be limiting if it is used for a purpose other than that for which it was originally developed. A study by Gamache et al. [6] found a subset of LOINC codes branded the "Top 2000" excluded a third of tests routinely performed for detecting communicable diseases that are required to be reported to public health authorities. The original value set was developed to help clinical labs standardize commonly used clinical methods performed for routine patient care. Yet the new use case focused on capturing all potential lab tests of interest to public health authorities. Therefore, the purpose and granularity of data exchange must be considered when selecting one or more standard terminologies or value sets for a given use case.

In addition to the context of use and the scope of data for exchange, HIE leaders must consider the workflow that either generates the data to be exchanged or how the data will be requested. In this case, given the static nature of the query by a public health authority, we consider the workflow around how the data are generated. Administration of vaccines are performed by nursing staff and included in their documentation at a clinic. NDC terms, however, are voluminous and complex, and many NDC identifiers are similar to one another. This makes clinical documentation using NDC terms challenging for nurses and physicians. Therefore, HIE leaders may need to implement an *interface terminology* in addition to NDC, a standard terminology. An *interface terminology* is one that is user-facing and consists of a set of words, terms, or phrases used in a point-of-care application. It may be a locally based terminology, or it could be a national or international reference terminology; however, reference terminologies are rarely presented to end users to select from in clinical workflows. Most often interface terminologies are locally based and mapped to a reference terminology to facilitate adoption. Of note, if workflows use interface-reference maps, the use of a subset—rather than the complete standard—occurs at the interface terminology level rather than the reference terminology level.

Additionally, decisions regarding terminology selection should be made with long-term use in mind. Frequent changes to the selected terminology and term mappings can be expensive and time-consuming. Such changes also can result in a loss of historical data compatibility.

Finally, technical, political, cultural, and economic factors must be taken into account when selecting a standard. This is necessary to ensure the standard's feasibility and sustainability in each HIE's unique context. To help guide this process, it may be beneficial to seek out information on successful implementation in similar settings [7]. In other cases, policy may dictate or guide selection processes. In the United States, the Office of the National Coordination for Health Information Technology publishes an annual Interoperability Standards Advisory that provides guidance on the selection of available terminology standards recommended for use in various contexts [8]. Other nations may create similar lists that may provide guidance or outline required terminologies.

CURRENT USE OF STANDARD TERMINOLOGIES

As previously described, a wide variety of reference terminologies are in a mature state of development and are readily available for use in health information systems [9]. However, despite availability, actual use in the real-world is reported to be limited, and local terms remain highly prevalent. For example, Dixon et al. [10] examined the use of LOINC and SNOMED CT coding in more than 7 million electronic laboratory messages exchanged in two states between 2010 and 2011. The researchers found that fewer than 17% of all messages reported by laboratories to public health authorities utilized a LOINC term to identify the test performed or a SNOMED CT term to identify the test result.

A separate but similar study, conducted by Dhakal et al. [11], investigated 63 non-federal hospitals' use of LOINC and SNOMED CT terms in electronic laboratory messages sent to a national surveillance system managed by the CDC. Analysis of over 14 million messages from various states and jurisdictions found that 23% of test orders and 33% of test results had missing or non-informative codes. Lack of standardized terms limited CDC's ability to classify results and analyze patterns across jurisdictions at a national level.

There can be many reasons why terminology standards fail to be implemented widely. In many instances, this is because the local requirements for documentation or workflow did not align with the standard, or the standard required complicated technology which was not implementable by the developers or users. It may also be the case that stakeholders do not perceive a value to implementing a reference terminology (eg, lack of business drivers). To facilitate implementation of reference terminologies and to address the ongoing challenge of situations such as these, a complex and resource-intensive linking process from one terminology to another, called mapping, may be necessary for implementation of the selected HIE standards.

MAPPING

Linking terms from one terminology to another is a process called *mapping*. Mapping can be defined as a correspondence between the concepts or terms in two different terminologies [3]. In mapping, the *source code* is the origin of the map (ie, the dataset from which one is mapping). The *target code* is that in which the relationship, or equivalence, is being defined [12]. In other words, the target code is that into which the source code is being translated. For example, mapping can be done to link terms from an interface terminology to a reference terminology. In this situation, the interface terminology would be considered the source, and the reference terminology the target.

It is important to note that while the use of mapping to a target terminology facilitates downstream data analysis and communication from a repository, *both* the original (verbatim) data element and the mapped (equivalence) element should be saved so as to always maintain fidelity to the original clinical information.

Equivalence

It should be noted that mapping does not always result in a 1-to-1 linkage from the source code to the target. Instead, many types of equivalence, or correspondence, can be observed [12–14], including:

- *1-to-1 exact*, where a single source code is mapped to a single target code with identical clinical meaning;
- *1-to-1 approximate*, where a single source code is mapped to a single target code with similar but not identical clinical meaning;
- *1-to-many*, where a single source code is mapped to multiple target codes with similar clinical meaning; and
- *Many-to-1*, where multiple source codes are mapped to a single target code with similar clinical meaning.

Variations and combinations of these may also occur. An illustration of the various types of mapping equivalence is presented in Fig. 9.1.

At times, it may occur that a source code may not be translatable or "mapped" to a target code, resulting in an *orphan code*. Such an occurrence may be due to various causes, which have been elucidated by Lin and colleagues [15], including:

- no equivalent concept for the source code exists in the target code;
- the source code has an ambiguous meaning, and this lack of meaning precludes any linkage into a meaningful target code;
- the source code is overly specific, preventing linkage to a less-specific target code;
- the data are narrative "free" text with no meaning outside a specific clinical case; or
- the source code is institution-specific, such as one related to internal processing procedures, and therefore may have no meaning outside its specific setting.

Mapping Process

The process of mapping between two terminologies is iterative, complex, and can be labor-intensive. Much like selection of terminology standards, it is context-specific and highly dependent on the use case necessitating HIE as well as the characteristics of the two terminologies. Furthermore, variations in interpretation of data standards are possible, requiring significant effort to harmonize approaches prior to implementation [16]. For this reason, it is

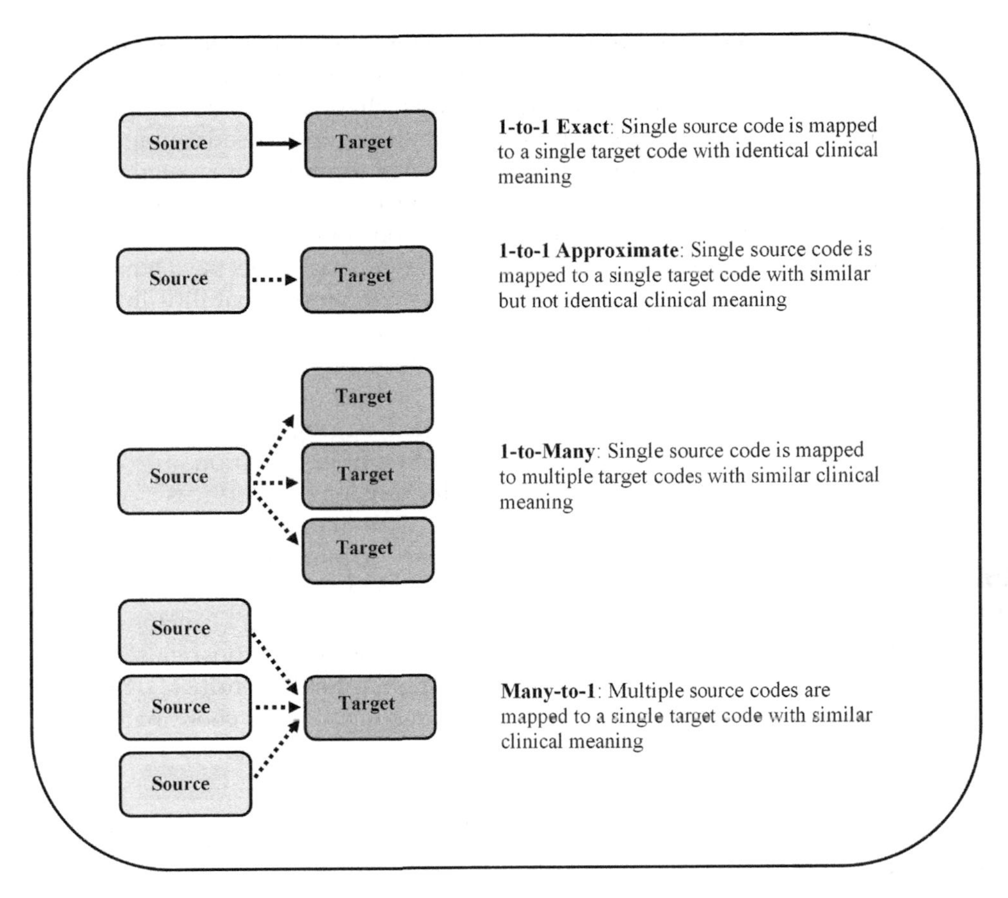

FIGURE 9.1 Types of mapping equivalence.

essential to establish a set of mapping rules to guide the entire process prior to undertaking subsequent steps [17,18] in order to ensure an efficient and effective process. The American Health Information Management Association published a set of best practices that offer guidance on mapping that might be of use [12].

Use of previously developed maps when possible is recommended, as this greatly reduces internal map development and maintenance burdens on the HIE [3]. A variety of mapping tools developed by SDOs, government entities, and commercial institutions are available for use [12]. It must be noted, however, that mapping cannot be fully automated [19]. Most participants in HIEs have some locally developed interface terminologies or ad hoc dictionaries [17] that must be mapped to the HIE's selected standards, and as such, local mapping will still be required.

A common requirement for mapping involves translation from pre-coordinated interface terms (commonly used clinical phrases or concepts) and post-coordinated reference terminologies (which require multiple reference concepts to capture the entire meaning of the source concept). Classifiers are available to assist in post-coordination, but this is an area of substantial effort if the interface terminology being used as a source does not already provide a reference terminology map for each pre-coordinated concept [20].

Regardless of mapping strategy used, all maps require clinical or subject matter expert review and curation before finalization to ensure accuracy and completeness [3]. For example, most maps involve some interpolation, as they may not be one-to-one. This requires subject matter experts to interpret and make value judgments on the maps. In addition, due to the dynamic nature of health care, such as the development of new laboratory tests, identification of new diseases, and advent of new procedures, no clinical map can be static. It will need to be revisited and revised over time.

TERMINOLOGY SERVICES

In the chapter "The Evolving Health Information Infrastructure" we introduced the Open HIE architectures, which includes a *Terminology Services* component. This component consists of server software and management tools, server and operating system software, database software, and associated hardware [3]. It integrates and manages terminology standards and definitions, including terminologies, ontologies, dictionaries, code systems, value sets, and mappings, across an HIE network or enterprise. It provides a centralized resource for key data structures that can ensure incoming data are normalized and stored using defined standards. It also provides a set a common service interfaces, or application programming interfaces, so that terminologies and other data structures can be accessed in a reliable, reproducible way.

Terminology Services can be focused either on central curation and distribution of interface and reference terminologies that are pushed out to the point of service, or the services can be used to dynamically translate point of service local or interface terminologies to reference terminologies for storage. The choice of architecture is beyond the scope of this chapter, but both options have their advantages and disadvantages. Standardized reference terminologies available in the point-of-service systems allow for sharing of data collection objects, clinical decision support, and reporting objects. Dynamic translation allows for more flexibility in point of service systems and other HIE components which can use these services to normalize clinical data. Both architectures allow for consistent measurement, aggregation, analysis, evaluation, and reporting of information.

Terminology Services enable compliance with national standards for health-care delivery. Ultimately, the result is an accurate exchange of information among members of the HIE community, including laboratories, clinics, pharmacies, hospitals, imaging centers, and public health entities. This exchange can enhance health care coordination and improve patient care decisions.

Implementation of Terminology Services

The implementation of Terminology Services within an HIE is a multistep process that begins with an assessment of available resources and the development of a project plan. To do so, the following types of activities must be addressed [3]:

- Choosing, acquiring, installing, and configuring software and hardware.
- Populating the Terminology Service with the required dictionaries and terminologies.
- Enhancing the point-of-care systems, insurance systems, and/or national registry systems that will interact with the Terminology Services so that they can communicate with the Terminology Service through the Interoperability Layer of the architecture.

- Documenting the technical information required to support the system.
- Testing the system to ensure that it is operating as planned.
- Developing and implementing policies and procedures required to support the system and business processes, and training users on these topics. These include processes for system maintenance and backup as well as processes, such as loading dictionary updates.

Once the project plan is in place, it is necessary to select and implement the Terminology Services software and hardware based on economic, technical, and standard-specific considerations. The software needs, the high-level system constraints, and the architecture will drive hardware needs.

After the software and hardware have been put into place, the next step is to load the interface terminologies, reference terminologies, and mappings that were identified using methods discussed earlier in this chapter. This should then be followed by establishing, testing, and verifying the interfaces between HIE components to ensure the connections required to support use cases and workflows are effective. Finally, all software used should then be tested and validated to ensure the Terminology Services can maintain and support terminologies, and that the interactions with other OpenHIE architecture components and interfacing systems are supported [3].

Terminology Service Support

Implementation of a Terminology Service is just the beginning. Once in place, ongoing, iterative support is necessary to meet the needs of the evolving field. Common types of support include:

- *Operations support*: This includes the development and maintenance of policies and procedures that are necessary to support business and technical processes for the Terminology Service. It may also comprise tasks such as evaluating adherence to the selected terminology standards.
- *Terminology support*: Standards are modified and improved over time. Newer versions of standards may impact previous mappings due to new concepts, retired concepts, or structural changes [21]. Because of this, the Terminology Services must have an ongoing analysis of impact of any terminology or mapping changes. In addition, the Terminology Service should maintain a history (versions, effective dates, etc.) of all the terminologies supported so that references to historical data can be normalized and longitudinal analyses performed.
- *Help desk support*: As more and more users and organizations utilize the Terminology Services, it may become important to identify, document, and triage responses to types of requests from the various users. For each request, it may be necessary to track who requested it, why it was requested, and when it was requested. Detailed information of how the issue was resolved should also be documented for reference purposes.
- *Training of support personnel*: Successful implementation of the support plan is grounded in effective training of all personnel charged with overseeing it.

Evaluation of Terminology Services

Once implemented with necessary support services in place, it becomes essential to conduct ongoing evaluation of the HIE's Terminology Services to ensure efficiency and effectiveness of the operation. Appropriate timing of these evaluations will be determined by the HIE, depending on need as well as data and resource availability. For example, they may be conducted annually, quarterly, or on a real-time basis. Varying aspects of the service can be assessed, including but not limited to: frequency of codes' use; correctness of methods of code validation; frequency, types, and causes of errors; and prevalence of redundancy/over-coding [3]. Any concerns or areas of weakness regarding these features or others should be referred to administrators for correction.

EMERGING TRENDS

Internationally, data standards have matured substantially in the 21st century, in no small part due to the growing cooperation among SDOs, as well as adoption of standards on a national level [22]. As such, substantial progress toward harmonization and practical applications has occurred. From here, continued growth in several areas is anticipated, including genetic data standardization [23], bidirectional public health data transfer [24], and the development of metadata standardization for interoperability of systems that include heterogeneous interacting components [22,25–27]. Another emerging area is the management, curation, and distribution of value sets, such as those available from the US NLM [5] and HL7 [28]. Additionally, as standards continue to be implemented, evaluation of their ability to achieve harmonization must be conducted to ensure their real-world effectiveness [29]. Changing regulations will also continually require data to be synchronized with new regulatory expectations [27].

In addition to data standards, interface (communication) standards have increased their focus on terminology and semantic consistency. Organizations such as HL7 [30] and IHE [31] have identified specific use-cases and profiles to address terminology query, normalization, and mapping. It is expected that this focus will continue and new interface protocols will need to be supported by Terminology Services implementations [32].

SUMMARY

Data standardization is an ongoing challenge but is key to facilitating semantic interoperability in HIE. Through the mapping of local terminologies to reference standards, effective exchange of clinical data between various entities in the health care ecosystem can occur, allowing for accurate and consistent measurement, analysis, and communication of information. The implementation of standards and Terminology Services is a complex undertaking that requires consideration of context-specific economic, political, social, and technological factors. Despite challenges, the field of data standardization is currently at a stage of rapid advancement due to increasing cooperation and international guidance. While much work remains, the future is promising for semantic interoperability.

QUESTIONS FOR DISCUSSION

1. Reference terminologies are the foundation of semantic interoperability in an HIE. Describe some of the potential beneficial outcomes that result from having comparable, structured language among the differing systems participating HIE.
2. What considerations must be taken into account when selecting an HIE terminology standard? Should the entire standard be utilized or only a subset?
3. Describe some types of equivalence that may be observed when mapping. What might cause a source code to go unmapped?
4. What is the purpose of a Terminology Service? What considerations must be taken into account when selecting the appropriate software and hardware of the Terminology Service?
5. Terminology Services require ongoing, iterative support and assessment. Explain why continuous evaluation and updates are necessary.

References

[1] Zafar A, Dixon BE. Pulling back the covers: technical lessons of a real-world health information exchange. Stud Health Technol Inform 2007;129(Pt 1):488–92.

[2] Giannangelo K. Healthcare code sets, clinical terminologies, and classification systems, 3rd ed. Chicago, IL: American Health Information Management Association; 2015.

[3] OpenHIE. OHIE terminology services: planning and implementation guide [Internet]; 2014 [cited June 15, 2015]. Available from: https://ohie.org/terminology-service/.

[4] Centers for Disease Control and Prevention. PHIN Vocabulary Access and Distribution System (VADS) [Internet]; 2011 [cited July 15, 2015]. Available from: https://phinvads.cdc.gov/vads/SearchVocab.action.

[5] U.S. National Library of Medicine. Welcome to the NLM Value Set Authority Center (VSAC) [Internet]; 2012 [cited July 15, 2015]. Available from: https://vsac.nlm.nih.gov/.

[6] Gamache RE, Dixon BE, Grannis S, Vreeman DJ. Impact of selective mapping strategies on automated laboratory result notification to public health authorities. AMIA Annu Symp Proc AMIA Symp AMIA Symp 2012;2012:228–36.

[7] Cimino JJ, Hayamizu TF, Bodenreider O, Davis B, Stafford GA, Ringwald M. The caBIG terminology review process. J Biomed Inform 2009;42(3):571–80.

[8] Office of the National Coordinator for Health Information Technology 2015 interoperability standards advisory [Internet]. Washington, DC: U.S. Department of Health and Human Services; 2015. [cited July 2, 2015]. Available from: http://www.healthit.gov/sites/default/files/2015interoperabilitystandardsadvisory01232015final_for_public_comment.pdf.

[9] Bodenreider O. Biomedical ontologies in action: role in knowledge management, data integration and decision support. Yearbk Med Inform 2008:67–79.

[10] Dixon BE, Gibson PJ, Grannis SJ. Estimating increased electronic laboratory reporting volumes for meaningful use: implications for the public health workforce. Online J Public Health Inform 2014;5(3):225.

[11] Dhakal S, Burrer SL, Winston CA, Dey A, Ajani U, Groseclose SL. Coding of electronic laboratory reports for biosurveillance, selected United States hospitals, 2011. Online J Public Health Inform 2015;7(2).

[12] AHIMA Data mapping best practices. J AHIMA 2011;82(4):46–52.

[13] Bronnert J, Clark J, Cook J, Fenton S, Scichilone R, Williams M, et al. Data mapping best practices. J AHIMA Am Health Inf Manag Assoc 2011;82(4):46–52.

[14] De S. 8 steps to success in ICD-10-CM/PCS mapping: best practices to establish precise mapping between old and new ICD code sets. J AHIMA Am Health Inf Manag Assoc 2012;83(6):44–9. quiz 50.

[15] Lin MC, Vreeman DJ, McDonald CJ, Huff SM. A characterization of local LOINC mapping for laboratory tests in three large institutions. Methods Inf Med 2011;50(2):105–14.

[16] McCarthy DB, Propp K, Cohen A, Sabharwal R, Schachter AA, Rein AL. Learning from health information exchange technical architecture and implementation in seven beacon communities. EGEMS (Wash DC) 2014;2(1):1060.

[17] Abhyankar S, Demner-Fushman D, McDonald CJ. Standardizing clinical laboratory data for secondary use. J Biomed Inform 2012;45(4):642–50.

[18] Vreeman DJ, McDonald CJ. Automated mapping of local radiology terms to LOINC. AMIA Annu Symp Proc AMIA Symp AMIA Symp 2005:769–73.

[19] Saitwal H, Qing D, Jones S, Bernstam EV, Chute CG, Johnson TR. Cross-terminology mapping challenges: a demonstration using medication terminological systems. J Biomed Inform 2012;45(4):613–25.

[20] Cimino JJ. Desiderata for controlled medical vocabularies in the twenty-first century. Methods Inf Med 1998;37(4-5):394–403.

[21] Wade G, Rosenbloom ST. The impact of SNOMED CT revisions on a mapped interface terminology: terminology development and implementation issues. J Biomed Inform 2009;42(3):490–3.

[22] Richesson RL, Chute CG. Health information technology data standards get down to business: maturation within domains and the emergence of interoperability. J Am Med Inform Assoc 2015;22(3):492–4.

[23] Deckard J, McDonald CJ, Vreeman DJ. Supporting interoperability of genetic data with LOINC. J Am Med Inform Assoc JAMIA 2015;22(3):621–7.

[24] National Committee on Vital and Health Statistics. Electronic standards for public health information exchange [Internet]; 2014. Available from: http://www.ncvhs.hhs.gov/.

[25] AHIMA Data standards, data quality, and interoperability [Updated]. J AHIMA 2013;84(11):64–9.

[26] Marcos C, González-Ferrer A, Peleg M, Cavero C. Solving the interoperability challenge of a distributed complex patient guidance system: a data integrator based on HL7's Virtual Medical Record standard. J Am Med Inform Assoc JAMIA 2015;22(3):587–99.

[27] HIMSS Health Information Exchange Committee. The future of HIE: HIMSS HIE thought leadership brief [Internet]; 2012. Available from: http://www.himss.org/.

[28] HL7. Value sets defined in FHIR—FHIR v0.0.82 [Internet]; 2014 [cited July 31, 2015]. Available from: http://www.hl7.org/implement/standards/fhir/terminologies-valuesets.html.

[29] Gold MR, McLaughlin CG, Devers KJ, Berenson RA, Bovbjerg RR. Obtaining providers' "buy-in" and establishing effective means of information exchange will be critical to HITECH's success. Health Aff (Millwood) 2012;31(3):514–26.

[30] HL7 International. Introduction to HL7 standards [Internet]; 2015 [cited July 17, 2015]. Available from: http://www.hl7.org/implement/standards/index.cfm.

[31] IHE International. IHE resources [Internet]; 2015 [cited July 17, 2015]. Available from: http://www.ihe.net/Resources/.

[32] HL7. FHIR: terminology service [Internet]; 2015 [cited July 10, 2015]. Available from: http://hl7.org/implement/standards/fhir/2015Jan/terminology-service.html.

CHAPTER

10

Shared Longitudinal Health Records for Clinical and Population Health

David Broyles[1], *Ryan Crichton*[2], *Bob Jolliffe*[3], *Johan Ivar Sæbø*[4] *and Brian E. Dixon*[5]

[1]Indiana University Richard M. Fairbanks School of Public Health, Indianapolis, IN
[2]Jembi Health Systems, Cape Town [3]Department of Informatics, University of Oslo, Norway [4]Department of Informatics, University of Oslo, Norway [5]Indiana University Richard M. Fairbanks School of Public Health; and the Center for Biomedical Informatics, Regenstrief Institute, Inc., Indianapolis, IN

OUTLINE

LEARNING OBJECTIVES

By the end of the chapter, the reader should be able to:

- Identify and describe the differences among an electronic medical record, electronic health record, and a shared heath record.
- Explain the role of a shared health record in a health information exchange.
- List and describe the components of a shared health record.
- Discuss the role and benefits of a health management information system within a health information exchange.
- Define a population health indicator.
- Identify and describe application domains for a health management information system.
- Define a database management system.
- Compare the implications of implementing a shared health record using an electronic health record system versus a database management system.
- Discuss emerging trends likely to shape the evolution of shared health records and health management information systems.

INTRODUCTION

Health-care systems are organized differently around the globe. Systems vary in the proportion of care delivered by public versus private facilities, in their emphasis on primary, secondary and tertiary care, in the levels and sources of funding, by the populations they serve, in the burden of disease faced by their populations, and in the level of development of the environments of human and technological infrastructure. Nevertheless, there is consensus that health information systems may have a pivotal role to play in improving quality and efficiency in all of these contexts [1], though the nature of such technological systems as well as the roles and relative importance of their individual components and their sequence of emergence will be conditioned by sociopolitical, historical, and geographical realities.

Electronic medical record (EMR) systems can streamline the delivery of health care within an individual organization by archiving, monitoring, and facilitating operations [2]. These systems assemble a digital representation of patient's legal medical record within a single health organization or network [2]. A patient's EMR contains information such as medical history, immunization records, physician notes, laboratory test results, and vital signs [2]. In the fragmented health-care system of the United States, many autonomous health networks coalesce to provide care for an individual patient [3]. Consequently, it should not be assumed that the EMR from an individual organization contains a complete medical history for an individual patient [2]. Key pieces of a patient's medical history such as a diagnosis or laboratory result that occurred in a different health network may not be available to a physician providing care.

In contrast, an electronic health record (EHR) system is designed to promote continuity of care across numerous health-care networks within a region through collaborative data sharing [4,5]. An EHR system consolidates health datasets that were collected from an array of different sources into a person-centric health record in order to provide a more complete and longitudinal portrayal of an individual's medical history [4,5]. However, this information may only be useful within the network of collaborating organizations. A national or regional health information exchange (HIE) must be able to harmonize the clinical information that is being collected from multiple EHR systems into a single shared longitudinal health record. These comprehensive, longitudinal records are intended to decidedly enhance the quality and productivity of health care through reductions in medical errors, decreased redundancies in testing, and averted costs [5–9]. Additionally, longitudinal records can be aggregated to provide population-level indicators of health outcomes to support public health practice, disease surveillance, health systems management, and clinical research.

TABLE 10.1 Common Data Elements Included in a Shared Longitudinal Health Record

Data Type	Description
Structured Data	Clinical observations
	Care summaries
	Allergies
	Prescribed medications
	Laboratory reports
	Immunizations
	Medical histories
	Mental health assessments
	Nutritional assessments
	Action Plans
	Quality of life indicators
Unstructured data	Medical imaging documents (eg, X-rays)
	Narrative text

SHARED LONGITUDINAL RECORDS FOR CLINICAL HEALTH

The OpenHIE model includes a component system called the shared health record (SHR) that compiles a longitudinal, person-centric record of a patient's clinical encounters that are being shared among the organizations participating in HIE. The SHR system provides a permanent, centralized repository to store and manage the health information that are shared by the heterogeneous information systems of a regional or national health system. Contributing applications could include anything from a robust EMR system to a small-scale mobile application (recall the point-of-care applications from the model in the chapter: The Evolving Health Information Infrastructure).

The SHR component of OpenHIE facilitates a variety of interactions between the internal components and external point-of-service applications with the goal of supporting the delivery of clinical care. The SHR enables point-of-service applications (eg, EMRs or pharmacy information systems) to store key clinical data such as a summary of care, laboratory test results, or vitals. The SHR can manage both structured data that is reconcilable with standard exchange formats (eg, discrete clinical observations) and unstructured data such as a digital image with associated patient information. Additionally, point-of-service systems can update existing patient records in the SHR with new information while preserving a version history. However, the data stored in the SHR should be restricted to include only information that is deemed relevant for sharing within the implementing nation or region [10]. The SHR should not necessarily contain a complete dump of information from all point-of-service systems in the nation or region, but rather contain relevant information that when shared gives a complete view of a patient's medical history. Table 10.1 provides a list of some of the pertinent types of clinical data that may be stored in an SHR.

An SHR also enables client services to retrieve clinical information from the repository as needed to improve the delivery of care. The SHR can provide end users with a complete longitudinal medical history for a particular patient. In addition, client systems can query the SHR to retrieve a partial subset of a patient's medical history that has been restricted to a specific time frame or a unique type of observation. For example, a physician caring for a patient with a high diastolic blood pressure may want to know if the elevated blood pressure is a trend or just an isolated occurrence in order to determine the appropriate approach for treatment. The physician could acquire this information by querying the SHR to retrieve a list of the patient's blood pressure during each previous encounter.

An SHR is also designed to semantically understand certain sections of the information that it receives from point-of-service systems. This is enabled through the use of standardized representations of the clinical information which support semantic descriptions of the data in the SHR. It is important for the SHR to semantically understand certain clinical information for a few main reasons. First, this enables the SHR to produce and return an accurate summary of a patient's clinical history and second it enables population health indicators to be produced more easily. Finally, semantic understanding of clinical information enables other, secondary uses of the clinical data, such as medical research.

SHARED LONGITUDINAL RECORDS FOR POPULATION HEALTH

In addition to improving the delivery of individual clinical care, sharing longitudinal health records also cultivates opportunities to improve health outcomes at the population level [11,12]. The OpenHIE model contains a component called the Health Management Information System (HMIS) that stores and distributes cumulative population level information. The HMIS primarily supports management or administration of a health system, and it contains a wide range of aggregate level data. The HMIS aggregates individual clinical records that are shared within an HIE in order to provide indicators that characterize the health of the underlying population at the provider, facility, state, or national level. In addition, the HMIS should contain data on human resource distribution, population figures, service availability, and service quality such as the efficiency of the supply chain. This opens up for added value analysis of the aggregated clinical data. The information in the HMIS is available for reporting purposes and is intended to improve the administration and development of public health programs rather than the delivery of clinical care [11]. Aggregated health information can benefit the health of a society by enhancing surveillance capacities, promoting advancements in medical research, and supporting the development of effective health policies.

Dashboard of Indicators

The aggregation of individual clinical records through the HMIS component of OpenHIE provides a dashboard of health indicators that can improve understanding of community health status. A health indicator is a metric that is routinely reported to provide insight into the characteristics of a population or the performance of a program [13]. An accurate assessment of the current health status of the population and influential factors within the community is essential for elevating the overall health of the community [14]. Important health indicators may constitute clinical outcomes (eg, mortality rates for cancer) or the prevalence of important health risk factors such as obesity or smoking [14]. These health indicators can be leveraged to drive public health action such as policy changes or interventions to address significant health issues [15]. Programs such as Healthy People 2020 use health indicators to help direct their agendas [13]. Aggregated health indicators allow Healthy People 2020 and other programs to identify crucial public health issues (eg, increasing prevalence of cardiovascular disease), institute goals for improving the issue (eg, reduce the mortality rate for cardiovascular diseases by 15% within 10 years), and then evaluate progress toward those goals (eg, compare the baseline mortality rate to the current mortality rate) [13].

Disease Surveillance

Recent threats to population health globally, including Ebola Virus (EBV), influenza (H1N1), Middle East Respiratory Syndrome (MERS-CoV), and severe acute respiratory syndrome (SARS), illustrate the importance of building capacities within countries to detect the presence of infectious diseases at an early stage of an outbreak [16,17]. Compiling information from individual clinical records can provide insight into the patterns and trends of disease throughout a population [11,15]. Integrating the information from the SHR and HMIS systems with traditional surveillance strategies, such as vital records reports, can provide a more complete picture of the prevalence and spatial distribution of important diseases [11,18].

Electronic, shared health records also offer the opportunity to conduct disease surveillance in real-time [18]. Clinical information in the SHR can potentially be actively monitored for symptoms that may indicate the emergence of important diseases rather than waiting for confirmation through test results [18]. Real-time information about disease trends increases the capability of public health organizations to detect emerging outbreaks at an early stage and implement appropriate control measures before the disease becomes widespread [19]. Capabilities that can integrate and monitor emerging patterns of disease would be transformative to public health surveillance practice [20].

Medical Research

Available, semantically interoperable information contained in the SHR and HMIS could be leveraged to advance medical research [12,15,21]. Analysis of the cumulative clinical data that is available in the HMIS can be especially useful for the generation of hypotheses and when performing comparative assessments [6]. Currently, population health in the United States is predominantly assessed through nationally funded health surveys such as the National Health Interview Survey (NHIS) [6,11,22]. The information collected in these surveys is self-reported, and may be unreliable or lack critical information [6]. Incorporating the cumulative information from the HMIS that was collected as a part of routine care can complement and strengthen the value of existing data sources [6].

SHRs also have the potential to identify eligible participants for clinical trials [11]. Clinical trial participants have traditionally been recruited through advertisements, notices, or contacting physicians [11]. An SHR system can be designed to simplify the process by adding optional alerts that can be relayed to candidates eligible for clinical trials by their physicians [11]. The Indiana Health Information Exchange, described in "The Indiana Health Information Exchange", is the only HIE known to routinely leverage its SHR for study recruitment, observational research, and comparative analyses.

IMPLEMENTATION

Due to differences in organizational needs and health information infrastructures, the most appropriate solution for the implementation of an SHR will vary across health systems and over time. In some cases, an EHR-based solution may be the most acceptable approach for implementing an SHR, while other implementations may require that an SHR is developed on a database management system (DBMS) platform with tailored services. In order for an SHR to be supportive of the requirements of consumers and local contexts, a thorough assessment of the goals, systems, data, standards, and challenges associated with the pertinent health system should be conducted prior to implementation.

SHR Implemented as an EHR

The OpenHIE model implements the SHR system as an independent component within a larger infrastructure. The interoperability layer (IL; described in the chapter: The Evolving Health Information Infrastructure) receives transactions from the disparate point-of-service systems exchanging information and facilitates the interaction between the internal components of the HIE. The OpenHIE infrastructure includes client registry (see the chapter: Client Registries: Identifying and Linking Patients), health worker registry (see the chapter: Health Worker Registries: Managing the Health-Care Workforce), and facility registry (see the chapter: Facility Registries: Metadata for Where Care Is Delivered) components to verify that the patients, providers, and facilities involved in a transaction request are known to the HIE. A complete shared record must also reconcile the unique terminologies and coding used by different point-of-service applications interacting with the HIE [23]. The OpenHIE uses a terminology service to map local codes to the standardized internal format (see the chapter: Standardizing Healthcare Data Across an Enterprise).

The SHR component of the OpenHIE was developed on a modified version of an EHR platform called OpenMRS (www.openmrs.org) to serve as the centralized repository for the storage and management of clinical data within the OpenHIE infrastructure. The capacity to manage discrete values effectively, and a powerful API, made OpenMRS a favorable SHR solution for OpenHIE [10]. OpenHIE provides three different types of modules that facilitate the processing and storage of data using the OpenMRS platform including interface modules, a content handler module, and processing modules (depicted in Fig. 10.1). The interface modules provide service interfaces that enable an external application to access the data in the SHR. A content handler module is used to receive data from the service interfaces, and pass the information on to the proper processing module for storage. Processing modules provide the capacity to decipher information in a specific format so that it can be stored in or retrieved from the OpenMRS system. For example, a robust HIE may require a processing module that accommodates Health Level Seven (HL7) version 2 documents, processing modules for multiple types of clinical document architecture (CDA) documents, and a processing module that supports unstructured documents. Fig. 10.1 illustrates the architecture of the components that would enable OpenMRS to be implemented as the SHR for OpenHIE.

The flexibility of the OpenHIE architecture permits implementers to replace or expand the storage model supporting the SHR as necessary. The most appropriate EHR platform for an SHR may vary based on the requirements and idiosyncrasies of the particular implementation [24–26]. Potentially more than one data storage model could be used for a single SHR. For example, OpenMRS could manage the discrete data within the SHR, whereas OpenXDS could manage the document store. The following EHR platforms could also be considered for use as a SHR:

- Mohawk EHRS
- RAMRS
- OpenXDS
- OpenEMR
- OSCAR
- HIEOS
- OpenVista

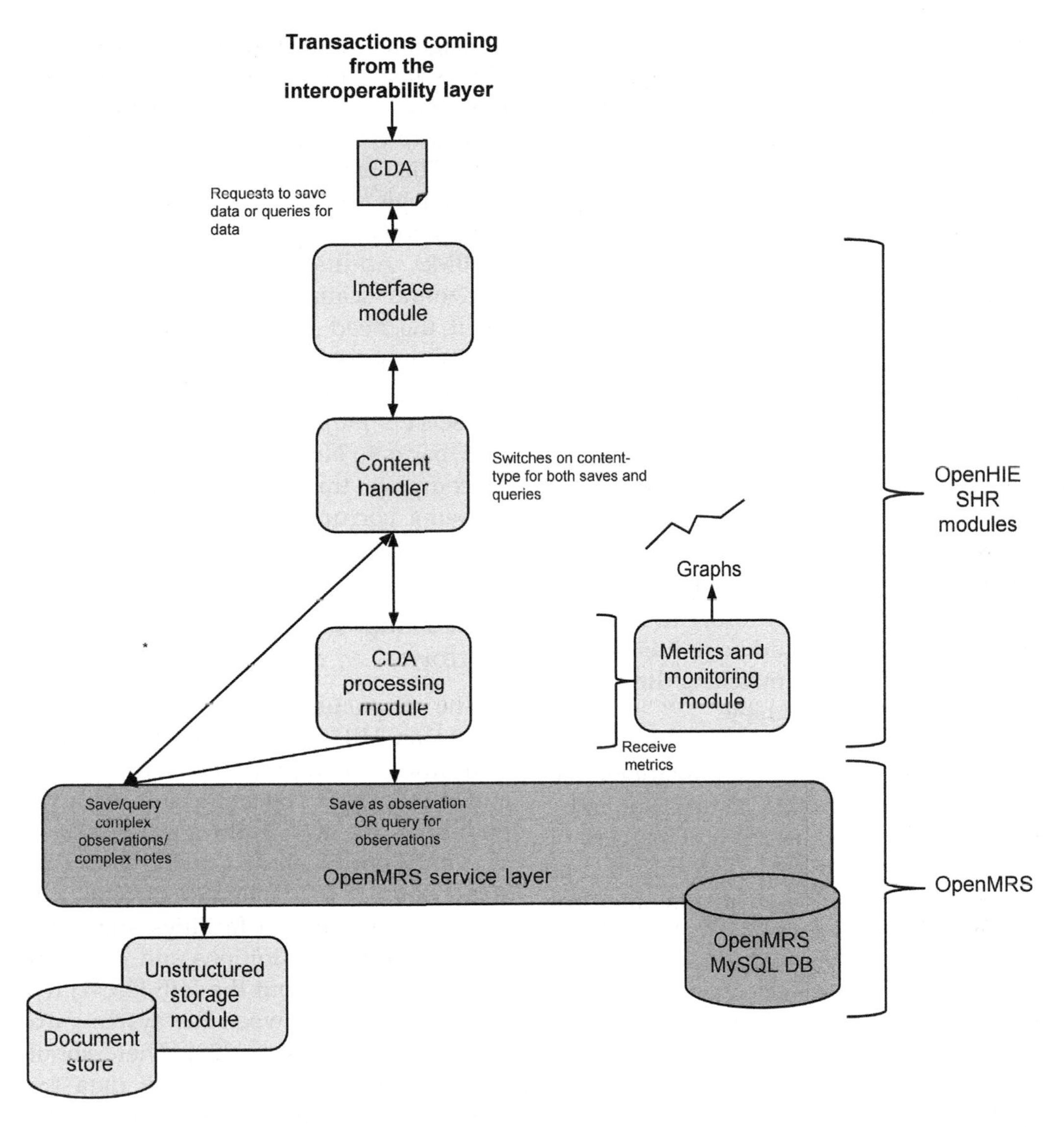

FIGURE 10.1 Architectural representation of the components of the shared health record as they could be implemented using the OpenMRS software.

SHR Implemented as a Database

An SHR can be operationalized as a database instead of an EHR system in order to provide a method of storing, organizing, and managing the clinical records. In this case, a database management system (DBMS) would be used to empower users or other applications to interact with the SHR. A DBMS allows users or applications to perform tasks such as saves, queries, and updates to the database. Relational database management systems (RDBMSs) and NoSQL DBMSs are two of the most common DBMS models [27].

RDBMS

An RDBMS model manages a database by allowing users to define and ascertain relationships between multiple tables within a repository. A standard language called Structured Query Language (SQL) is used to communicate with and manipulate the database [27,28]. SQL allows users to perform complex queries and analysis with relatively basic syntax [28]. A relational database has tables that consist of rows that represent records and columns that contain descriptive characteristics such as heart rate, age, or gender. Assigning a unique identifier to each row enables the table to be linked to rows from other tables in the database that share the same identifier. For example, if a researcher needed to combine a table that contained patient heights with a table that contained patient weights in order to calculate BMI, an SQL statement could be written to link the two tables together by matching the unique patient identifier from each table.

However, using an RDBMS to manage and store clinic databases has some limitations that must be considered. An RDBMS does not easily support documents such as medical imagery or free text [27,29]. In addition, clinical databases often contain a large number of fields that primarily remain unpopulated [27]. An RDBMS managing an SHR with an excessive number of blank fields may experience substandard performance and inefficiencies [27].

NoSQL DBMS

The limitations of relational databases led to a demand for an alternative approach to database management [27]. There has been a recent shift toward the use of NoSQL data stores to manage large clinical databases [27]. NoSQL stands for "Not only SQL" and refers to a category of DBMSs that were developed with a contrasting approach to traditional relational databases [27]. NoSQL DBMSs do not depend on predefined relationships for the management and storage of clinical data which allows faster processing [27]. NoSQL also supports structures such as key-value, document, and graph in addition to relational databases [27]. This flexibility allows a NoSQL DBMSs to manage the diversity of formats associated with medical data more easily than a traditional RDBMS. Additionally, NoSQL DBMSs enable horizontal scaling to increase system capacity if the need arises [27,30]. Horizontal scalability describes the capability of the DBMS to disburse the data and workload among multiple servers [30]. However, there are also some drawbacks to NoSQL DBMSs. RDBMSs are able to complete transactions without losing data or being corrupted with more reliability than NoSQL DBMSs [27].

HMIS Implemented as Data Analysis Platform

The implementation of an HMIS system within an HIE requires the standardization of indicators, an appropriate software platform, and methods of collecting and evaluating the quality of the data from a variety of sources. The indicators included in the HMIS must be standardized to facilitate meaningful comparison across health facilities and geographic areas. Indicator definitions and codes must be consistent throughout the HIE [25,31] to enable interoperability between the systems exchanging health information [32]. There should also be cohesion of the aggregated data from the facility level on up to the national level [25].

A challenge facing HMIS/EHR interoperability is the lack of development of mature data exchange standards in this domain—certainly in comparison with other domains of HIE. In 2009, the World Health Organization (WHO) led an effort to develop a standard called SDMX-HD for representing indicators and aggregate datasets [25,31] aimed primarily at global health reporting. The SDMX-HD standard never saw significant uptake.

In the same year, the HL7 consortium published the first edition of a standard for quality indicator reporting from EHR systems called QRDA (Quality Reporting Document Architecture). QRDA documents are contained within HL7 CDA documents (see the chapter: Standardizing and Exchanging Messages) and include a type (QRDA category 3) designed specifically for the representation of aggregate data. QDM (Quality Document Measure) is an HL7 standard for representation of indicator sets and their detailed definition and mappings into the EHR. QRDA together with QDM provide standards-based building blocks for automatic extraction of quality data—including aggregated indicators [33].

From the HMIS perspective, there are two challenges with QRDA. The first is that it is a complex, verbose, and difficult standard. The second is that it is premised on the fact that the data originate in an EHR (hence its encapsulation as a clinical document). The OpenHIE HMIS described below has its origins in a context of use where EHR systems have been thin on the ground. Aggregate health data messages could originate in an HL7 compliant EMR system, but are just as likely to be mined from the logistics management system for cold chain management data or from simple community health worker mobile phone applications. For this reason, the HMIS community within OpenHIE is actively driving the development of a new profile in the QRPH (Quality Research and Public Health) committee of IHE called ADX (Aggregate Data Exchange). ADX is not a CDA document, owing more of its ancestry to SDMX-HD. EHR systems which can and do produce QRDA should be readily able to map that content onto ADX (though the reverse mapping would not be possible).

The software platform that is used to collect, manage, and dispense aggregated health information for an HMIS can be a DBMS or a more flexible and customizable open-source model [25]. The OpenHIE HMIS was built on an open-source platform called the District Health Informative Software (DHIS) v2. DHIS v2 enables implementing nations or regions to tailor the HMIS system to meet their requirements without the need for extensive programming [25]. The aggregated information captured by the SHR is imported into the DHIS v2 system to produce reports on a regular basis that can be disseminated through the HIE [25].

Of major importance to DHIS v2 is the flexibility to also rely on manual data entry, as the HMIS should contain a wide range of data for combinatorial analysis. In a majority of developing countries, an OpenHIE architecture is not supported by interoperable software applications, and data beyond the clinical encounter at the facility level is collected through a wide range of paper-based forms. Due to different maturity levels, it is important that the HMIS, given its importance for overall health service management, is able to function as a wholly or partly independent electronic system. The variation in contexts around the world calls thus not only for standardization of data exchange but also for flexibility in data collection to respond to a mix of electronic and manual processes.

Data Quality Challenges to Implementation

In order for the HMIS to provide a reliable method of measuring population health outcomes and evaluating the performance of public health programs and policies, it is critical that data quality is assessed effectively [34]. A high degree of data quality can be attained by regulating processes, identifying the underlying sources of errors, and correcting processes to eliminate failures [35]. A quality assessment should consider the data itself, the use of the data, and the collection process [34]. Many healthcare organizations have adopted a total quality management (TQM) approach to consistently improve the quality of their data

[36,37]. The TQM approach pursues quality improvement through the continuous refinement of existing systems and processes based on evaluations and feedback [36]. While originally used in the business sector, recent work has adapted it for use in health care [37].

Studies are revealing significant challenges in realizing the automatic extraction of indicators from EHR [38,39] in practice. This stems partly from a dominant institutional logic of EHR implementations driven by the needs of transactional use case requirements rather than quality reporting and the related consequences in completeness and quality of data. The study from the Netherlands [38], for example, shows that the accuracy of indicator data derived from EHR is not necessarily better than that which was obtained from the paper registers. This result is also consistent with what the authors have seen in implementations in Rwanda and has been described in India [40]. The results are also consistent with other studies examining the quality of data in EHR-captured clinical documentation [41] as well as HIE transactions [42,43]. With the increasing focus on quality reporting from EHR in OECD countries coupled with the continued growth of EHR in countries of the global South, we can expect these challenges to receive greater and urgent attention.

EMERGING TRENDS

The creation and management of SHR and HMIS components within HIE infrastructures in the United States as well as other nations are likely to both influence and be influenced by two emerging trends. First, the movement toward creating learning health systems that enable learning feedback loops on a national scale will ultimately benefit from SHRs and real-time calculation of population level indicators. Similarly, efforts to better understand the social determinants of health will benefit from HIE components that can efficiently and effectively gather information across a wide range disparate sources. Yet these movements are also likely to influence design changes to the SHR and HMIS as they evolve.

Clinical databases are important sources of evidence that can be used to analyze and improve the quality, safety, and efficiency of medical care [44–46]. The Institute of Medicine (IOM) is working toward the development of a learning health-care system that harnesses this evidence to provide a patient with the best possible care, and then capture the results in order to enhance future treatment [44,46]. Physicians are currently forced to treat patients through medical procedures and pharmaceuticals that have a relatively small amount of evidence to document their effectiveness [45]. Leveraging the vast amount of information about diseases and patient encounters available in EHR systems could enable the optimization of treatment strategies for conditions such as cancer or coronary artery disease [45]. Supplying physicians as well as patients with this information could make a substantial difference health outcomes [45]. A future goal of the IOM is to ensure that at least 90% of all clinical decisions will be based on high quality, up-to-date evidence by the year 2020 [44,46].

Efforts to create learning health systems will therefore not only benefit from the SHR and HMIS components but also shape their evolution. Many learning health system initiatives are just now emerging, and their data needs are similar in nature to traditional observational and comparative research. Yet, given the broad scope of the IOM's vision, these efforts are likely to expand dramatically in the next 5–10 years. As they expand, data and analytical needs will morph which may require changes to the scope of both the SHR and HMIS components as we might envision them today.

The Robert Wood Johnson Foundation (RWJF) is seeking to promote a culture that considers the impact of factors beyond clinical care on the collective health of a community or nation as a whole [47]. Social determinants, such as income level, educational attainment, family environment and crime rate, have a significant influence on both health outcomes and health disparities [47]. The increasing availability of large, up-to-date clinical datasets that bridge organizational boundaries, such as those in an SHR or HMIS, enables analyses that can reveal patterns of health outcomes and their underlying factors [48].

However, such analyses require integration not only of clinical data but also data from sources well beyond the health system. A report from IOM highlights that EHR systems in the United States currently do a poor job of capturing data on the social determinants of health. Therefore, for SHR and HMIS components to support analyses of social determinants, new types of data will need to be added to Table 10.1. Additional indicators will also need to be defined as they emerge in various nations (eg, which social determinants will be of highest priority will vary by nation). Pilot efforts in Indiana as well as Oregon are just starting to gather, integrate, and analyze social determinants in combination with data from EHR systems [49,50]. As these efforts grow, and others evolve both in the United States and globally, the requirements for the SHR and HMIS will need to be updated. Yet these components hold much promise for enabling the kind if integration and analysis envisioned by IOM and RWJF.

SUMMARY

Patient care is a multifaceted process that can involve a range of tasks such as personal consultations, blood tests, and X-rays [29,51]. As a result, clinical data are collected in many different formats including structured observations, image documents, transcribed notes, or laboratory results [29,51–53]. This information often resides in numerous heterogeneous information systems. The ability to successfully assemble the data that are stored in disparate formats and systems into a single, integrated and longitudinal patient health record can benefit the individual patient, the healthcare organizations participating in the HIE, and the community as a whole [9,54,55]. An SHR simplifies interoperability between information systems by providing a centralized repository that stores the information moving throughout the HIE in order to improve the quality and efficiency of clinical care [56]. Shared, longitudinal health records can also be aggregated at the population level through systems such as the OpenHIE HMIS, and subsequently distributed through an HIE to promote the advancement of community health outcomes through policy changes, surveillance, and research [11].

QUESTIONS FOR DISCUSSION

1. What kind of stakeholders benefit from shared, longitudinal health records in a health system? What benefits do these stakeholder receive from access to SHRs?
2. How would the implementation of an SHR system in the United States differ from an implementation in other countries around the world?
3. What advantages does an HMIS component offer over traditional sources of health indicator data such as population-based surveys?
4. What are some of the benefits of NoSQL DBMS in comparison to an RDBMS for managing clinical data?

References

[1] Walsham G, Sahay S. Research on information systems in developing countries: current landscape and future prospects. Inf Technol Dev 2006;12(1):7–24.
[2] Healthcare Information and Management Systems Society. Electronic medical records vs. electronic health

records: yes, there is a difference; 2006. Available from: <https://app.himssanalytics.org/docs/WP_EMR_EHR.pdf>.

[3] Coiera E. Building a National Health IT System from the middle out. J Am Med Inform Assoc 2009;16(3):271–3. Epub May 2, 2009.

[4] Katehakis DG, Sfakianakis SG, Kavlentakis G, Anthoulakis DN, Tsiknakis M. Delivering a lifelong integrated electronic health record based on a service oriented architecture. IEEE Trans Inf Technol Biomed 2007;11(6):639–50. Epub December 1, 2007.

[5] Healthcare Information and Management Systems Society. Electronic health records; 2015. Available from: <http://www.himss.org/library/ehr/>.

[6] Miriovsky BJ, Shulman LN, Abernethy AP. Importance of health information technology, electronic health records, and continuously aggregating data to comparative effectiveness research and learning health care. J Clin Oncol 2012;30(34):4243–8. Epub October 17, 2012.

[7] Gand K, Richter P, Esswein W. Towards lifetime electronic health record implementation. Stud Health Technol Inform 2015;212:225–32. Epub June 13, 2015.

[8] Krist AH. Electronic health record innovations for healthier patients and happier doctors. J Am Board Fam Med 2015;28(3):299–302. Epub May 10, 2015.

[9] Gunter TD, Terry NP. The emergence of national electronic health record architectures in the United States and Australia: models, costs, and questions. J Med Internet Res 2005;7(1):e3. Epub April 15, 2005.

[10] Mamlin BW, Biondich PG, Wolfe BA, Fraser H, Jazayeri D, Allen C, et al. Cooking up an open source EMR for developing countries: OpenMRS—a recipe for successful collaboration. AMIA Annu Symp Proc 2006:529–33. Epub January 24, 2007.

[11] Kukafka R, Ancker JS, Chan C, Chelico J, Khan S, Mortoti S, et al. Redesigning electronic health record systems to support public health. J Biomed Inform 2007;40(4):398–409. Epub July 17, 2007.

[12] Wu AW, Kharrazi H, Boulware LE, Snyder CF. Measure once, cut twice—adding patient-reported outcome measures to the electronic health record for comparative effectiveness research. J Clin Epidemiol 2013;66(Suppl. 8):S12–20. Epub July 17, 2013.

[13] Office of Disease Prevention and Health Promotion. About healthy people; 2015 [cited July 1, 2015]. Available from: <http://www.healthypeople.gov/2020/About-Healthy-People>.

[14] Centers for Disease Control and Prevention. Community health assessment for population health improvement: resource of most frequently recommended health outcomes and determinants; 2013. Available from: <http://wwwn.cdc.gov/CommunityHealth/PDF/Final_CHAforPHI_508.pdf>.

[15] Menachemi N, Collum TH. Benefits and drawbacks of electronic health record systems. Risk Manag Healthc Policy 2011;4:47–55. Epub February 9, 2012.

[16] WHO Ebola Response Team Ebola virus disease in West Africa—the first 9 months of the epidemic and forward projections. N Engl J Med 2014;371(16):1481–95. Epub September 23, 2014.

[17] Paterson BJ, Durrheim DN. The remarkable adaptability of syndromic surveillance to meet public health needs. J Epidemiol Global Health 2013;3(1):41–7. Epub July 17, 2013.

[18] Zeng DCH, Lynch C, Eidson M, Gotham I. Infectious disease informatics and outbreak detection Medical informatics. New York, NY: Springer Science + Business Media, Inc.; 2005.359.95

[19] Foldy S, Grannis S, Ross D, Smith T. A ride in the time machine: information management capabilities health departments will need. Am J Public Health 2014;104(9):1592–600. Epub July 18, 2014.

[20] McNabb SJ, Conde J, Ferland L, Macwright W, Okutani S, Park M, et al. Transforming public health surveillance. Elsevier; 2015.

[21] National Institutes of Health. Electronic health records overview; 2006 [cited May 22, 2015]. Available from: <http://www.himss.org/files/HIMSSorg/content/files/Code%20180%20MITRE%20Key%20Components%20of%20an%20EHR.pdf>.

[22] Centers for Disease Control and Prevention. About the national health interview survey; 2012 [cited June 25, 2015]. Available from: <http://www.cdc.gov/nchs/nhis/about_nhis.htm>.

[23] Dixon BE, Vreeman DJ, Grannis SJ. The long road to semantic interoperability in support of public health: experiences from two states. J Biomed Inform 2014;49:3–8. Epub April 1, 2014.

[24] Mohammed-Rajput NA, Smith DC, Mamlin B, Biondich P, Doebbeling BN. OpenMRS, a global medical records system collaborative: factors influencing successful implementation. AMIA Annu Symp Proc 2011;2011:960–8. Epub December 24, 2011.

[25] Braa J, Kanter AS, Lesh N, Crichton R, Jolliffe B, Saebo J, et al. Comprehensive yet scalable health information systems for low resource settings: a collaborative effort in sierra leone. AMIA Annu Symp Proc 2010;2010:372–6. Epub February 25, 2011.

[26] Seebregts CJ, Mamlin BW, Biondich PG, Fraser HS, Wolfe BA, Jazayeri D, et al. The OpenMRS implementers network. Int J Med Inform 2009;78(11):711–20. Epub January 23, 2009.

[27] Lee KK, Tang WC, Choi KS. Alternatives to relational database: comparison of NoSQL and XML approaches for clinical data storage. Comput Methods Programs Biomed 2013;110(1):99–109. Epub November 28, 2012.

[28] Jamison DC. Structured Query Language (SQL) fundamentals Baxevanis Andreas D, editor. Current protocols in bioinformatics/editoral board; 2003 [Chapter 9,Unit9.2. Epub April 23, 2008].

[29] Cios KJ, Moore GW. Uniqueness of medical data mining. Artif Intell Med 2002;26(1–2):1–24. Epub September 18, 2002.

[30] Cattell R. Scalable SQL and NoSQL data stores. ACM SIGMOD Rec 2011;39(4):12–27.

[31] World Health Organization. WHO indicator registry; 2015. Available from: <http://www.who.int/gho/indicator_registry/en/>.

[32] World Health Organization. Developing health management information systems; 2004 [cited June 16, 2015]. Available from: <http://www.wpro.who.int/health_services/documents/developing_health_management_information_systems.pdf>.

[33] Fu Jr. PC, Rosenthal D, Pevnick JM, Eisenberg F. The impact of emerging standards adoption on automated quality reporting. J Biomed Inform 2012;45(4):772–81. Epub July 24, 2012.

[34] Chen H, Hailey D, Wang N, Yu P. A review of data quality assessment methods for public health information systems. Int J Environ Res Public Health 2014;11:5170–207.

[35] Canadian Institute for Health Information. The CIHI data quality framework; 2009 [cited July 2, 2015]. Available from: <http://www.cihi.ca/CIHI-ext-portal/pdf/internet/DATA_QUALITY_FRAMEWORK_2009_EN>.

[36] Kim PS, Johnson DD. Implementing total quality management in the health care industry. Health Care Superv 1994;12(3):51–7. Epub February 7, 1994.

[37] Dixon BE, Rosenman M, Xia Y, Grannis SJ. A vision for the systematic monitoring and improvement of the quality of electronic health data. Stud Health Technol Inform 2013;192:884–8. Epub August 8, 2013.

[38] Dentler K, Cornet R, ten Teije A, Tanis P, Klinkenbijl J, Tytgat K, et al. Influence of data quality on computed Dutch hospital quality indicators: a case study in colorectal cancer surgery. BMC Med Inform Decis Mak 2014;14:32. Epub April 12, 2014.

[39] Garrido T, Kumar S, Lekas J, Lindberg M, Kadiyala D, Whippy A, et al. e-Measures: insight into the challenges and opportunities of automating publicly reported quality measures. J Am Med Inform Assoc 2014;21(1):181–4. Epub July 9, 2013.

[40] Jolliffe B, Mukherjee A, Sahay S. Heterogeneous interoperable systems as a strategy towards scaling: the case of hospital information systems in India. In: The 12th international conference on social implications of computers in developing countries (IFIP Working Group 94); 2013. p. 456–466.

[41] Liaw ST, Chen HY, Maneze D, Taggart J, Dennis S, Vagholkar S, et al. Health reform: is routinely collected electronic information fit for purpose? Emerg Med Australas 2012;24(1):57–63. Epub February 9, 2012.

[42] Dixon BE, Siegel JA, Oemig TV, Grannis SJ. Electronic health information quality challenges and interventions to improve public health surveillance data and practice. Public Health Rep 2013;128(6):546–53. Epub November 2, 2013.

[43] Dixon BE, McGowan JJ, Grannis SJ. Electronic laboratory data quality and the value of a health information exchange to support public health reporting processes. AMIA Annu Symp Proc 2011;2011:322–30. Epub December 24, 2011.

[44] Institute of Medicine Roundtable on Evidence-Based Medicine The National Academies Collection: Reports funded by National Institutes of Health. Leadership Commitments to Improve Value in Healthcare: Finding Common Ground: Workshop Summary. Washington (DC): National Academies Press (US) National Academy of Sciences; 2009.

[45] Robert Wood Johnson Foundation. Creating a rapid-learning health system; 2014 [cited July 12, 2015]. Available from: <http://www.rwjf.org/content/dam/farm/reports/program_results_reports/2014/rwjf72101>.

[46] Institute of Medicine. The learning health system and its innovation collaboratives; 2011 [cited July 3, 2015]. Available from: <https://www.iom.edu/~/media/Files/Activity%20Files/Quality/VSRT/Core%20Documents/ForEDistrib.pdf>.

[47] Robert Wood Johnson Foundation. Building a culture of health; 2014 [cited July 10, 2015]. Available from: http://www.rwjf.org/content/dam/files/rwjf-web-files/Annual_Message/2014_RWJF_AnnualMessage_final.pdf.

[48] Plough AL. Developing new systems of data to advance a culture of health. eGEMs (Generating Evidence & Methods to improve health outcomes) 2014;2(4):9.

[49] Comer KF, Grannis S, Dixon BE, Bodenhamer DJ, Wiehe SE. Incorporating geospatial capacity within clinical data systems to address social determinants of health. Public Health Rep 2011;126(Suppl. 3):54–61. Epub August 13, 2011.

[50] Bazemore AW, Cottrell EK, Gold R, Hughes LS, Phillips RL, Angier H, et al. "Community Vital Signs": incorporating geocoded social determinants into electronic records to promote patient and population health. J Am Med Inform Assoc 2015 Epub July 16, 2015.

[51] Castellani B, Castellani J. Data mining: qualitative analysis with health informatics data. Qual Health Res 2003;13(7):1005–18. Epub September 25, 2003.

[52] Hayrinen K, Saranto K, Nykanen P. Definition, structure, content, use and impacts of electronic health records: a review of the research literature. Int J Med Inform 2008;77(5):291–304. Epub October 24, 2007.

[53] Johnson SB, Bakken S, Dine D, Hyun S, Mendonca E, Morrison F, et al. An electronic health record based on structured narrative. J Am Med Inform Assoc 2008;15(1):54–64. Epub October 20, 2007.

[54] Barbarito F, Pinciroli F, Barone A, Pizzo F, Ranza R, Mason J, et al. Implementing the lifelong personal health record in a regionalised health information system: the case of Lombardy, Italy. Comput Biol Med 2015;59:164–74. Epub November 19, 2013.

[55] Iakovidis I. Towards personal health record: current situation, obstacles and trends in implementation of electronic healthcare record in Europe. Int J Med Inform 1998;52(1–3):105–15. Epub December 16, 1998.

[56] Healthcare Information and Management Systems Society. HIE technical information overview; 2011 [cited May 20, 2015]. Available from: <https://www.himss.org/files/HIMSSorg/content/files/HIMSSHIETechnicalOverview.pdf>.

CHAPTER

11

Client Registries: Identifying and Linking Patients

Timothy D. McFarlane[1], *Brian E. Dixon*[2] *and Shaun J. Grannis*[3]

[1]Indiana University, Richard M. Fairbanks School of Public Health, Indianapolis, IN [2]Indiana University Richard M. Fairbanks School of Public Health; and the Center for Biomedical Informatics, Regenstrief Institute, Inc., Indianapolis, IN [3]Indiana University, School of Medicine and the Center for Biomedical Informatics, Regenstrief Institute, Inc., Indianapolis, IN

OUTLINE

LEARNING OBJECTIVES

At the end of the chapter, the reader should be able to:

- Define a client registry and describe why such registries are needed in health information exchange.
- Detail common strategies for implementing a client registry.
- Discuss common challenges encountered when implementing a client registry.
- Highlight the critical role a unique identifier plays in implementing a client registry.
- Distinguish between the common methods of patient matching.

INTRODUCTION

Uniquely identifying patients is an essential task for both the delivery and administration of health care and doing so accurately is deceptively difficult, yet crucial, to delivering the right care to the right patient. Patient data moving within and between organizations, as in the case of health information exchange (HIE), further motivates a need to accurately describe who these data represent.

Simply transmitting (or routing) information from point A to point B does not require knowing about whom the information pertains. Participants in HIE networks, however, seek not only to move information about the network but also to create services that aggregate information about patients and populations to support a range of tasks in clinical and public health. These services rely on *patient-centric data*: a set of data (eg, diagnoses, prescriptions, visits, demographics, symptoms) pertaining to a single, unique individual who has utilized the health system. Patient-centric data are often scattered across multiple facilities, including health care organizations and providers, pharmacies, urgent care clinics, and mental health professionals, where each institution or system typically uses proprietary identifiers that are largely meaningless outside of the assigning organization.

Fully functional, patient-centric HIE services must uniquely identify patients through record linkage. Community-based HIEs (defined in the chapter: What is Health Information Exchange?) need to link patient records across multiple health systems, and private HIEs (defined in the chapter: What is Health Information Exchange?) need to link patient records across facilities within their network or enterprise. In many cases, a single hospital or clinic also needs to link records across different sources, including clinical laboratory, radiology, pharmacy, and admitting services. Furthermore, record linkage is not unique to the health care environment. In 1946, Dunn first described record linkage as a method of bringing together pages in the book of life [1]. By the 1950s, record linkage was used in matching vital records for individuals and families [2]. Today, record linkage is ubiquitous with applications in business (eg, mailing lists), research (eg, database management and merging), and government agencies (eg, US Census), and health care [3,4].

Integration of separate, patient-centric data sources facilitates timely access to an individual's continuum of health while also adding a rich data source to improve health through clinical and population research, as well as public health. Regardless of the use, all data are patient-centric and at some point the identity of the patient must be determined. Even in countries where citizens are assigned a national identifier, there remains a need to ensure the unique identity of an individual among the myriad fragmented information systems that collectively represent a person's electronic health record (EHR). A client registry (CR) is a software application designed to support uniquely identifying individuals who receive health care services from multiple sites and collate these records into a single, longitudinal health record.

This chapter begins by introducing techniques used for identifying patients within organizations, followed by a discussion of unique patient identifiers (UPIs)—how they are constructed, which attributes contribute to their efficacy, and what options currently exist. The topic of unique identifiers precedes an overview of key considerations for a CR, including emphasis on data quality and techniques for matching patient records.

PATIENT IDENTIFIERS

EHR systems manage records. Much of the information maintained in EHR systems pertains to patients—or clients—who receive health care services from a clinic or hospital. In order to effectively manage information about patients, EHR systems must assign and use patient identifiers, such as a medical record number (MRN), when performing tasks such as creating a new record, updating an existing record, or deleting a record. Identifiers (or IDs) ensure that the correct record is added, updated, or deleted.

Patient identifiers can be thought of as belonging to two general classes: (1) a unique code or set of codes specifically designed to uniquely identify a patient in a given system and (2) an aggregate set of demographic and related attributes used to describe a patient uniquely, such as name, sex, date of birth, address, etc. Whether utilizing existing or creating new patient identifiers, it is prudent to understand the context in which the identifiers will be deployed.

Strategies that rely upon unique identifiers vary based on the country of implementation and availability of certain identifiers, such as a national health ID number or national ID number. If a national ID exists, it is important to understand the attributes of the identifier. Are all individuals given an identifier at birth, or later in life? Does every person, including immigrants, possess an identifier?

Within the context of each country, demographic attributes vary based on naming conventions, geographic data (eg, village vs city), and other cultural practices. Additionally, the collection of certain demographic attributes may be more complete based on cultural differences (eg, withholding for privacy), health care infrastructure, and the presence of civil registration systems. Adding to the difficulty, the format, completeness, and accuracy of demographic attributes often vary between organizations, even within the same region, state, or country.

Due to both the assortment of available identifiers and inconsistent use of these identifiers across health care institutions, for both unique codes and demographic attributes, there exists a need to understand how identifiers are created, what makes a good identifier (ie, ideal attributes), and what identifiers are currently available. As will be detailed, the CR uses a combination of unique identifiers and demographic attributes to establish patient identity. The CR must deal with issues of data quality in order to make use of personal identifiers, in particular demographic attributes.

UNIQUE PATIENT IDENTIFIERS

Strategy for Assigning UPIs

A UPI requires a sequence allocation sufficiently large to cover an entire population over time, theoretically for as long as the number will be in use. Sequencing schemes available for development of a UPI generally fall into three numbering systems: (1) serial, (2) derived, and (3) composite.

1. In serial numbering systems, each individual is assigned a number from a central location. These numbers are automated and do not assimilate any nonunique characteristics of the individual. England's National Health Service number is an example of serial numbering system, with some added functionality [5].
2. As the name suggests, derived numbering systems create a number based on, or derived from, a personal trait of the individual. In contrast to serial numbering, assignment of a derived number can take place anywhere but runs the risk of failing to be unique when derived from a personal trait which is shared by other individuals.
3. Composite numbering systems assign part of the number from a central location and the other part is derived from personal traits, thus represents a combination of the serial and derived systems [6].

Regardless of the allocation methodology, errors can occur during entry, transcription, and preparation. The incorporation of check digits limits errors by implanting one or more nonidentifying numbers or characters within the UPI that are checked against an algorithm to validate the number [7,8]. Check digits improve accuracy of identifiers during data entry and retrieval, improving the reliability and accuracy of patient identification.

Attributes of Ideal Identifiers

Much of the concern around utilizing a universal identifier for health care, particularly in the United States, is fear of malicious intent in the event of a data breach. The only true way to prevent the possibility of confidentiality breaches is to exclude personal information; such as name, social security number (SSN), date of birth, etc., and to eliminate the possibility of linking the health care identifier to databases which contain personal information [9]. At the time of writing, and for the foreseeable future, no identifier exists which will perfectly ascertain all individuals uniquely across all scopes of health care; at least not one that is neither physically invasive (eg, implanted device) nor invasive of a citizen's right to privacy.

Health care identifiers are often assigned within individual information systems (eg, laboratory, radiology) as well as organization-wide (eg, MRN). However, as discussed, these identifiers are meaningless outside of the domain in which they operate. One solution to this identity challenge is to establish a unique identifier that crosses organizational boundaries. The American Society for Testing and Materials (ASTM), which is a standards development organization accredited by the American National Standards Institute (ANSI), describes 30 criteria which should be used to evaluate the efficacy of a candidate identifier [10]. Meeting all of the proposed criteria would lead to a UPI that achieves the following:

- positively identifies patients,
- automatically links and collates patient records from disparate electronic sources, creating a longitudinal care record,
- protects patient's personal health information and privacy, and
- effectively minimizes the cost of patient record management.

No identifier exists which could meet all of the criteria proposed by the standard because some ideal attributes conflict with each other. For example, a ubiquitous and easily accessible identifier may not adequately preserve privacy. The following is a description of selected

TABLE 11.1 Attributes of Ideal Unique Personal Identifiers

Attribute	Description	Examples
Unique	An identifier which can only be associated with a single individual or entity	Fingerprints, retinal scans, DNA, national identifiers
Ubiquitous	A durable and constantly available identifier which is accepted across the healthcare spectrum	Name, date of birth, sex, eye color, smart cards, fingerprints, retinal scans
Unchanging	The identifier is permanently associated with the individual and will not change over time	Date of birth, sex, DNA
Uncontroversial	The potential for malicious use of the identifier must be limited	Identifier not derived from personal attributes such as serial numbering system.
Uncomplicated	The identifier should be simple to implement, use, and recall	SSN
Inexpensive	The implementation and maintenance should be reasonable within the context of healthcare costs	Existing identifiers: Name, date of birth, sex, SSN

ideal UPI attributes; for succinct definitions and examples, refer to Table 11.1.

- A *unique* identifier, by definition, can never be associated with more than one individual. That is, once assigned, the possibility of another person being assigned the same number must be eliminated, or infinitely minuscule.
- A *ubiquitous* identifier is available and accepted across the health care spectrum. For example, a nonubiquitous identifier would identify a patient for a hospitalization but not the subsequent primary care visit. Ubiquity also requires the identifier to be durable and made readily available at the time of service.
- *Unchanging*. In order for an individual identifier to be effective, every individual should have an identifier that applies only to that individual and does not change over time. This requires foresight on the part of the issuing agency because enough numbers must be generated to support the population throughout the life span of the identifier.
- *Uncontroversial*. The identifier should help minimize the opportunities for crime and abuse and should not contain substantive information about the individual. Similarly, the various stakeholders must perceive the identifier to be minimally invasive. The subjectivity of what is and is not invasive makes universal acceptance difficult, if not impossible.
- *Uncomplicated*. An identifier or identifier system that is not practical to implement or that does not meet the requirements of administrative simplification must be deemed unacceptable.
- *Inexpensive*. The costs of implementation and use of the identifier must be within an acceptable range. Analysis of costs across all health care settings should be considered including, patients, providers, payers, and government agencies. For example, it has been estimated that a national health identifier implemented in the United States would cost between $4.9 and $12.2 billion to deploy and $1.5 billion per year, which many view as unsustainable [11].

Existing Unique Patient Identifiers

The Health Insurance Portability Accountability Act of 1996 (HIPAA) recognized the need to uniquely identify patients for managing care and administrative purposes, thus proposing a unique health identifier for all individuals [12]. UPIs have been implemented in several international health care systems but have yet to come to fruition in the United States for a number of reasons: a funding embargo imposed by Congress; costs to implement such a system; privacy concerns; difficulties in conforming existing information systems to utilize the identifier; and a lack of consensus on selection of an identifier [11,13,14].

The interested reader is referred to a 1998 Health and Human Services white paper, developed prior to a congressional ban on government funded UPI discussion, which discusses relevant legislation, privacy and confidentiality concerns, as well as strengths and weaknesses of several proposed implementations of a national UPI [15]. The following is a discussion centered on commonly broached UPIs—SSN, biometric identifiers, and a voluntary universal health care identifier.

Social Security Number

The SSN has been advanced as a candidate for a UPI in the United States because it is theoretically unique, ubiquitous, unchanging, most adults can recite it from memory, and would not require additional infrastructure to implement (ie, inexpensive and uncomplicated). However, in reality, the SSN is sometimes shared by multiple individuals, not all people are eligible for an SSN, in rare circumstances an individual may possess more than one SSN, SSNs are not universally available at birth, and there is no legal protection for maintaining SSN confidentiality in nongovernment organizations [15]. Using the SSN also comes with controversy, largely as a result of its universality. At its inception, the SSN was for use only within the context of the Social Security program and intended to identify an account, not a person. Today, the SSN has become tightly linked to an individual's credit score, among other things, and is now largely viewed as a nonconfidential identifier [16].

A common concern surrounding UPIs is the belief that improper linkage of an individual's information becomes easier with a single identifier, as compared with using multiple separate identifiers at each organization. The concern of inappropriate linkage is further exemplified in the case of the SSN because of the associated credit, employment, government activities (eg, Internal Revenue Service), and consumer behavior data linked to the identifier. Despite these concerns, the SSN is already incorporated in health care to a great extent and is frequently included in patient matching algorithms, as will be discussed later in this chapter.

Biometric Identifiers

Biometric identifiers such as fingerprints, iris scans, voice recognition, and facial shapes offer unique, ubiquitous, and relatively unchanging identifiers. In developed nations, implementation of biometrics has been scarce, mainly because of concerns with privacy and the potential for law enforcement to use these data [17]. However, underdeveloped nations often lack universal coverage by civil registration systems leading to an identification problem that reaches far beyond health care. Recent technological advances are allowing cheaper, more accurate identification using biometric indicators such as fingerprints and iris scans. In a report for the Center for Global Development, Gelb and Clark [18] found that 160 countries have deployed biometrics to address the identify gap covering over 1 billion people.

While highly discriminatory, biometric identifiers do not eliminate the need for sophisticated matching algorithms to uniquely identify an individual. Measurements of a person's fingerprint or iris will possess variability within persons, due to changes in age, environment, disease, stress, and occupational factors, as well as variability due to hardware (eg, sensor calibration and age of the device). In the case of fingerprints, any single individual can produce several distinct images depending on the angle of depression, pressure, presence of dirt, moisture, and sensor characteristics [19].

Voluntary Universal Healthcare Identifier

ASTM established two international standards, E1714 and E2553, which specified the architecture and implementation, respectively, for a Universal Healthcare Identifier (UHID) [10,20]. Privacy and confidentiality concerns, in large part, have led to hesitance surrounding establishing a government-facilitated, national UHID.

Hieb (2006) therefore proposes that assignment of a Voluntary Universal Health Identifier (VUHID) from a not-for-profit or a government–private partnership would alleviate concerns around a central government-managed database. Furthermore, patients have the control by opting in or out, allowing them to weigh the benefits and potential privacy risks [21,22].

An example of VUHID was deployed by Global Patient Identifiers, Inc. (GPII) and attempts to completely eliminate patient matching errors by augmenting existing probabilistic matching algorithms with a VUHID [23]. The patient may request one open voluntary identifier (OVID), which as the name suggests shares all information with all providers, and multiple private voluntary identifiers (PVID) that will only disclose information to patient-selected providers.

A key design element for the VUHID proposed by GPII is that once a patient requests to participate through their provider, they are assigned a unique identifier that, unlike the SSN, is used only to identify them in the health care setting. The VUHID then routes the unique identifier back through the HIE CR to be associated with the patient's records. The unique identifier (implemented by barcode, magnetic strip, smart card, etc.) is given to the patient and presented when visiting a provider. Drawbacks of the proposed VUHID include the complexity introduced by the PVID, which assumes that patients will understand when it is clinically important to share information from one provider with another, and concerns that the failure to share all records may impede hospitals from producing complete billing records [24].

International Unique Patient Identifiers

UPIs have been developed and implemented in low-, middle-, and high-income countries. Details on the purpose, formats, validation methods, technical architectures, and lessons learned from UPI implementations in England, Newfoundland and Labrador, Australia, New Zealand, and Germany may be found in a review from 2010 by the Health Information and Quality Authority [25]. Specific use cases for implementing a UPI in Denmark, Botswana, Kenya, Brazil, Malawi, Ukraine, Thailand, and Zambia are discussed in a UNAIDS white paper addressing developing and using individual identifiers for health services including HIV [26].

Although no single identifier currently exists with each of the ideal attributes, Figure 11.1 depicts the degree to which the examples discussed meet the expectations of an ideal identifier. As will be discussed, a key strength of the CR is the ability to utilize multiple identifiers through matching algorithms to positively identify a patient. That is, the CR does not rely on the necessity to produce an ideal UPI; however, when a UPI is available, matching efficiency is improved.

UPIs hold promise for simplifying patient identification, but even in the case a UPI is in use, there is a need to match patients using other attributes, such as demographics, when a UPI is unavailable at the time of service (eg, forgot card or emergency situations). Similarly,

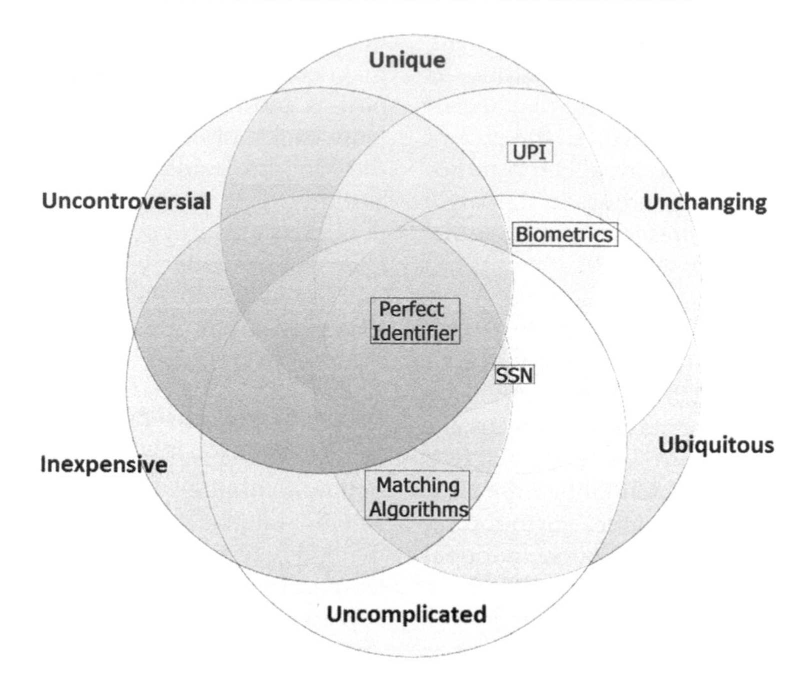

FIGURE 11.1 The ideal attributes of unique personal identifiers, highlighting where commonly used identifiers exist within this framework. UPI, unique patient identifier; SSN, social security number.

if a temporary identification must be issued, the central authority will need to utilize other identifiers, such as demographics, to link a patient's UPI to the temporary ID to prevent record fragmentation. In general, the implementation of a UPI will improve the accuracy of matching procedures but will not replace the need for demographic attributes.

THE ENTERPRISE MASTER PATIENT INDEX

To more fully explore the need for unique patient identification and record linkage, let us consider a scenario applicable to both clinical and population health. Diabetes mellitus is an example of a complex, chronic medical condition that requires coordination between primary care and specialist physicians; uncontrolled diabetes can result in high emergency department (ED) as well as hospital utilization. Patients with diabetes often have an entire health care team consisting of the primary care provider, dietician, endocrinologist, ophthalmologist, mental health professional, and podiatrist, among others [27]. Furthermore, the health care team is often scattered across multiple physical locations and some providers may not be part of the same integrated health care system.

Consider the scenario in which a diabetic patient, Bob, is having difficulty controlling his blood sugar levels, experiences frequent foot ulcers and blurred vision. As a result, Bob's primary care physician refers him to an endocrinologist, a podiatrist, and an ophthalmologist. Between visits, Bob experiences an episode requiring a visit to the ED. Before his next primary care visit, Bob's physician retrieves the results of each specialist visit. Despite data being entered at four different locations (specialist offices and ED), all of Bob's results are linked together within an enterprise EHR system used at all the locations in which Bob received care. Linking records on the same patient to create an integrated and complete medical record is accomplished by an *enterprise master patient index (eMPI)*. The eMPI is software that assigns a unique identifier to each patient and ensures that the patient is represented only one time within the enterprise EHR system or private HIE. But what if Bob's ED encounter occurred within another, competing health care system?

Each health care organization's eMPI associates its own unique identifier with patient data; thus, a single patient may have several "unique" eMPI identifiers, one within each organization where care occurred. The lack of a shared identifier across organizations makes integration of patient data difficult. So if Bob visits an ED outside his usual integrated health care system, data about the visit would not be integrated into the EHR system record utilized by his primary care physician and, unless Bob discloses this information, his primary care physician may never be aware of the incident. The unique identifier problem has an intuitive solution that creates a unique identifier to span all health care organizations.

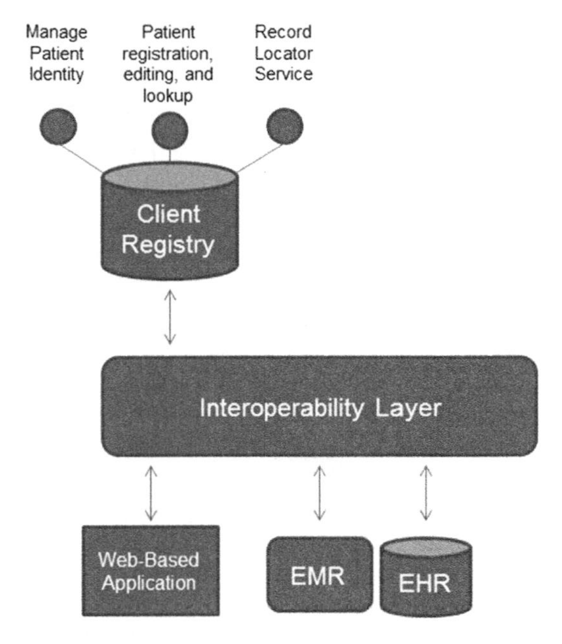

FIGURE 11.2 The client registry architecture within the OpenHIE model. EMR, electronic medical record; EHR, electronic health record.

THE CLIENT REGISTRY

The eMPI uniquely identified and linked each of Bob's specialty care visits because they were within the same network or enterprise, but data from an ED visit outside Bob's usual integrated health care system would remain in a silo. A natural, logical solution might be the use of an UPI that could span all of Bob's health care services and allow for positive identification and linkage of Bob's ED visit to his other health care data. However, no single UPI is currently available that would facilitate linking all of Bob's records. Thus, in order to link data across the health system, we must rely upon an assemblage of existing identifiers.

A CR operates by adjudicating the assemblage of demographic attributes and other personal identifiers from each data supplier (eg, hospitals, clinics, etc.) to create a single record for each patient within the HIE. Figure 11.2 demonstrates how the CR fits into the scheme of the HIE model. Organizational EHR systems and point-of-care applications interact with the CR through the interoperability layer allowing users to retrieve, add, and edit patient records. Once positive identification is made, the CR associates each patient's records with a unique number called the *master patient index (MPI)*. Although similar in concept to the unique number assigned by an eMPI, the MPI—in the context of the CR—acts as the controller for all other local identifiers that may be associated with the patient, including one or more MRNs assigned by individual facilities and

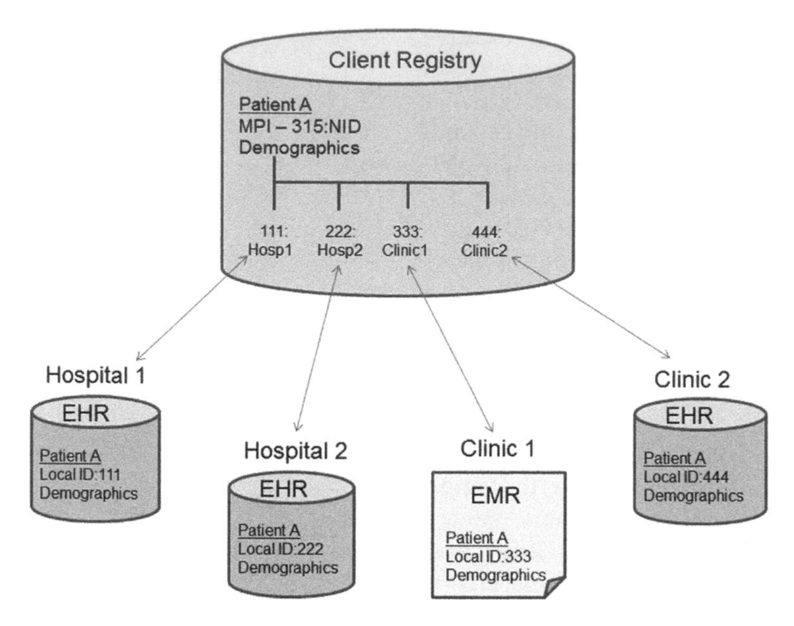

FIGURE 11.3 The relationship between the client registry and EHR systems of participating organizations within an HIE network. HIE, health information exchange; EHR, electronic health record.

eMPI identifiers assigned by integrated health care networks; this relationship is depicted in Figure 11.3. The MPI of the CR, therefore, bridges the gap for interorganizational patient identification, allowing creation and maintenance of patient-centric records that contain all clinical information regardless of the source.

The relationship between each organization and the CR is depicted in Figure 11.3. Each hospital and clinic identifies the patient using a set of demographic attributes and identifiers (eg, name, SSN, date of birth, etc.) and a local unique code identifier (eg, MRN, eMPI) and communicates these data to the CR. As will be discussed later in this chapter, the incoming data are subjected to a matching algorithm that establishes positive patient identity and links the new record to any previous records, when applicable. If the patient is new to the HIE, the CR assigns a new MPI for future record linkage. Once an MPI has been established, the CR becomes the source of truth for identity of individuals.

TABLE 11.2 Example of Attributes for Patient Identification Within the Client Registry

Local patient identifier	Social security number
Patient name	Facility identifier
Date of Birth	Universal identifier, if applicable
Sex	Admission date
Race	Discharge date
Ethnicity	Service type
Address	

In order for the CR to resolve patient identity, facilities must send sufficiently discriminating demographic attributes. Examples of common data elements used for resolving identity are listed in Table 11.2. As the source of truth about identity, the CR can communicate with myriad EHR systems and point-of-service applications to update and sync patient identity for future encounters. Strength of the

CR is the ability to perform linkage of patient demographics when the patient is registered with slightly different demographic attributes as a result of receiving care from multiple sites. For example, our hypothetical diabetic patient, Bob, could still be identified if his podiatrist included last name, date of birth, and sex, while his endocrinologist included first and last name, SSN, and address.

Establishing the identity of a patient within the CR and communicating this identity consistently across participating organizations enables the implementation of a *record locator service (RLS)*. The RLS queries HIE records to identify all locations where a patient may have data. This is particularly useful for rapid retrieval if a clinician is seeking a specific piece of information, such as a primary care physician searching for an emergency room discharge summary [9].

The CR is inordinately impacted by data quality; the limiting factor of any matching algorithm is the data used to match records. Because the goal is to match based on a collection of demographic attributes and personal identifiers, multiple incomplete or inaccurate identifiers decrease the confidence of positive patient identification. Poor data quality can arise from any point in the care process. The next section will discuss common data-related errors as well as solutions in the form of metadata and standards (ie, data format), after which the discussion shifts to how the CR handles inconsistent data across participating organizations and common approaches to algorithmic patient matching used by the CR.

DATA QUALITY

Data quality represents a challenge for CR because the integration of health care data largely depends on matching a number of personal identifier attributes, such as demographics. The accuracy and reliability of the CR is largely determined by the quality of data captured at the point-of-care. This is particularly challenging, yet important, when an organization first joins the HIE network and their historic patient data must be cleaned prior to being exported. Often organizations do not have the resources or the foresight to effectively prepare these data, leading to future matching difficulties. However, as will be discussed in the next section, the CR may standardize incoming data to improve identity resolution and facilitate integration of patient data.

Errors affecting data quality typically occur during data collection, entry, and query. For example, data quality can suffer during collection from incorrect patient recall, data collectors making assumptions or incorrect observations (eg, race), or simply failing to collect relevant patient demographics. More often than not, recording errors take one of the following forms: (1) phonetic misrepresentations; (2) typographical inaccuracies; and (3) morphological confusion [24].

1. A phonetic error occurs when a spoken word or name has multiple "correct" handwritten representations. For example, a woman named Lindsey who lives on Neely Avenue represents at least 35 phonetically similar but incorrect combinations: Lindsy, Lindsay, Linsea, Lyndsey, Lyndsay, Lyndsy, Lynzay, who lives on Neeley, Nealy, Nealey, Kneely, or Kneeley.
2. Typographical errors are another common recording error that occurs as a result of omitted, inserted, or transposed characters (eg, Lndsey, Linndsey, and Lnidsey, respectively).
3. Characters that appear similar, such as the number 0 (zero) and capital letter O or lowercase L and capital I, can be mistakenly interchanged leading to a morphological error [24].

Although errors are more numerous during data entry, a provider querying the HIE for a patient may encounter similar errors as those committed during data entry, thus failing to locate the patient's data.

Erroneous or omitted data will continue to be a challenge in patient identification but can be limited by providing adequate and continuous training for staff that register patients and establishing a data quality monitoring program to identify and resolve problems. The CR provides solutions to data recording errors through the implementation of phonetic transformations and string comparators, which will be discussed in more detail later in the section on algorithmic matching.

In contrast to errors related to data entry, which are at least in theory preventable, data accuracy may not be as amenable to improvement by adherence to procedures and standards alone. Personal traits are often unstable, such as address, employer, marital status, and surname. In the United States, there are more than 2 million marriages and 900,000 divorces each year, which are likely to result in a number of demographic changes to the individuals involved [28]. Furthermore, roughly 11%–15% of the US population changes their address in a given year [29,30]. Since patients are not required to update providers when a change occurs, it is imperative to request updates at each point of care. Demographic updates should be communicated to CR and subsequently sent out to other organizational EHR systems to maintain consistent identification.

Differences in culture may also impact the semantic meaning, or interpretation, of patient data. For example, Hispanic cultures may use multiple family names. Consider the daughter of a Hispanic couple named Carlos Lopez and Isabella Gonzalez, Maria Lopez Gonzalez. Maria's name should be entered as either Maria Lopez or Maria Lopez Gonzalez, but not Maria Gonzalez [24]. Other cultural practices to consider include the order of names (surname listed before given name), usage of particles (eg, de, da, dos) and hyphens or other special characters in names, religious names, and different practices of listing date of birth (DD/MM/YYYY vs MM/DD/YYYY) [13]. In some cases, an encounter may correctly match to an individual but the data were generated from a different person, such as the case in identity theft and when individuals share identifiers. For these and many other reasons, patient data must be normalized through metadata and standards.

METADATA AND STANDARDS

As discussed throughout the book, interoperability is achieved through universal and consistent implementation of standards, including HL7 or X12 for data transactions (see the chapter: Syntactic Interoperability and the Role of Standards). The same need exists for patient identification. The health care industry needs to develop and adhere to standards for the various data fields used to identify patients, or at the very least provide adequate descriptions of fields (also referred to as metadata). Although syntactic data field standards exist, such as MM/DD/YYYY for date of birth, usage may differ from one EHR system to another. Furthermore, the meaning or semantics of data may differ by organization and the individual entering the data. Consider the example of Ms. Lopez Gonzalez. By name alone, it is quite possible that she could be entered into an EHR system under three different names. The lack of precise standardization can hinder accurate linkage of disparate records originating from the same patient, resulting in incomplete data sharing and fragmented records.

The CR seeks to overcome barriers of syntactic and semantic heterogeneity by standardizing identifier fields, based on the context of health care delivery in a particular country. Examples of standard specifications provided by national or international bodies include the following:

- HL7 Patient Identifier Cross-Reference (PIX) [31],
- HL7 Patient Demographic Query (PDQ) [31],

- Philippines National Health Data Dictionary [32,33],
- ISO (International Standards Organization)/ IEC 5218—identification of gender [34],
- ISO/TS 22220:2011—Identification of subjects of healthcare [35], and
- ISO 21091:2013: Health informatics—Directory services for healthcare providers, subjects of care, and other entities [36].

In addition to coding standards, the CR can improve the linkage of patient records by the following: controlling the type of data allowed in a field (eg, only numbers for a lab result); parsing out components; and standardizing attributes. For example, addresses may be parsed into street number, street name, city, zip code, country, etc., and standardized by mapping different inputs (eg, road, rural route, rd) into one commonly stored abbreviation, RD [4].

Parsing components may help complete missing or incorrect data fields. For example, if an error was made in the spelling of city, the street name, street number, and zip code can be used to resolve the error. Another commonly encountered example is the storage of patient sex. Male could be stored as M, 0, 1, or 2 and female as F, 0, 1, or 2 depending on the protocols established at the registering organization. Some description of these data (metadata) would need to accompany the message, but these data can rather simply be converted to a standardized format for identification purposes within the CR. Although, to fully achieve interoperability, the generating facility should transmit these data in a standardized form (eg, ISO IEC 5218) such that the CR would be able to receive and interpret data without instructions.

ALGORITHMIC MATCHING

The crux of the CR is its use of matching algorithms to determine whether the client (patient) already exists in the registry, subsequently linking records regardless of the source, when applicable. The CR can accommodate differences between the data sources by the following sequential processes:

- preparing (cleaning) data,
- using programs that detect errors and deviations (field comparators),
- separating likely matches from unlikely matches (blocking), and
- configuring matching algorithms to classify record pairs as reflecting the same individual or entity.

Generally, CR algorithms can be described as deterministic, probabilistic, or a combination of both. Many algorithms are available for matching, but no single method has emerged as universally appropriate for every situation [37]. Figure 11.4 provides a simple representation of matching methodologies with increasing complexity from left to right. In the absence of an ideal UPI, matching can be accomplished using one or more patient traits. Unlike algorithms that rely on UPIs, which are fundamentally simple by comparison, matching methods that use demographic attributes are more complex and rely upon sufficient data quality (eg, accuracy, completeness) of multiple attributes and, intuitively, the accuracy of the matching algorithm increases with the number of (high-quality) identifiers used [4]. Using an improperly tuned algorithm may result in a higher rate of duplicate records; therefore, it is recommended that the HIE develop a process to determine the appropriate matching scheme. Furthermore, because patient attributes as well as populations change over time, CR matching schemes should be reexamined, and possibly recalibrated, at regular intervals.

Basic Concepts of Matching

Common personal traits or identifiers such as names, SSN, date of birth, address, parent's

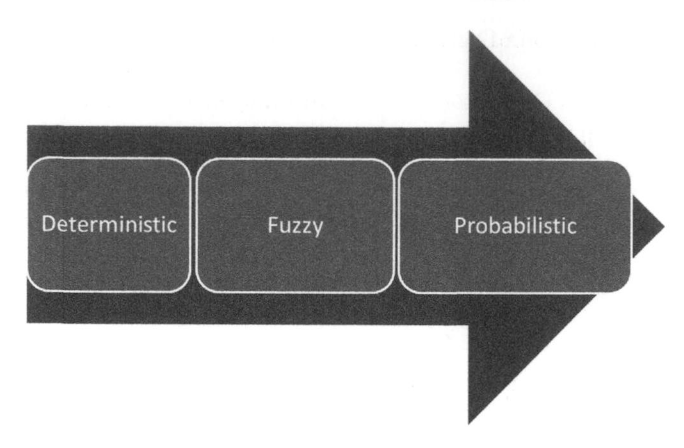

FIGURE 11.4 Graphical representation of the sophistication spectrum of client registry patient matching techniques. The least sophisticated techniques are on the left with the most sophisticated techniques on the right.

names, and sex are often used as matching variables. When choosing matching variables, it is important to consider their discriminating power or ability to distinctly identify a patient. For example, SSN possesses more discriminatory power than sex because sex can only take the form of two values, male or female. The discriminatory power of matching variables will differ based on the context of the CR implementation. In some countries, a relatively small number of given names will represent a large segment of the population, limiting the usefulness for matching purposes. Put simply, any CR implementation is highly specific to the population and cannot simply be replicated in other contexts.

The decision rule, or match determination, is established by the algorithm employed—generally deterministic, fuzzy, or probabilistic—and the matching variables selected. A pair is evaluated based on the prescribed decision rule, which will delineate the pair as a match, a possible match, or a nonmatch. Possible matches that lack sufficient information to enable the decision rule to assign the pair to the match or nonmatch group typically require human review, or are simply labeled as a nonmatch when the cost of human review is prohibitive. The resulting matched pairs will fall into one of the following four groups [4]:

1. true match—the decision rule matched records which are indeed the same person;
2. false match—the decision rule matched records which are not the same person;
3. true nonmatch—the decision rule correctly did not match records which are not the same person; and
4. false nonmatch—the decision rule failed to match records which are truly the same person.

Data Preparation

The ability of the CR to reliably identify pairs as matching or nonmatching is critically dependent upon a balance between data quality and matching algorithms. A simple algorithm with complete and standardized data will perform well, but as data degrade more sophisticated algorithms will be necessary. In general, high-quality data are preferred over a sophisticated algorithm. The data preparation phase is where the CR addresses the concerns of heterogeneity of data, as discussed in previous sections of this chapter, by parsing and transforming (standardizing) potential matching variables.

Field Comparison Methods

The occurrence of typographical and phonetic errors limits the ability to compare two strings for exact matches. If matching, or blocking, depended on exact character matches, the algorithms may erroneously exclude true matches due to variant spellings or transposed keystrokes. Several coding systems have been created which loosen the constraints around the argument and allow approximate agreement between fields. For example, a "fuzzy match" may be employed to apply semantic logic or allow some range of disagreement among fields, such as date of birth (eg, within 3 months) or a name which agrees on a defined number of characters (eg, Alex Smith vs Alexander Smith).

The fuzzy matching technique is similar to a probabilistic method but without the statistical complexity. Rather, the intent of a fuzzy match is to apply meaningful terms to data fields to resemble human reasoning [38]. Several phonetic transformation systems are available that limit the disruption caused by errors from similar sounding words and match these homophones even though minor variations in spelling exist, such as the following: the New York State Identification and Intelligence System (NYIIS); soundex; metaphone; and double metaphone.

Approximate string comparators, such as Levenshtein edit distance, Jaro–Winkler comparator, and longest common subsequence, act to improve matching efficiency by computing a comparator score, or measure of similarity, between the strings of two records within a field. If the comparator score exceeds a specified threshold, the two records are considered a match. Grannis and colleagues (2004) have shown that Jaro–Winkler can achieve sensitivities exceeding 97%, which is approximately 10% greater than requiring exact matches for linkage [39].

The details of the algorithms are beyond the scope of this text, but readers who are interested in comparators are referred to the appendix of Gill (2001) "Methods for automatic record matching and linkage and their use in national statistics" for a nice review of methodology and applications of phonetic transformations as well as the article by Grannis and colleagues (2004) for a review of approximate string comparators.

Blocking

Imagine the scenario where an organization newly joins the HIE and, based on their eMPI, has 100,000 unique patients in their private database. Say, for instance, the CR contains 1,000,000 unique patients. In all likelihood, some of the 100,000 patients from the organization are already uniquely identified within the CR from encounters at other organizations. Therefore, each unique record in the organization's eMPI must be compared to each unique record in the CR's MPI, leading to (100,000× 1,000,000) 100 billion possible pairs to evaluate. A naive approach would attempt to make these computationally infeasible comparisons. To increase the efficiency of the matching process, regardless of the matching algorithm to be deployed, records are often considered for comparison only if they match on a few specific identifiers, such as the last four digits of SSN or zip code combined with age. The datasets are then separated into blocks, or subsets, and candidate matches are only evaluated within each block.

People perform blocking to assist them in tasks on a daily basis. For example, if you are searching the phone book for Timothy McFarlane, you may first mentally block based on those with the last name beginning with Mc, then the first name Tim or Timothy. Intuitively, this process is much more efficient than starting at the A's and searching each name until you find the one for which you are looking. CR blocking fields should be those which are least prone to recording errors, have high discriminatory power, and have uniform distributions in the population [40]. Generally, it is advisable to perform multiple passes of blocking, with different blocking criteria, to catch false nonmatches or missed matches that failed to agree on the previous blocking criteria [41].

Deterministic Matching

Also known as heuristic, rule-based, exact, and all-or-none algorithms, deterministic matching techniques typically use a set of rules based on either exact matching of two records or the use of field comparators and phonetic transformations for near matching. Deterministic models are best when both records contain a field that is highly discriminatory. The UPI, organization-specific MRN, and to a lesser degree, SSN, represent examples of fields often used in deterministic matching. In fact, most information systems implement a basic deterministic matching algorithm using exact (MRN or SSN) or partial matching (name and date of birth) [42]. However, basic deterministic models are severely limited by the quality and completeness of data and by the discriminatory power of the identifier. Accuracy can be improved by first matching on a ubiquitous and highly discriminatory identifier (eg, SSN) and then further confirming with additional traits such as sex, name, and date of birth [43]. Because of the need for precision and accuracy, and heterogeneous nature of data across entities, purely deterministic algorithms are not typically well-suited for a CR. Even in instances where UPIs have been distributed nationwide, such as in the United Kingdom, it is advisable to supplement with additional patient traits [44].

Probabilistic Matching

The reality that data moving across entities often do not contain complete, error-free data fields, or universal UPIs necessitates the usage of probabilistic record linkage techniques. Contrasting with deterministic methods, probabilistic models do not require an exact match and the allowance of partial matches (or nonmatches) is quantified in a more statistically rigorous manner. The most widely adopted method was developed by Fellegi and Sunter (1969), based on the ideas introduced by Newcombe (1959), which draws from maximum likelihood theory to produce probabilities that two records represent the same person [2,45]. At a basic level, a weight, or probability, is calculated for each matching variable and these weights are summed to create a score representing the degree to which a pair of records is believed to be a correct match. If these scores are greater than an appointed upper threshold they are deemed a true match, if they fall below a lower threshold they are deemed a true nonmatch, and if they are in between the thresholds the pair represents a possible match. Although in practice possible matches often require human review, more sophisticated decision rules have been shown to perform at a high level when human intervention is not feasible [46,47].

The performance of a decision rule can be simply quantified by:

- $\text{Sensitivity} = \dfrac{\text{True Match}}{\text{True Match} + \text{False NonMatch}}$
  $= \text{The true positive rate (aka recall)}$

  and $1 - \text{sensitivity} = \text{false-negative rate}$

- $\text{Specificity} = \dfrac{\text{True Non-Match}}{\text{True NonMatch} + \text{False Match}}$
  $= \text{The true negative rate}$

  and $1 - \text{specificity} = \text{false-positive rate}$

A false negative occurs when a pair of records match in reality but the decision rule declared them as a nonmatch. On the other hand, a false positive occurs when two truly nonmatching records are erroneously linked together. In health care, it is usually desirable to

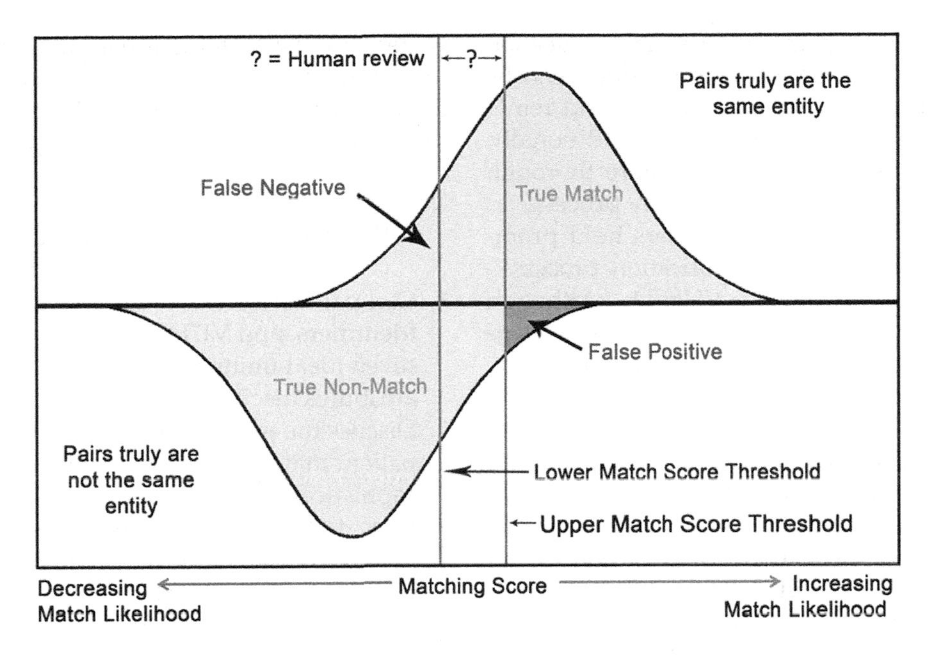

FIGURE 11.5 Decision rules and results of probabilistic matching techniques.

control the rate of false positives because erroneously linking together data from two different patients may result in significant morbidity and mortality from inappropriate treatments. False negatives may also lead to incomplete information regarding medical conditions, medications, or allergies, but these errors are analogous to the fragmented nature of health care without HIE, and therefore perceived by many as less severe [11].

It is not possible to eliminate all false positives because there is an inverse relationship between false-negative and false-positive rates; as one measure decreases, the other increases proportionately. That is, there is no free lunch—one can only achieve a false-positive rate of 0% by drastically increasing the rate of false negatives. This concept is illustrated in Figure 11.5 by two distributions; the top represents the distribution of pairs which are actually the same entity, the bottom represents the distribution of pairs which are truly not the same entity, and the area underneath the curves represents the true positive rate and true negative rates. Despite the give-and-take relationship of false positives and negatives, the CR will typically utilize enough reliable and stable matching variables to limit false positives. Implementers of CRs must set a balance between the two errors by tuning the threshold/s which indicate a match based on the available data within the context of their implementation.

EMERGING TRENDS

As reverberated throughout this chapter, data quality is the primary limiting factor for accurate record linkage. In order to improve and simplify linkage, focus must be placed on the data gathering process. From a technical level, data may be improved by implementing standards for data capture (eg, HL7, SNOMED). However, standards will not alleviate all data entry errors or omissions. One method of enhancing data gathering is to continually train personnel for data collection and entry. Once trained, accountability can be established by keeping an error log and remediating users when errors occur. Additionally, users can be incentivized to be more thorough during the data collection and entry process.

Two unique personal identifiers hold promise for simplifying the identification process—biometric identifiers and VUHIDs. Although biometric identifiers have yet to gain acceptance in many developed nations, the technology is becoming more affordable and amenable to daily use. As society becomes more acquainted with biometrics, such as using a fingerprint to unlock their cellular phone, these identifiers may gain acceptance for use in health care settings. Increasing awareness and usage of VUHIDs will simplify patient matching because they represent a UPI issued specifically for health care which can span the entire health system within a country. Issuance from a nongovernment associated central body may alleviate consumer concerns of providing the government with all the details of their health. Furthermore, patients govern usage of their data by using multiple VUHIDs, improving the consumer perception of privacy.

SUMMARY

Health care data are generated from numerous clinical sites, often by different EHR systems. Each organization has its own method of uniquely identifying patients, but these identifiers are incapable of identifying patient records from outside organizations. Currently, no single unique patient identifier is capable of spanning the entire health care environment, and record linkage must rely upon multiple patient attributes and identifiers. The CR handles inconsistent completeness and quality of identifying data by standardizing incoming data and employing statistical matching algorithms to link data from separate organizations for the same patient. Once identified, a single, unique identifier (the MPI) is associated with the patient, allowing HIE networks to create and maintain patient-centric records and services.

QUESTIONS FOR DISCUSSION

1. Compare and contrast SSN, Biometric Identifiers, and VUHIDs in terms of the seven ideal unique patient identifier attributes discussed in the chapter.
2. Discuss the impact data quality has on CR patient matching. Is it preferable to have a sophisticated algorithm or high-quality data?
3. How do CRs limit the number of potential matches before deploying matching algorithms? Describe how this is achieved.
4. What are the differences between deterministic and probabilistic matching algorithms? Is one preferred to the other?

References

[1] Dunn HL. Record linkage. Am J Public Health Nations Health 1946;36(12):1412–6.

[2] Newcombe HB, Kennedy JM, Axford SJ, James AP. Automatic linkage of vital records. Science (New York, NY) 1959;130(3381):954–9.

[3] Herzog TH, Scheuren F, Winkler WE. Record linkage. Wiley interdisciplinary reviews. Comput Stat 2010;2(5):535–43.

[4] Winkler W. Matching and Record Linkage Washington DC. Available from: <http://www.census.gov/srd/papers/pdf/rr93-8.pdf>; 1993.

[5] Department of Health. The operating framework for the NHS in England 2012–2013. London, England; 2011.

[6] Gill L. Methods for automatic record matching and linkage and their use in national statistics. Norwich: National Statistics. Her Majesty's Stationary Office; 2001.

[7] Wild WG. The theory of modulus N check digit systems. Comput Bull 1968;12:308–11.

[8] Fernandes L., Schumacher S. Universal health identifiers: issues and requirements for successful patient information exchange. IBM Software, 2010.

[9] Markle Foundation Working Group on Accurately Linking Information for Health Care Quality and

Safety. Linking health care information: proposed methods for improving care and protecting privacy; 2005.
[10] ASTM E1717-07 Standard guide for properties of a Universal Healthcare Identifier (UHID). West Conshohocken, PA: ASTM International; 2013.
[11] Hillestad R, Bigelow J, Chaudhry B, Dreyer P, Greenberg M, Meili R, et al. Identity Crisis: an examination of the costs and benefits of a unique patient identifier for the U.S. Health care system. Santa Monica, CA: RAND Corporation; 2008.
[12] 42 U.S.C. 1320d-2(b)(1). Available from: <http://www.gpo.gov/fdsys/pkg/USCODE-2011-title42/pdf/USCODE-2011-title42-chap7-subchapXI-partC-sec1320d-2.pdf>.
[13] HIMSS Patient Identity Integrity Work Group. Patient identity integrity white paper; 2009.
[14] Public Law 105-277 106th Congress. Available from: <http://www.gpo.gov/fdsys/pkg/PLAW-105publ277/pdf/PLAW-105publ277.pdf>.
[15] U.S. Department of Health and Human Services. White paper on unique health identifier for individuals. Washington, DC; 1998: Revised 2011.
[16] Fernandes L, O'Connor M. Patient identification in three acts. J AHIMA 2008;79(4):46–9. quiz 51-2.
[17] Prabhakar S, Pankanti S, Jain AK. Biometric recognition: security and privacy concerns. IEEE Secur Priv 2003;1(2):33–42.
[18] Gelb A, Clark J. Identification for Development: The Biometrics Revolution. Center for Global Development; 2013.
[19] Pato J, Millett L. Biometric recognition: challenges and opportunities. Washington DC: The National Academies Press; 2010.
[20] ASTM E2553-07 Standard guide for implementation of a voluntary universal healthcare identification system. West Conshohocken, PA: ASTM International; 2013.
[21] Netter WJ. Curing the unique health identifier: a reconciliation of new technology and privacy rights. Jurimetrics. 2003;43(2):165–86.
[22] Hieb BR. The case for a voluntary national healthcare identifier. J ASTM Int 2006;3(2).
[23] Hieb B, Macmillan R. Moving toward zero: how to solve the United States healthcare person matching challenge. : Global Patient Identifiers, Inc. 2013.
[24] Dimitropoulos L, Grannis S, Banger AK, Harris DH. Privacy and security solutions for interoperable health information exchange. Chicago, IL: RTI International; 2009.
[25] Health Information and Quality Authority. International review of unique health identifiers for individuals; 2010.
[26] Beck E, Santas X. Developing and using individual identifiers for the provision of health services including HIV. Montreux, Switzerland: UNAIDS; 2009.
[27] American Diabetes Association. Your health care team Alexandria, VA2015 [cited August 17, 2015]. Available from: <http://www.diabetes.org/living-with-diabetes/treatment-and-care/whos-on-your-health-care-team/your-health-care-team.html?referrer=https://www.google.com/>.
[28] National Center for Health Statistics Marriage and divorce. Atlanta, GA: Centers for Disease Control and Prevention; 2011. Available from: <http://www.cdc.gov/nchs/fastats/marriage-divorce.htm>.
[29] Schacter J. Why people move: exploring the March 2000 current population survey. Washington, DC: United States Census Bureau; 2001.
[30] United States Census Bureau. Migration/Geographic mobility 2014 [updated March 2015]. Available from: <http://www.census.gov/hhes/migration//data/cps/cps2014.html>.
[31] Health Level Seven International Standards. Available from: <http://www.hl7.org/implement/standards/index.cfm?ref=nav>; 2015.
[32] Alcantra A. PhilHealth health data dictionary: Philippine Health Insurance Corporation; n.d. [cited June 15, 2015]. Available from: <http://www.aehin.org/Portals/0/AeHIN%20Hour/Bonus%20Session/PhilHealth%20HDD.pdf>.
[33] Republic of Philippines Department of Health. Unified health management information system, national health data dictionary version 2 2011 [cited 2015 06/15]. Available from: <http://uhmis.doh.gov.ph/downloads/forms/135-national-health-data-dictionary-version-2.html>.
[34] International Standards Organization. ISO/IEC 5218:2004—codes for the representation of human sexes 2004. Available from: <http://www.iso.org/iso/catalogue_detail.htm?csnumber=36266>.
[35] International Standards Organization. ISO/TS 22220:2011—Identification of subjects of healthcare 2011. Available from: <http://www.iso.org/iso/home/store/catalogue_tc/catalogue_detail.htm?csnumber=59755>.
[36] International Standards Organization. ISO 21091:2013: Health informatics—Directory services for healthcare providers, subjects of care and other entities. 2013. Available from: <http://www.iso.org/iso/home/store/catalogue_tc/catalogue_detail.htm?csnumber=51432>.
[37] Winkler W. Overview of record linkage and current research directions. Washington, DC: U.S. Census Bureau Statistical Research Division; 2006.
[38] Zadeh L. Commonsense knowledge representation based on fuzzy logic. Computer 1983;16(10):61–5.
[39] Grannis SJ, Overhage JM, McDonald C. Real world performance of approximate string comparators for use in patient matching. Stud Health Technol Inform 2004;107(Pt 1):43–7.

[40] Jaro M. Advances in record-linkage methodology as applied to matching the 1985 Census of Tampa, Florida. J Am Stat Assoc 1989;84:414–20.
[41] Mason CA, Tu S. Data linkage using probabilistic decision rules: a primer. Birth defects research Part A. Clin Mol Teratol 2008;82(11):812–21.
[42] Bartschat W, Burrington-Brown J, Carey S, Chen J, Deming S, Durkin S, et al. Surveying the RHIO landscape. A description of current RHIO models, with a focus on patient identification. J AHIMA 2006;77(1) 64a–64d.
[43] Grannis SJ, Overhage JM, McDonald CJ. Analysis of identifier performance using a deterministic linkage algorithm. Proc AMIA Symp 2002:305–9.
[44] Lichtner V, Wilson S, Galliers JR. The challenging nature of patient identifiers: an ethnographic study of patient identification at a London walk-in centre. Health Inform J 2008;14(2):141–50.
[45] Fellegi IP, Sunter SB. A theory of record linkage. J Am Stat Assoc 1969;64(328):1183–210.
[46] Grannis SJ, Overhage JM, Hui S, McDonald CJ. Analysis of a probabilistic record linkage technique without human review. AMIA Annu Symp Proc 2003:259–63.
[47] Winkler W. Using the EM algorithm for weight computation in the Felligi-Sunter model of record linkage. In: Division USCBSR, editor. Washington, DC; 2000.

CHAPTER

12

Facility Registries: Metadata for Where Care Is Delivered

Timothy D. McFarlane[1], *Scott Teesdale*[2] *and Brian E. Dixon*[3]

[1]Indiana University, Richard M. Fairbanks School of Public Health, Indianapolis, IN
[2]InSTEDD [3]Indiana University, Richard M. Fairbanks School of Public Health and the Center for Biomedical Informatics, the Regenstrief Institute, Indianapolis, IN

OUTLINE

LEARNING OBJECTIVES

By the end of this chapter, the reader should be able to:

- Define the concept of a facility registry.
- Differentiate between a master facility list and health facility registry.
- Recognize the value of health facility registries in supporting health care systems as well as reform.
- Discuss various methods of generating unique identifiers for health care facilities.
- Recommend facility registry signature and service domain components based on local context.
- Describe how metadata enable facility data integration and harmonization.

INTRODUCTION

In the previous chapter, we discussed how to identify each unique individual to link patient-centric data, answering the question: who do these data represent? The focus now shifts to identifying and describing the facilities where care is delivered. A facility can be defined "as a concept which represents multiple dimensions of care delivery location" including its name, location, clinical services, organizational hierarchy, and infrastructure [1]. Health care delivery is scattered among thousands of facilities, and the rapid pace of evolution in the health care environment results in frequent changes to facility services, resources, staffing, and ownership. In the absence of regular, systematic identification and description of facilities, it is difficult, if not impossible, for stakeholders to grasp the complete nature of services in a community or country. Comprehensively identifying facilities establishes a connection for linkage of secondary data and a means of primary data collection, which enables the determination of factors that may be used for decision-making and planning, such as what care services are provided, how services are funded, population access to care, quality of services, and the state of health care infrastructure [2].

Although related, it is important to note that the facility where care is delivered and the provider of said care are, in fact, distinct. Many providers, of different specialties, will deliver services at a single facility, and a single provider may practice at multiple facilities. Furthermore, business processes make distinguishing between providers and facilities acutely important. For example, identifying a provider at a given facility does not provide insight as to the conditions and resources of the facility in which they practice nor would it detail all of the services offered at the facility. Identification of health workers, including providers, is the focus of the chapter "Health Worker Registries: Managing the Health Care Workforce."

FACILITY REGISTRY BACKGROUND

Integrated and interoperable health information systems are critical to improve the quality

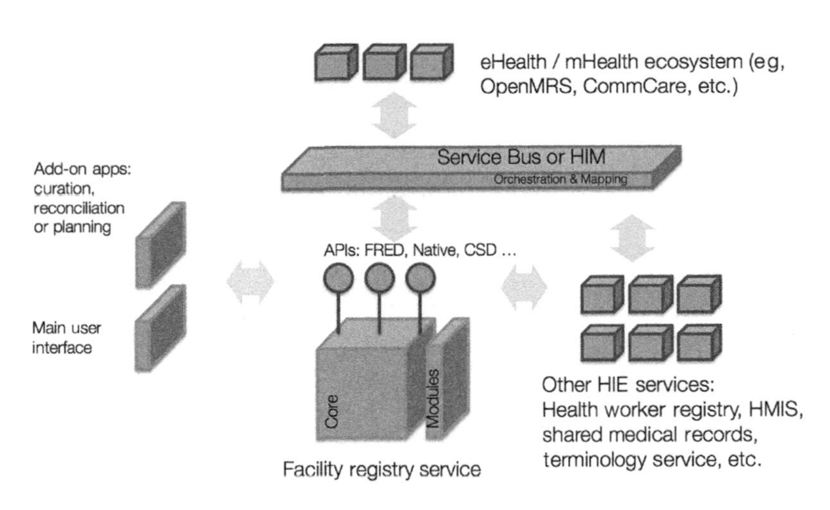

FIGURE 12.1 Facility registry conceptual model. *Source: Provided by the OpenHIE facility registry community.*

and continuity of health care. Improved data sharing among electronic health (eHealth) tools can serve to reduce both redundancy and cost associated with each system. Despite the potential value of health information exchange (HIE), many eHealth systems continue to be highly fragmented. One example of this challenge can be observed among systems that collect and store separate lists of health facilities with divergent levels of standardization, curation, quality, and completeness. Registries are fundamental to addressing the challenges related to normalizing reference data sets and facilitating interoperability. The purpose of a *health facility registry (FR)* is to act as the central authority to collect, store, and distribute an up-to-date and standardized set of facility data. The resulting current, canonical facility data set stored in the registry is called a *master facility list (MFL)* and is the key to linking disparate data sources.

While closely related, an FR can be understood as the technology that manages and shares facility data, while an MFL is the standardized data stored in the registry. Accordingly, an FR acts as a source of truth to collect, store, and share facility data. To further differentiate between the FR and MFL, refer to Fig. 12.1, a basic conceptual model of an FR, and Fig. 12.2, a depiction of the data stored in the MFL. As Fig. 12.1 details, the FR includes the technical infrastructure necessary to integrate MFL data with external information systems (eg, eHealth point-of-service applications), user interfaces, and applications to facilitate data contribution and consumption. On the other hand, the simple schema of the MFL displayed in Fig. 12.2 pertains only to the facility-related data. These data will be the primary focus of this chapter; however, core FR functionalities will be introduced.

From a technical point of view, an FR is relatively simple. The difficulties with implementation are often sociopolitical; feasibly balancing the needs and interests of private, public, and governmental facilities or agencies, and consumers is complex. Thus, facility data contribution and consumption should mirror the diversity of the users.

The strategy for implementing an FR is heavily influenced by local contexts, largely because health care administration, health care infrastructure and governance, and resources for developing the registry will differ by country, region, or state. The first step of the process is

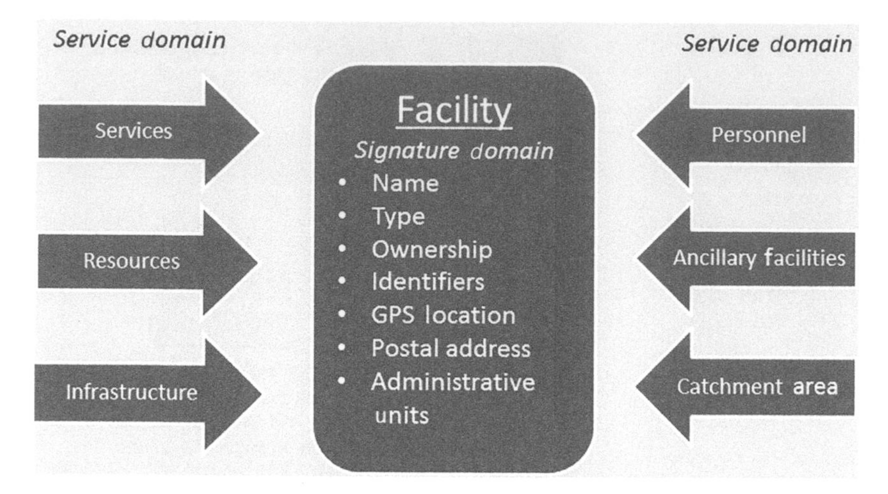

FIGURE 12.2 Master facility list domains and data elements.

to understand the landscape, stakeholders, and assets for the planned implementation area. Do all facilities have some form of electronic data storage, and if so, is connectivity (eg, web-based services) available? Are there current means of identifying facilities, and if so, what gaps need to be filled by the FR?

The key to any successful implementation is understanding stakeholder needs and motivations. Because an FR may span a diverse network of stakeholders, with various types of information systems, it is critical to unite entities interested in facility data to ensure concordance of data standardization, thus promoting interoperability and benefits. Local stakeholders may hold the key to understanding what data sources or assets are already established and available for amalgamation into the registry.

Requirements of the FR must be established to address what the registry will achieve and how it will operate. Requirements should be the result of a collaborative effort between FR implementers and key stakeholders. The requirements will be met by appointing data specifications based on both existing metadata and data collected specifically for the purposes of the FR, when necessary.

Development of an FR should be an iterative process to recognize, prioritize, and address stakeholder needs or use cases, as well as add new stakeholders or use cases as they develop over time. The iterative process allows the registry to grow by continuously adding entities that provide or consumer facility data, maximizing value to the health care community.

Throughout this chapter, we will reference two examples of FR implementations in the countries of Rwanda and Tanzania. The FR in these countries utilized the open-source reference implementation, Resource Map [3]. Resource Map was developed by InSTEDD, a nonprofit technology organization that focuses on solutions which support health, safety, and sustainable development.

THE VALUE OF FRs

The FR serves as a consistent list across all information systems that track health care activity and therefore should serve as a reference for point-of-service applications to facilitate care coordination by managing, for example, referrals and tracking of patient services. As the demand for data-driven decision-making has increased, so has the need to understand where facilities are and what services are available in governing, planning, strengthening, and monitoring the health care environment. Facility-based data enable researchers and planners, from both governmental and nongovernmental agencies, to monitor and evaluate how factors like service availability and delivery, health workforce, health information systems, medical products and technologies, financing, and leadership are related to improved health outcomes, responsiveness, social and financial risk protection, and improved efficiency [4]. For example, health service research often depends on identification of specific facilities to analyze how idiosyncratic nuances in governance, policies, leadership, etc., translate into services and outcomes.

The Veterans Access, Choice, and Accountability Act of 2014 enables greater access to care outside of the Veterans Affairs (VA) health system and requires VA facilities to conduct independent assessments of their eHealth systems, among other directives [5]. Each legislative component in the new law will require facility identification. Outside, non-VA facilities need to be identified for care coordination as well as billing purposes, and health services researchers will need to identify VA facilities for evaluation and quality improvement (QI) of eHealth systems.

In addition to use by professionals and policy makers, facility registries can be made publically available for patients to find a facility that matches their health care needs. For example, in the United States, the Health Resources and Services Administration publishes their facility data warehouse online [6]. The website allows users to find health facilities by name or by entering an address to display nearby facilities with Google maps.

Care Coordination

Due to the nature of health care professional specialization and relatively limited interaction with patients, each provider may be cognizant of only a small piece of the complexity of a patient's overall health status, leading to fragmented perspectives of patient health [7]. This is particularly true in the case of treating and managing chronic diseases, which may require several specialists and frequent encounters in emergency departments (EDs) and hospitals. Bringing together each specialized view of patient's health status, through care coordination, allows for a complete and up-to-date medical history and can improve patient outcomes [8].

An FR provides the means by which care for a patient can be coordinated across the health service environment, supporting policy goals including meaningful use (MU) regulations in the United States [9]. A study by O'Malley and colleagues (2010), which surveyed US physicians, office staff, chief medical officers, electronic medical record (EMR) vendors, and US national experts found the perception that implementation and use of an EMR facilitates within-office care coordination but not coordination between clinicians or settings (facilities). A survey by Schoen and colleagues (2011) revealed that external care coordination is a challenge in multiple nations [10]. This is because eHealth tools, such as EMRs, are necessary but in sufficient, because information systems often lack interoperability [11].

As discussed throughout the book, HIE operates to resolve the discordance between the languages of information systems through application of standards to assimilate data from disparate sources into a shared and longitudinal record (see the chapter: Shared Longitudinal Health Records for Clinical and Population Health). This process brings together the specialized views of patient health but still does not ensure coordination. Furthermore, the contemporary health care consumer is mobile. One study, in the US State of Indiana, found that 40% of ED patients possessed data at multiple institutions and the majority of EDs shared patients with more than 80 other EDs, putting to rest the commonly held belief that "all health care is local" [12]. In order for primary care physicians to facilitate coordination with and between specialists, emergency care, and hospital encounters, they must be able to accurately identify the location and contact information for where all care is delivered, whether within or across health care facilities.

Quality Improvement

Quality, according to the Institute of Medicine, is "the degree to which health services for individuals and populations increase the likelihood of desired health outcomes and are consistent with current professional knowledge" [13]. Under this working definition of quality, Quality Improvement (QI) consists of obtaining measurable improvement in health care services and the health outcomes of those receiving services, with the operative word being measurable [6]. At the facility level, this may consist of projects that improve some workflow process or implementing clinical decision support for access to up-to-date clinical practice guidelines. However, both the scope of QI projects and measureable results often differ from facility to facility; therefore, standardization of quality assessment and improvement is often lacking. It is important to understand how health care facilities are improving at an aggregate level in order to achieve national and global goals for health services (eg, primary cancer prevention) and health outcomes (eg, surveillance and control of communicable diseases). Currently, few countries possess the data necessary to strengthen their health services by evaluating the quality of health services and monitoring temporal changes [14,15]. Of course, crucial to the process is the ability to comprehensively identify all facilities where patient care is delivered.

The FR maintains the MFL, which establishes a standardized identification process and regular point of contact for each facility. Once established, the FR provides an avenue for accurate data collection and analysis over time, as well as improvement in data harmonization by linking different databases pertaining to the same facility. These data may be used to assess goals at any scale, such as access to health services goals set forth by Healthy People 2020 [32]. These goals not only seek to improve access to care but also to understand the determinants of inadequate coverage and explore emerging issues [15].

Public Health

During a public health crisis, a short amount of time could mean the difference between containing the spread of a disease and catastrophic sequelae. The ability to identify and communicate with facilities for information dissemination, coordination, assessment, and utilization of facility-based resources is crucial to rapid response and control of communicable disease outbreaks and other public health emergencies (eg, natural disasters) [16]. For example, if susceptible (ie, unvaccinated or never exposed), nine out of 10 individuals who come into close contact with a measles patient will subsequently develop measles [17].

Intuitively, rapid response to suspected measles cases is pivotal to preventing widespread transmission. Consider the recent outbreak of measles tied to Disney theme parks in Southern California where 39 measles cases occurred among park patrons between December 17, 2014, and December 20, 2014. By February 8, 2015, an additional 86 cases from seven states (mostly California) and three countries were identified as linked to this outbreak, demonstrating the ease at which the disease is transmitted even among a largely vaccinated population [18]. The threat of catastrophic outbreaks of communicable disease is much greater in many developing nations, where the causative organisms are more common and health care infrastructure is often deficient, thus, specifically highlighting the need to know where facilities are located and what services they can handle during a public health emergency.

Yet the issue of identifying facilities is suboptimal even in the United States. In the case of communicable disease reporting, a study by Dixon and colleagues (2011) found the data field indicating the name of the submitter (eg, physician, hospital, or clinic) in electronic laboratory messages was complete for only 57.4–66.5% of transactions and the address of the submitter was complete for only 84.6% of transactions [19]. Incomplete facility data can impede the ability of public health professionals to perform surveillance and manage a disease outbreak or public health emergency in a timely and effective manner.

COMPONENTS OF AN FR

An FR consists of primarily an MFL and the functional components to facilitate contribution to and consumption of the MFL (Fig. 12.1). However, what constitutes a facility in the MFL will vary based on contextual factors and stakeholder needs. After assessing such requirements for the MFL, the HIE can define or customize the following attributes of the MFL as depicted in Fig. 12.2:

- Data specification—technical specification document outlining the data elements to be included in the signature and service domains that define a facility.
- Signature domain—collection of attributes which identify both private and public facilities.
- Service domain—information about the facility with respect to infrastructure, workforce, and/or types of services offered.

In the remainder of this section of the chapter, we briefly introduce the functionality of an FR then discuss the MFL attributes, offering guidance on their design and implementation.

FR FUNCTIONALITY

Similar to other registry components, the functionality of an FR will depend on the needs of stakeholders in a given context. The functionality will iteratively evolve over time as the scope of the registry is expanded. Regardless of scope, several core FR functionalities exist, and are presented in Table 12.1. Briefly, the FR functional components include the following:

- managing the MFL by adding, editing, deleting fields and records;
- creating custom queries through free text searches, filtering, and grouping;
- importing and exporting data in various formats for ease of contribution and/or consumption;
- geospatial mapping of the physical location and attributes of facilities;
- integrating or interfacing an FR with other systems or applications, using SOA or APIs, for interoperability and graphical user interfacing (see the chapter: The Evolving Health Information Infrastructure); and
- managing user authentication for MFL access and layering authorization for MFL capabilities (eg, read/write).

The user stories in Table 12.1 are all examples of successfully implemented FR requests from various stakeholders in Rwanda and Tanzania, and further elucidate how the same functionality can be implemented to serve various needs based on the context.

TABLE 12.1 User Stories of Core Facility Registry Functionalities

Facility Registry Function	User Story for Facility Registry Functions
Managing the MFL	• Collecting and storing an MFL so that users and systems can access and update trustworthy facility information. • Easily editing and adapting the data dictionary of the facility data to remain agile as system requirements change. • Creating fields with single and multiple select lists that can predefine the options available for user selection.
Searching, filtering, and grouping	• Finding a facility by looking up a specific name, identifier, or other field. • Filtering facilities by multiple attributes, such as ownership and facility type, to determine the catchment area served by the area managed by the user. • The ability to view a group of facilities based upon their administrative zone. • Identifying empty fields in order to curate and complete data as needed.
Importing and exporting	• Exporting a list of facilities into a spreadsheet for use outside the FR. • Importing data contained in CSV format to quickly get started with an existing list.
Mapping and visualization	• Establishing the ability to find facilities and visualize administrative zone boundaries. • Establishing the ability to measure the distance between facility locations on a map. • Distinguishing different types of facilities from one another graphically while looking at a map (eg, hospitals from medical clinics, one partner from another)
Integration and API	• Establishing the ability to consume and provide data between the registry and other systems using an API. • Specifying codes to fields, and to options in lookup fields, so that the information exposed in APIs have a stable schema that is not dependent on labels and internationalization. • Creating a notification mechanism around changes to data, metadata, permissions, etc.
Authentication and authorization	• Creating accounts, managing credentials, resetting passwords, etc. • Specifying public collections/layers, to allow for public users to perform searches, and access the API for specified. • Specifying explicit permissions for users to view and/or edit data in different layers.

DATA SPECIFICATION

A data specification document is a technical tool describing the MFL data elements or the information to be managed in the FR. This is a similar concept to a data dictionary where the contents and format of data elements in the system are documented. Critical to the process of data specification is input from a representative group of stakeholders who will use the FR. A number of recommendations for data specification have been proposed but stakeholder input and iterative development is necessary to ensure that the FR is responsive to the users' needs and applicable to the local context. The basic layout of a specification document includes:

- *Variable Name*—The short name and/or the database code used to describe the data element.
- *Definition*—A simple description of the data element, along with any relevant context.
- *Data Type*—Predefined data types are helpful to understand the formatting associated with a data element. Some common data types that have been used in other FRs include

text, numeric, yes/no, select one, select many, hierarchy, date, site, user, identifier, email, and phone.

- *Hierarchy or List Metadata*—Hierarchical, single, and multiple select data elements will have additional categorical or leaf metadata which should also be documented in the data specification.
- *Data Rules*—A description of constraints or conditions that should be applied to a data elements to improve accuracy and clarity. A single select variable, numerical, text field, or a specific algorithm for an identifier such as the Luhn algorithm.
- *Data Source*—A description of the individual, group, and system where this information is generated from. Often an FR will collect partial updates from other systems and it is helpful to understand the source of each data element.
- *Standards*—Documenting any semantic standards or common code sets used as metadata. Documenting these will help with interoperability with other systems.

Signature Domain

The signature domain is a collection of attributes which identify both private and public facilities. In many cases, such as facility name, a single attribute is not sufficient for canonical identification. However, implementation of a unique identifier will, in most cases, provide sufficient discriminatory power for positive facility identification. Recommendations of exemplar data elements by the Health Facility Assessment Technical Group and World Health Organization (WHO) are described in Table 12.2, but may not be applicable in all countries or contexts [15,20].

To respond to the need for current and standardized facility data, the OpenHIE Facility Registry Community recommends proven tools, processes, and technologies to implement facility registries. These resources have been derived from existing reference implementations in Tanzania and Rwanda. As an example of the signature domain, the Rwanda health facility registration form is presented in Fig. 12.3. Although the structure of the form could be used in many contexts, the content will differ based on each country's facility nomenclature and hierarchical structure.

Service Domain

The service domain contains information about the facility in terms of infrastructure, workforce, and types of services offered. Ideally, these data should depict a more granular view of the facility, allowing for assessments of the facility's resources, understanding if the needs of the facility catchment area are being met and planning for the future in terms of staffing and infrastructure. A catchment area is the population which a given facility routinely serves. For example, if there are four facilities in a particular district of a malaria-endemic country and only one offers malarial prophylaxis, diagnosis, and treatment, they may be overwhelmed by patients, from both an infrastructure and staffing point of view. Identifying the gap in services offered will allow for policy makers to make educated decisions about resource allocation.

The services offered section in the Rwandan health facility registration form is provided as an example in Fig. 12.4. In this case, data are captured using simple Boolean (yes/no) responses by asking respondents to check all services that apply. Types of services are binned as clinical, surgical, organ transplants and blood transfusions, pharmacy, prosthetics and medical devices, complementary actions to promote health, diagnostic, and health promotion and prevention. As one can see in Fig. 12.4, this is a simple method for collecting detailed data regarding services rendered at the facility.

The data regarding facility infrastructure can be at a high level, such as having inpatient or

TABLE 12.2 The Signature Domain: Suggested Data Fields from the World Health Organization [14] and Health Facility Assessment Technical Working Group [19]

Attribute	Description	Suggested Data Rules
Date of data collection	The date is invaluable when examining time trends and combining data sets.	Standardized entry based on countries' preferred presentation.
Health facility country registration code or unique identifier	If a district, state, or national ID exists, it should be associated with all data from a facility. This ID is the authoritative and unequivocal facility identifier and acts as the primary key to link data sources.	Should be unique, not vary over time, and be assigned in the same manner for all facilities within the country.
Facility name	The official (full) name of the facility.	A text field for the legal name of the facility, free of abbreviations, and with proper punctuation.
Facility type	The classification of the facility. Example: acute care hospital, clinic, free standing emergency room, long-term care, etc.	Standardization will vary by country of implementation. A central authority (eg, Ministry of Health) should provide facilities with a structured list for selection.
Facility ownership	Examples: military, private, government.	Standardization will vary by country of implementation. A central authority (eg, Ministry of Health) should provide facilities with a structured list for selection.
Facility location/address and contact information	The physical location of the facility. Other pertinent information includes main telephone and fax number, main email address, name of the director, and director's contact information.	Standardization will vary by country of implementation. The address should be given to the lowest possible administrative level and parsed into subparts (eg, street name, street number, ZIP, state/provenance).
Administrative units	Refers to the facilities location in terms of district, provenance, census tract, etc. This is useful for differentiating facilities with identical or similar names.	Avoid including facility name in the field and indicate designated level in hierarchy (eg, 0 = national, 1 = provincial, 2 = district).
Geographical coordinates	The physical coordinates of the facility.	Implementation should reflect the preferred national coordinate system. Generally latitude and longitude recorded in decimal degrees referencing the WGS84 system is often preferred.
Operational status	The operational status of the facility, such as operational, closed, licensed, pending licensure, etc.	Each country should provide operational statuses based on regulatory and licensing bodies.

1. Identification			
Health Facility Name :		FOSA ID: (HMIS unit only)	
Type of health facility :	☐ National Referral Hospital (HNR) ☐ Provincial Referral Hospital (PH) ☐ District Hospital (HD) ☐ Health Center (CS) ☐ Health Post (PS) ☐ Dispensary (DISP) ☐ Community Dispensary (FOSACOM)	☐ Prison Clinic (PRIS) ☐ Medical Clinic (CLIN) ☐ Military Hospital (HM) ☐ District Pharmacy (DP) ☐ Mutuelle/CBHI section (MU) ☐ Blood Bank (BB) ☐ Other, Specify : .	
Status :	☐ Active : ☐ Planned, specify probable opening date : ☐ Closed :		
Category:	☐ Public ☐ Agrée ☐ Private ☐ Community owned ☐ Parastatal (e.g. Military, Police, Prison, State run dispensaries)		
Date inaugurated :			
Name of titulaire/director :		NID #	
email of titulaire/director:		Cell phone #	
Name of primary referral/reporting facility[1]			
Implementing partner organization:			
2. Geographic Coordinates			
Province:		Latitude:	
District:		Longitude:	
Sector:		Catchment area population (list villages in section 5):	
Cell:		Source of population data :	
Village:		Year of population estimate :	
PO box:			
Street:		Number	Complement

FIGURE 12.3 Identifying facilities with the Rwanda health facility registry form signature domain.

maternity beds, or described in more detail by including the types of rooms and beds, vehicles own by the facility, physical barriers for infection control and personal protective equipment, and facility sanitation, among other things. The data elements captured regarding infrastructure are largely country-specific. In Rwanda and other developing countries, it is pertinent to collect fundamental information that may not be relevant to developed countries, such as facilities' power source (if applicable), water source, internet connectivity, modes of transportation, and x-ray capabilities (Fig. 12.5). In addition to basic services, such as x-ray and laboratory testing, stakeholders of developed countries may be more interested in advanced technologies, such as digital imaging, clinical decision support, Da Vinci surgical robotics, smart patient rooms, and robotic drug dispensing.

The final data element captured in the service domain relates to the types and number of staff the facility employs. Although more detailed data may be available from the health worker registry, as will be discussed in the chapter "Health Worker Registries: Managing

4. Services offered (check all services that are offered)					
03		**Clinical services**	**06**		**Pharmacy**
0301		Primary Outpatient Curative Consultation (CPC)	0601		Pharmacy
0302		Hospitalization	**07**		**Prosthetics and Medical devices**
0303		Emergency care	0701		Prosthetics
0304		Dentistry	0702		Other medical devices
0305		General Ophthalmology	**08**		**Complementary actions to promote health**
0306		Integrated Management of Childhood Illness	0801		Hygiene and environmental health
0307		Management of gender violence	0802		Medico-Legal documentation
0308		Mental Health Services	0803		Pre-marital Consultation
0309		Physical therapy	0804		Vector and Zoonosis control
0310		Nutritional Rehabilitation	0805		Epidemiological Surveillance and Response
0311		Cardiovascular care and treatment	**02**		**Diagnostic services**
0312		TB care and treatment	0201		Laboratory
0313		Care and treatment for persons living with HIV/AIDS	0202		Voluntary Counseling and Testing
0314		Diabetes care and treatment	0203		Ultrasound
0315		Other Non Communicable disease (NCD) care and treatment	0204		Medical Imagery (x-ray)
0316		Management of dystocic pregnancies	**01**		**Health promotion and prevention**
0317		Post-abortion care	0101		Ante-natal consultation
0318		Deliveries - high risk	0102		Behavior Change Communication/Health Education
0319		Deliveries – normal	0103		Community mobilization
0320		Newborn care	0104		Family Planning
04		**Surgical services**	0105		Post Natal Consultation
0401		Major surgical interventions	0106		Growth Monitoring/Nutrition Surveillance
0402		Minor surgical interventions	0107		Vaccination
05		**Organ transplants and Blood transfusions**	0108		Psychosocial support
0501		Blood bank	0109		General Health Promotion Activities
0502		Organ transplants			

FIGURE 12.4 Capturing facility health service availability with the Rwanda health facility registry form.

3. Infrastructure				
Number of rooms (clinical and administrative) :			Number of patient beds:	
Transport available : (and functional)	# of ambulances		Principal water source:	☐ National piped water supply ☐ Local piped water supply ☐ Protected well ☐ Open well ☐ Surface water (river, lake, etc.) ☐ Rain water reservoir ☐ Water truck ☐ No regular water source
	# of cars			
	# of motorcycles			
Principal electricity source :	☐ National grid ☐ Generator, specify KVA : ☐ Solar panels ☐ No electricity			
Cold chain:	# of functional refrigerators/freezers:		Computers :	# functioning
Communication: (belonging to FOSA)	☐ Fixed telephone	N°	Internet connetion:	☐ Cell modem ☐ Fixed line (ADSL, fibre) ☐ Satellite (VSAT) ☐ Wireless (WIMAX, etc.) ☐ No internet connection
	☐ Mobile telephone	N°		
	☐ Radio			

FIGURE 12.5 Assessment of facility infrastructure using the Rwanda health facility registry form.

TABLE 12.3 Possible Facility-Specific Data Elements for Services, Infrastructure, and Workforce for the Service Domain

Services Offered	Infrastructure	Workforce
General clinical services (inpatient/outpatient care)	Types of rooms	Primary care physicians
Malaria diagnosis and treatment	Types of beds	Specialist physicians
TB diagnosis, care, and treatment	Ambulances	Subspecialist physicians
Cardiovascular care and treatment	Cars	Physician assistants
HIV/AIDS prevention	Motorcycles	Nurse practitioners
HIV/AIDS care and treatment	Sterilization and infection control	Nurses
Therapeutics	Referral point	Radiology technicians
Prosthetics and medical devices	Source of energy	Laboratory technologists
Health promotion and disease prevention	Mobile networks	Respiratory therapists
Diagnostic services	Source of water	Midwives
Reproductive and child health care services	Toilet facility	Clinical nursing assistants
Growth monitoring/nutrition surveillance	Toilet remarks	Medical assistants
Oral health service (dental services)	Waste management	
ENT services		
Emergency preparedness		

the Health Care Workforce," it is important to maintain an aggregated list of personnel for each facility for emergency preparedness and assessing facility-specific workforce needs. A nonexhaustive list of proposed data elements for the service domain is listed in Table 12.3.

CREATING UNIQUE IDENTIFIERS

The long-term goal of the FR should be to develop and uniformly implement unique identifiers for facilities. Furthermore, as discussed above, it is often challenging to uniquely identify facilities by their names alone. Many techniques are available for generating and assigning unique facility identifiers for the signature domain. Regardless of the method employed, manual generation is discouraged because of the increased likelihood of error and duplication. The intent is to create and disseminate a standardized unique identifier which serves as the primary, authoritative, and unequivocal identifier for a given facility. Thus, once assigned, the identifier must be permanently attached to a facility regardless of changes in physical location, ownership, and name.

We now discuss two sets of candidates that an HIE or country might consider when considering the design of its MFL. The first set is derived from a report by the WHO. The second comes from a US-based case study involving HIE to improve disability determination.

WHO Candidate Identifiers

Three types of identifiers are described in a WHO report on creating MFLs, each with their own merits and pitfalls: integer codes, facility codes, and universally unique identifiers (UUIDs) [15]. An example of a fourth unique identifier is the facility identification number used in the Tanzania, Africa, FR.

Integer codes

Integer codes are automatically generated and managed by a central authority. The numbers generated are considered information-free because they do not contain any facility-specific attributes, such as an administrative unit prefix. For this reason, integer codes can stand the test of time when facilities relocate or alter their affiliations, and they are guaranteed to be unique when generated by a central authority. When implemented in decentralized architectures, a range of numbers can be assigned to each administrative unit. For example, District A corresponds to a combination of three integers from 000 to 100 and district B is represented by 101 to 200.

Facility codes

Identifiers containing a combination of numbers and letters that frequently include some piece of facility-specific information, which may or may not be human readable, are referred to as facility codes. For example, the code in Fig. 12.6 can be segmented into three letters for country code, followed by three numbers for first administrative district, the next three identify the lower level district, then a series of numbers identifying the facility. The primary difficulty of facility codes is they would need to be updated if a facility was to move or the country restructured their districts.

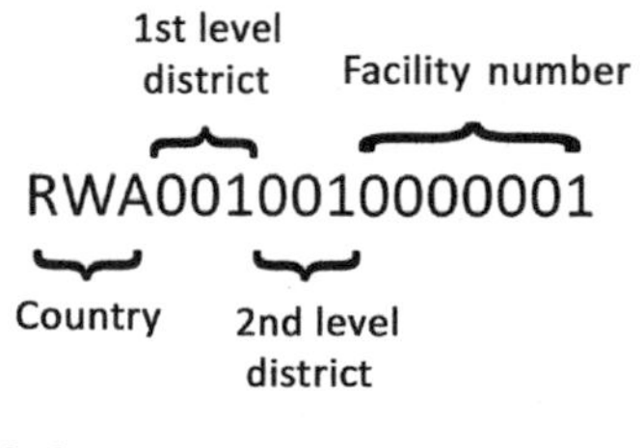

FIGURE 12.6 Components of a facility code.

Universally Unique Identifiers (UUIDs)

Also known as globally unique identifiers, UUIDs represent a standard identifier that is ubiquitous throughout computer applications. UUIDs are a 128-bit value, for example, 261a7f40-1f9f-11e5-adfc-0002a5d5c51b, that can be uniquely generated by a standard algorithm regardless assigning entity's location. As such, UUIDs are well-suited for decentralized architectures where no central issuing authority is designated.

The Tanzanian Facility Identifier Number

The Tanzanian FR identifies facilities using an autogenerated sequential number allocated to each facility when it is added to the MFL. It is generated by the central FR and provided back to the health community for subsequent use, replacing the old registration ID. The ID follows the format: xxxxxx-y, where xxxxxx is a six-digit numeric code and y is a one-digit check digit, generated via the Luhn Algorithm. The Luhn algorithm, an ISO standard, is a modulus 10 "double-add-double" algorithm which is used to generate check digits in numerous identification systems including the US Centers for Medicare and Medicaid Services (CMS) National Provider Identifier (NPI) [21].

Other Candidates for Creating Unique Identifiers

In search of unique identifiers for facilities in a US-based HIE, Dixon and colleagues (2014) considered the following candidates: object identifiers (OIDs), NPIs, and health industry numbers (HINs) [1].

Object Identifiers (OIDs)

OIDs are globally unique identifiers for objects in a distributed system, and they are an alternative to UUIDs. Many health care networks and facilities in the United States already possess OIDs, as they are required for HL7 CDA-based HIE transactions in compliance with MU to identify assigning authorities in messages. Unfortunately, OIDs are sometimes reused within a given health system network of facilities. Therefore, to be effective, unique OIDs would need to be created and maintained at a health system level making maintenance of an MFL for a community or nation challenging as health systems expand and contract.

National Provider Identifiers (NPIs)

Created by CMS, NPIs uniquely identify providers, but providers frequently practice at multiple medical facilities. CMS also allows health care organizations and facilities to request NPIs, so an alternative approach would be to require facilities to obtain an NPI if it did not already have one. However, many medical centers are large campuses composed of numerous and variable buildings, clinics, private offices, and other care delivery units. The NPI of a medical center can apply to multiple physical locations that vary greatly in the type(s) of care delivered (eg, intensive, acute, rehabilitation, chronic, long-term residential). Therefore, there would have to be consensus on the level of granularity of the lowest denominator NPI.

Health Industry Numbers (HINs)

The HIN is a unique identifier used in electronic data interchange transactions among health care trading partners for supply chain management [22]. These identifiers are maintained by the Health Industry Business Communications Council, an accredited international standards development organization which uses multiple sources to identify human health care facilities and assign each a unique identifier. A database of HIN identifiers is available for licensing. Current HIN licensees are predominantly pharmaceutical companies, medical device manufacturers, and wholesalers [23]. To date, there has been no use of the HIN database within HIEs despite the list of licensees including so-called data intermediaries.

The identifier chosen to uniquely represent facilities should reflect stakeholder consensus as well as governance and health care structures. Beyond unique identification, the FR provides the technology to standardize and manage data that describe the facility, and will be the focus for the remainder of the chapter. The 2014 Ebola virus outbreak in West Africa represents a prime example of the requisite need for data which goes beyond facility identification. It is essential to quickly ascertain facilities with personnel capable of handling the deadly potentially deadly virus and also have the infrastructure required to protect health care workers and other patients (eg, full body coverage and isolation rooms). Identifying well-equipped facilities allows public health to act fast in establishing centers to immediately provide care and prevent further transmission of the virus.

DATA SOURCES FOR CONSTRUCTING THE MFL

Limiting expenditures in the health care environment is often a top priority for policy makers. Therefore those implementing an FR should use existing data sources when possible. The initial goal in creating an FR should be to compile a complete MFL for the country or service area. If an MFL is already in place, this should be used to populate the FR. Even in the case where no MFL exists, most countries will have some type of facility list, with varying degrees of completeness and frequency of updates.

An MFL is often governed by the country's Ministry of Health although the list may be generated by a separate licensing regulatory body or health management information system, such as the International Health Information Systems Programmed (HISP) supported by the University of Oslo [24]. In the United States, several sources of facility data exist, including but not limited to: the CMS NPI, the Health Resources and Services Administration's health center data warehouse, the Social Security Administration (SSA), and governmental public health agencies. Furthermore, disease-specific registries (eg, cancer, HIV, and tuberculosis) may provide facility information where each patient received care.

Existing surveys, while not necessarily comprehensive, will assist in populating the MFL as well as obtaining additional service domain data. Examples of surveys include the WHO Service Availability and Readiness Assessment (SARA) and the Service Provision Assessment (SPA) by the US Agency for International Development [25,26].

As should be apparent by now, it is unlikely that a single source will populate all of the data elements desired, establishing the need to link data on a facility from multiple databases. The common identifiers in the signature domain of the MFL provide a mechanism to link disparate data sources to obtain more complete data for the services domain. However, just as the case in linking client-level data, in most cases, facility databases will not be inherently interoperable establishing the need for metadata and standards within the FR.

AN EXAMPLE FROM THE US SOCIAL SECURITY ADMINISTRATION

In 2010, approximately 18.7% or 56.6 million civilian, noninstitutionalized US citizens reported a communicative, mental, or physical disability to the US Social Security Administration (SSA) [27]. The SSA determines disability and awards benefits, including health insurance benefits, through a sequential process that incorporates the medical, legal, and vocational aspects of disabilities [28]. As a part of the claim submission process, individuals submitting claims are required to list the name and addresses for all health care providers and facilities from which they received care and these reported facilities should match health care records. Needless to say, the existing paper-based system is considered by researchers, the Institute of Medicine, and SSA advisory board to be inefficient, often incomplete, and outdated [28–30]. So, in 2010, SSA partnered with the Regenstrief Institute (RI) to facilitate evaluation of submitted claims using a statewide HIE. RI utilized the HL7 continuity of care document (CCD) standard (based on the Clinical Document Architecture or CDA) to populate a comprehensive EHR using information from various health care facilities [1].

In total, between May 2012 and June 2013, RI received over six million encounter transactions and delivered 7732 CCDs to SSA. However, SSA noticed the facility names contained within the CCDs differed from the claimant submissions and were uninterpretable by SSA case reviewers. Some facilities would include a full name (eg, xyz clinic) while others would be cryptic, such as "NORTH". For example, "WKRANC" represented a hospital cardiology service; a university hospital was simply named "UH"; and the surgical ward at a hospital was represented as "B2". Furthermore, the majority of transactions (60.4%) did not provide any value in the CCD field designated for facility identification.

When examining the issue, RI noted that HL7 CCD specifications allow virtually any information to represent a facility. Facilities can be represented by both free text as well as coded elements, yet the codes can be locally developed and maintained. In one case, a large 20 hospital health system used more than 9000 distinct facility identifiers, uniquely identifying every campus, floor, unit, and bed in its network. Other examples included different facility identifiers depending on the information system (eg, laboratory, pharmacy, radiology, etc.) which transmitted the message [1]. Clearly, such facility identifiers are not useful to SSA nor would they be useful for an FR.

This study highlights one of many use cases for a unique and universal facility identifier in the United States and that current systems not only lack standardized identifiers needed for interoperability but also are frequently uninterpretable and impossible to map to standards for data linkage. In order to support care coordination, public health, QI and assurance, research, policy making, and other use cases, the various stakeholders must agree and implement a standardized method for identifying facilities. Once the data specifications are agreed upon, an FR can be tasked with maintaining these data.

EMERGING TRENDS

Health care reform in the United States is having an effect on the number and type of facilities available in the United States health system. Hospitals as well as primary and specialty care practices are partnering to form new integrated delivery networks. Some of these networks are becoming accountable care organizations (ACOs) in which the network accepts shared financial responsibility for providing care to a population in addition to delivering care to individual patients who come in for services. Some ACO models involve multiple networks who partner to manage a population spread across geographic boundaries. These changes make facility identification increasingly important as names, ownership, and service offerings seem to change on a monthly basis. Uniquely identifying facilities would allow for name and service updates without impacting the ability of payers and/or researchers to longitudinally examine aspects of the facilities. Furthermore, ACOs must pay for care no matter whether their managed population receives the care in- or out-of-network. Therefore, ACOs have a need to identify the facilities where their predefined population is receiving care as well as the network or ACO with which that facility associates. Unique identification of facilities, MFLs for states or regions, and the capacity to effectively manage facility information would be a useful service for US-based HIEs. These system factors might become a driving force in creating value worthy of investment.

SUMMARY

Health care facilities are scattered by both geography and scope. Providing access to services, in terms of emergency or routine care, and strengthening appropriate and timely delivery of health care requires the capacity to identify facilities in an area as well as enumerate their menu of services and capabilities. An FR provides the technical infrastructure to develop and manage an MFL for identification, integration of data from various sources, and communication with information systems to harmonize facility data across the health care environment.

Acknowledgments

The authors thank Eduardo Jezierski, CEO of InSTEDD, for his contributions to the Implementation Guide for the OpenHIE FR [31], which served as a primary reference for this chapter. The authors further thank Ed and all those working to implement HIE and facility registries in countries around the world for their input in this chapter and the book.

QUESTIONS FOR DISCUSSION

1. Compare and contrast the different protocols for developing unique facility identifiers. Which method would be preferable for a

rapidly developing and changing health care environment? Which would be preferable for a well-established environment?

2. How can facility registries achieve true interoperability? What are some barriers to interoperability of facility-related data?
3. Discuss why it is important to go beyond facility identification and collect facility services and infrastructure or resources.

References

[1] Dixon BE, Colvard C, Tierney WM. Identifying health facilities outside the enterprise: challenges and strategies for supporting health reform and meaningful use. Inform Health Soc Care 2014;40(4):319–33.

[2] Ritz D., Althauser C., Wilson K. Connecting health information systems for better health: leveraging interoperability standards to link patient, provider, payor, and policymaker data. Seattle, WA. Joint Learning Network For Universal Health Coverage, 2014.

[3] InSTEDD. Resource map 2011 [cited July 30, 2015]. Available from: http://resourcemap.instedd.org/en.

[4] World Health Organization Everybody's business: strengthening health systems to improve health outcomes, WHO's framework for action. Geneva, Switzerland: WHO; 2007.

[5] Dixon BE, Haggstrom DA, Weiner M. Implications for informatics given expanding access to care for Veterans and other populations. J Am Med Inform Assoc 2015;22(4):917–20.

[6] Health Resources and Services Administration Quality improvement. Washington, DC: U.S. Department of Health and Human Services; 2011. [cited June 20, 2015]. Available from: http://www.hrsa.gov/quality/toolbox/methodology/qualityimprovement/.

[7] Office of the National Coordinator for Health Information Technology Benefits of EHRs: improved care coordination. Washington, DC: U.S. Department of Health and Human Services; 2014. [cited June 29, 2015]. Available from: http://www.healthit.gov/providers-professionals/improved-care-coordination.

[8] Bell B, Thornton K. From promise to reality: achieving the value of an EHR. Healthc Financ Manage 2011;65(2):50–6.

[9] Agency for Healthcare Research and Quality. Table 4. Meaningful use measures that assess care coordination: care coordination measures Atlas update. Rockville, MD 2014 [cited June 29, 2015]. Available from: http://www.ahrq.gov/professionals/prevention-chronic-care/improve/coordination/atlas2014/chapter4tab4.html.

[10] Schoen C, Osborn R, Squires D, Doty M, Pierson R, Applebaum S. New 2011 survey of patients with complex care needs in eleven countries finds that care is often poorly coordinated. Health Aff (Project Hope) 2011;30(12):2437–48.

[11] O'Malley AS, Grossman JM, Cohen GR, Kemper NM, Pham HH. Are electronic medical records helpful for care coordination? Experiences of physician practices. J Gen Intern Med 2010;25(3):177–85.

[12] Finnell JT, Overhage JM, Grannis S. All health care is not local: an evaluation of the distribution of Emergency Department care delivered in Indiana. AMIA Annu Symp Proc 2011;2011:409–16.

[13] Institute of Medicine. Crossing the quality chasm: the IOM health care quality initiative 2001. Available from: http://www.iom.edu/Global/News%20Announcements/Crossing-the-Quality-Chasm-The-IOM-Health-Care-Quality-Initiative.aspx.

[14] World Health Organization. Monitoring and evaluation of health systems strengthening: an operational framework. Geneva, Switzerland 2010.

[15] World Health Organization. Creating a master health facility list. Geneva, Switzerland 2012.

[16] Reeder B, Revere D, Hills RA, Baseman JG, Lober WB. Public health practice within a health information exchange: information needs and barriers to disease surveillance. Online Journal of Public Health Inform 2012;4:3.

[17] Centers for Disease Control and Prevention Measles (Rubeola). Atlanta, GA: National Center for Immunization and Respiratory Diseases, Division of Viral Diseases; 2015. [cited June 25, 2015]. Available from: http://www.cdc.gov/measles/hcp/index.html.

[18] Zipprich J, Winter K, Hacker J, Xia D, Watt J, Harriman K. Measles outbreak—California, December 2014–February 2015. MMWR 2015;64(06):153–4.

[19] Dixon BE, McGowan JJ, Grannis SJ. Electronic laboratory data quality and the value of a health information exchange to support public health reporting processes. AMIA Annu Symp Proc 2011;2011:322–30.

[20] Health Facility Assessment Technical Working Group The signature domain and geographic coordinates: a standardized approach for uniquely identifying a health facility. Chapel Hill, NC: Carolina Population Center, University of North Carolina; 2007.

[21] Department of Health and Human Services 45 CFR part 162 HIPAA administrative simplification: standard unique health identifier for health care providers; final rule Prevention CfDCa. Washington, DC: Federal Registrar; 2004.

[22] Health Industry Business Communications Council The health industry number system. Phoenix, AZ: Health Industry Communications Councel; 2012. [cited June 30, 2015]. Available from: http://www.hibcc.org/hin-system/.

[23] Health Industry Business Communications Council Health Industry Number Sytem (HIN) authorize licensees. Phoenix, AZ: Health Industry Communications Councel; 2014. [updated January 24, 2014; cited June 30, 2015]. Available from: http://www.hibcc.org/wp-content/uploads/2012/09/Current-HIN-Authorized-Licensees.pdf.

[24] Oslo Uo. Research: HISP Oslo, Norway; 2011 [updated June 24, 2015; cited July 7, 2015]. Available from: http://www.mn.uio.no/ifi/english/research/networks/hisp/.

[25] World Health Organization. Health statistics and health information systems: service availability and readiness assessment (SARA) Geneva, Switzerland 2015 [cited July 7, 2015]. Available from: http://www.who.int/healthinfo/systems/sara_introduction/en/.

[26] U.S. Agency for International Development The DHS program: service provision assessments (SPA). Rockville, MD: The Demographic and Health Surveys Program; 2015. [cited July 7, 2015]. Available from: http://dhsprogram.com/What-We-Do/Survey-Types/SPA.cfm.

[27] Brault MW. U.S. Department of Commerce Americans with disabilities: 2010. Washington, DC: U.S. Census Bureau Economics and Statistics Administration; 2012. p. 70–131.

[28] Social Security Advisory Board. Aspects of disability decision making: data and materials Washington, DC: U.S. Social Security Administration; 2012 [cited July 23, 2015]. Available from: http://www.ssab.gov/Publications/Disability/GPO_Chartbook_FINAL_06122012.pdf.

[29] Ni P, McDonough CM, Jette AM, Bogusz K, Marfeo EE, Rasch EK, et al. Development of a computer-adaptive physical function instrument for Social Security Administration disability determination. Arch Phys Med Rehabil 2013;94(9):1661–9.

[30] Institute of Medicine Improving the social security disability decision process Stobo JD, McGeary M, Barnes DK, editors. Committee on improving the disability decision process: SSA's listing of impairments and agency access to medical expertise. Washington, DC: The National Academies Press; 2007.

[31] OpenHIE. OpenHIE Health Facility Registry Implementation Guide. 2015 Feb [cited August 1, 2015] Available from: https://ohie.org/facility-registry/#pe-accordion-item-8-7.

[32] Office of Disease Prevention and Health Promotion 2020 topics and objectives: Access to health services. Washington, DC: Department of Health and Human Services; 2015. [cited July 23, 2015]. Available from: http://www.healthypeople.gov/2020/topics-objectives/topic/Access-to-Health-Services.

CHAPTER

13

Health Worker Registries: Managing the Health Care Workforce

Jennifer M. Alyea[1], *Dykki Settle*[2], *Carl Leitner*[3] *and Brian E. Dixon*[4]

[1]Indiana University Richard M. Fairbanks School of Public Health, Indianapolis, IN [2]PATH, Seattle, WA [3]IntraHealth International, Chapel Hill, NC [4]Indiana University Richard M. Fairbanks School of Public Health; and the Center for Biomedical Informatics, Regenstrief Institute, Inc., Indianapolis, IN

OUTLINE

LEARNING OBJECTIVES

By the end of this chapter, the reader should be able to:

- Define a health worker.
- Identify sources of health worker data and describe the limitations of their use.

- Define a health worker registry.
- Identify and describe potential uses for a health worker registry in the context of health information exchange.
- Explain the process of developing a minimum data set for a health worker registry.
- Identify syntactic and semantic standards to support a health worker registry.

INTRODUCTION

As described in earlier chapters, registries play an important role in health information exchange (HIE). Client registries, for example, facilitate patient-level data transfer and allow for continuous longitudinal patient care across episodic health care encounters (see the chapter: Client Registries: Identifying and Linking Patients). Facility registries provide a central authority to store, manage, and share health facility identification, services, and resource data across a community, state, or nation (see the chapter: Facility Registries: Metadata for Where Care Is Delivered). Here we present another type of registry—the health worker registry (HWR)—as an additional component of HIE for use across myriad contexts by multiple stakeholders.

The health care field consists of workers from a variety of professions, including clinical workers such as physicians and nurses, but also health sector and facility managers, pharmacists, pharmaceutical supply chain workers, ambulance drivers, and even volunteer community health workers, just to name a few. Harmonization of information about health care workers—such as licensure and employment data—across these various fields can allow for efficient workforce planning, identification of worker shortages, emergency response preparation, and improved coordination of care. However, the current patchwork of data sources and variations in content often preclude their use for these purposes. In this chapter, we discuss how the inclusion of an HWR within an HIE can help to address this gap and maximize information gained from the available health worker data sets.

NEED FOR COORDINATED HEALTH CARE WORKER DATA

Health care is a multifaceted field consisting of a diverse and multidisciplinary workforce. Indeed, the definition of who is a "health worker" is broad and extensive. According to the World Health Organization (WHO), health workers are "all people engaged in activities whose primary intent is to enhance health" [1, p. 2]. Given this inclusive definition, it is evident that health care workers are a diverse group with a variety of approaches to providing patient care. Physicians, nurses, health sector managers, pharmacy warehouse employees, and ambulance drivers are all just a few of the many health care workers in the field today [2]. But who are these individuals? Where and when were they trained? Where do they work now? Tracking such information has proven to be difficult.

Data on health care workers are currently available from a variety of disparate sources. In the United States, extensive data from state licensure records and surveys as well as professional organizations are available [3]; however, these are often inconsistent from source to source. For example, the North Carolina Health Professions Data System (HPDS) collects licensed health care provider data through a collaboration between a university-based policy center, state professional licensing boards, and an Area Health Education Centers (AHEC) program [4]. Some data, such as gender, birth year, home address, graduation year, school of attendance, and practice setting, are collected on all licensed professionals. Other data, such as place of birth and clinical practice area, are collected for some but not others. Additionally, data for health care workers who do not require licenses—such as medication aides, geriatric aides, and feeding assistants—are collected through an entirely separate system via North Carolina's Division of Health Service Regulation Health Care Personnel Registry Section [5]. Given the variety of sources and data collection methods, barriers to aggregation and analysis are inevitable. Internationally, similar challenges are present, with employment data often housed within a country's Ministry of Health and licensure data often housed within professional councils [6]. As such, whether in an entire country or within an enterprise such as an HIE, developing a single source of health worker data has proven to be a challenging and complex undertaking.

While challenges exist, efforts to create a master and canonical list of health workers can yield substantial benefits [2,3,6]. Access to such coordinated data can allow for efficient workforce planning. It can provide verification of employment, education, and other training. It can aid in understanding the geographic distribution of health professionals to identify areas of abundance as well as areas of shortages, allowing for worker deployment into areas of need for specific types of care. A master list of health care workers would also allow for rapid identification of professionals needed for emergency responses purposes. Additionally, such a list would allow for ease of referrals between providers, facilitating effective and comprehensive patient care. A canonical list would also support provider attribution or identifying a primary care provider for a given patient in a given context (eg, which provider delivered the majority of preventative services). Finally, making this list available to other health information systems would support interoperability and comparability of information across systems. For example, calculation of quality indicators or performance indices would be possible by physician, nurse, or allied health professional instead of clinic or hospital level only. Given its potential utility, a single canonical registry with complete and current data on all health workers is a valuable component of an HIE.

HEALTH WORKER REGISTRIES

An *HWR* is defined as a central, authoritative information system that captures, stores, and maintains the unique identities of health workers using a predefined canonical minimum data set (MDS) [6]. An *MDS* is a canonical list of names, definitions, and sources of data elements needed to support a specific purpose. In the context of an HWR, an MDS should contain the smallest, most basic set of data necessary to answer critical health workforce questions, including:

- How many practitioners do we have?
- Where are they practicing?
- Who is providing patient care?
- What types of care are practitioners providing?

MDSs facilitate the establishment of national databases with consistent core data elements covering demographic, educational, credentialing, and practice characteristics of health professionals. In the United States, several health professions' MDSs [7] are defined and maintained by the Health Services Resources Agency (HRSA).

Because there can exist numerous lists of health workers within a state or country, an

HWR seeks to merge various lists in accordance with a governance policy to be established by HIE stakeholders. The policy should ensure that as data are merged, the HWR creates a superset of health worker identities to enable deduplication across available individual data sets. WHO provides guidance on development of such policies as part of its national health workforce accounts [8].

Health Worker Registries Within an HIE

As noted, an HWR serves as a container for authoritative information on health workers within a nation or enterprise. In an HIE, an HWR component must easily communicate with other parts of the system, just as a client registry (see the chapter: Client Registries: Identifying and Linking Patients) and facility registry (see the chapter: Facility Registries: Metadata for Where Care Is Delivered) must do (see Fig. 13.1). The HWR allows queries to be conducted by a variety of client systems consisting of computer and human users, including mobile health (mHealth) tools, such as clinical decision support or health service directory apps; electronic medical record systems; training information systems; human resource (HR) management systems; licensure and qualification systems; health management information systems; and health workforce observatories, which cooperative organizations designed to promote, develop, and sustain a knowledge base for health-related HRs in a region [6]. Ultimately, any source system in the HIE should report the MDS for health worker data from the system it manages to the HWR, and any client system should be able to query the HWR for any information defined by the MDS.

Despite its potential usefulness, an HWR is generally considered to be a "nice to have" component in the United States and therefore

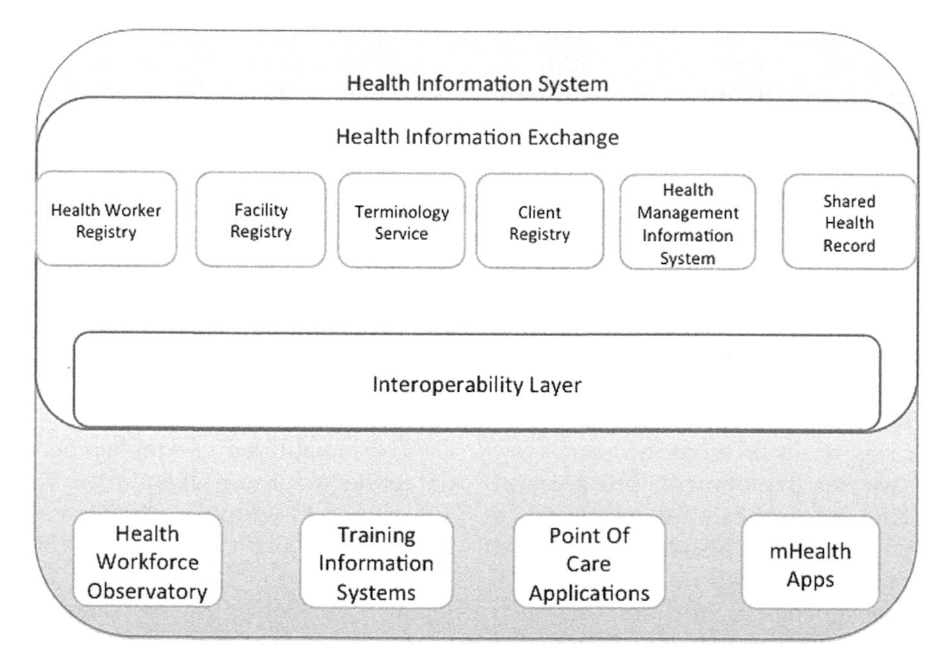

FIGURE 13.1 Illustration of the OpenHIE architecture highlighting the health worker registry and point-of-service applications that potentially interface with the registry. *Adapted from Ref. [6].*

not implemented by most HIEs. The closest analogs to an HWR in US-based HIEs are Health Information Service Providers (HISPs) created as part of the Direct Project [9,10]. However, this analogy is very weak as described below.

The Direct Project specifies a method for medical providers, government organizations, vendors, and others to send authenticated, encrypted health information directly to known, trusted recipients over the Internet [11]; a method often referred to as secure electronic mail (email) for providers. HISPs are the entities responsible for delivering messages between senders and receivers. HISPs must therefore create and maintain email addresses for each sender and receiver, who are most often licensed health workers. For example, the Indiana Health Information Exchange (IHIE) created a direct email address for each of them more than 25,000 DOCS4DOCS providers to help comply with meaningful use regulations in the United States [12]. The email addresses were yet another data element added to the MDS IHIE maintained for its DOCS4DOCS service. The list of health care providers participating in an HISP, therefore, is similar in concept to an HWR because it requires maintaining an MDS about each provider. However, HISP lists are incomplete and often represent only those providers who subscribe to a specific HIE service like DOCS4DOCS; therefore, HISPs should not be considered true HWRs.

Inclusion of an HWR within US-based HIEs requires consideration of economic factors. For example, should an HIE wish to offer an HWR service for a fee, this would require the participation of clients such as states and professional organizations to ensure access to robust and timely data, thereby justifying the expenditure of scarce financial resources. Additionally, an HWR would compete with existing workforce management systems and therefore must demonstrate cost-effectiveness to gain buy-in of HIE participants. As such, much work remains to make this an appealing and economical option.

Internationally, feasibility creating and maintaining an HWR could be more favorable than in the United States. In some countries, much of the data are centralized within a national Ministry of Health, which could make coordination less daunting. Yet in other nations, a Ministry might consist of federated units similar to the fragmented system in the United States. Fragmented nongovernmental organizations can also provide a significant portion of health workers in a nation, similarly making construction of an HWR complex. However, developing HWRs may still be valuable components to the implementation of national eHealth strategies.

Existing MDSs

As previously mentioned, an MDS is the cornerstone to the development of an HWR. An MDS identifies which data to collect from both the public and private sectors [6]. In the United States, HRSA currently maintains MDSs for several professions [13], including: dental hygienists, licensed professional counselors, nurses, occupational therapists, pharmacists, physical therapists, physician assistants, physicians, psychologists, and substance abuse/addiction counselors. However, each MDS is distinct and separate from the others, and they are not coordinated within an HWR. Additionally, the degree to which data collection and implementation is complete varies by state. As such, gaps remain and efforts to improve coverage continue.

WHO strongly supports the establishment of health care workforce MDSs and HWRs [2]. The organization has provided guidance to inform the process throughout the world [2]. Within this context, numerous international efforts for MDS development for a variety of health care workers have already been undertaken [13–18].

Creation of MDSs

The creation of an MDS for an HIE is a process that requires substantial stakeholder input [2,6]. In many cases, it will be necessary to conduct interviews of source system participants in order to identify data elements that currently exist or elements that users desire to have collected. From there, it is necessary to link the identified data elements to previously established use cases and user stories for the HIE. This will ensure that the scope of the MDS matches what users need with the most appropriate set of data elements.

To determine whether a data element should be included in an MDS, a good rule of thumb is the 80:20 rule. This states that if an element will be used by at least 80% of the source or client systems, it should be part of the MDS. Possible data fields to consider for inclusion are demographic, contact, employment, education, and license/certification information [2,6], with others included as indicated by user needs.

TABLE 13.1 Common Health Worker and Health Services Data Standards

Standard	Full Name	Responsible Organization
ANSI/ HL7 V3 HCSPDIR, R1-2010	HL7 Version 3 Standard: Healthcare, Community Services, and Provider Directory Service	HL7 (www.hl7.org)
CSD	Care Service Directory	Integrating the Healthcare Enterprise (IHE) (www.ihe.net)
FHIR	Fast Health Care Interoperability Resources	HL7 (www.hl7.org)
HPD	Health Care Provider Directory	Integrating the Healthcare Enterprise (IHE) (www.ihe.net)
ISO 21091:2013	Health Informatics—Directory Services for Healthcare Providers, Subjects of Care and Other Entities	International Organization for Standardization (ISO) (www.iso.org)

Standards to Support the MDS

As with any component of an HIE, interoperability is the goal. To accomplish this, an MDS must follow a set of standards. For example, standardized data lists that provide a reference terminology must be adopted in order to ensure the data can be effectively analyzed [6]. These lists are typically available through a terminology service (see the chapter: Standardizing Health Care Data Across an Enterprise). In addition to using reference terminologies, component interaction or technical standards must also be selected [6], including those for terminology services, such as Sharing Value Sets [19], Fast Health Care Interoperability Resources Value Sets [20], and Common Terminology Services 2 (CTS2) [21]. Standards for health worker and health services data also must be selected. Descriptions of such standards are included in Table 13.1.

EMERGING TRENDS

In the future, as the health care field adapts to accommodate an aging population as well as a shifting focus on prevention rather than treatment, the health care workforce will need to adapt [22]. Anticipated worker shortages, increasing specialization, and emphasis on multidisciplinary care will necessitate efficient coordination of health professionals to address the population's changing needs [23–26]. Further development of an HWR will be central to facilitating successful management of these needs. Ultimately, international stakeholders, under the guidance of WHO, will continue to advance the global cooperation and coordination of health worker data to meet growing workforce management demands [27].

SUMMARY

The health care field consists of a variety of workers from diverse specialties. Through the harmonization of numerous health worker data sets from varying sources, the development of an HWR utilizing an MDS within an HIE can allow for efficient and effective workforce planning and coordination. Challenges in the development of HWRs exist, particularly due to a patchwork of disparate data sources. However, the potential benefits of HWR likely justify their development and use in both United States and international efforts to support a range of services that allow health systems to assess and adapt to a rapidly changing health care landscape.

APPLICATION EXERCISE/ QUESTIONS FOR DISCUSSION

1. What are some of the major challenges in creating an HWR for an HIE? How do these vary by country?
2. Describe some of the benefits of implementing an HWR. Provide examples of situations where an HWR might improve workforce efficiency.
3. Who are some of the potential users of an HWR? Who may provide the data?
4. What considerations must be taken into account when developing an MDS? Who should participate? What data fields should be included?
5. How might future changes in health care influence the usefulness of HWRs?

References

[1] World Health Organization. Health workers [Internet] 2006 [cited June 22, 2015]. Available from: <www.who.int/whr/2006/06_chap1_en.pdf>.

[2] World Health Organization. Human resources for health information system: minimum data set for health workforce registry [Internet] 2015 [cited July 5, 2015]. Available from: <http://www.who.int/hrh/statistics/minimun_data_set.pdf?ua=1>.

[3] Hosenfeld C. Health professions minimum data set [Internet]. Health Resources and Services Administration. 2013 [cited June 20, 2015]. Available from: <http://bhpr.hrsa.gov/healthworkforce/data/minimumdataset/minimumdataset.pdf>.

[4] Cecil G. Sheps Center for Health Services Research, University of North Carolina at Chapel Hill. North Carolina Health Professions Data System (HPDS) [Internet]. Sheps Center. n.d. [cited July 24, 2015]. Available from: <https://www.shepscenter.unc.edu/programs-projects/workforce/projects/hpds/>.

[5] North Carolina Department of Health and Human Services. NC HCPR: About the NC Health Care Personnel Registry Section [Internet] 2011 [cited July 24, 2015]. Available from: <https://www.ncnar.org/about.html>.

[6] OpenHIE. OpenHIE health worker registry implementation guide [Internet]. 2014 [cited June 20, 2015]. Available from: <https://ohie.org/health-worker-registry/>.

[7] Health Resources and Services Administration. Health professions minimum data set [Internet]. [cited July 1, 2015]. Available from: <http://bhpr.hrsa.gov/healthworkforce/data/minimumdataset/index.html>.

[8] World Health Organization. WHO | POLICY BRIEF—National health workforce accounts [Internet]. WHO. 2015 [cited July 31, 2015]. Available from: <http://www.who.int/hrh/documents/brief_nhwfa/en/>.

[9] HealthIT.gov. DIRECT Project [Internet] 2014 [cited July 5, 2015]. Available from: <http://www.healthit.gov/policy-researchers-implementers/direct-project>.

[10] Morris G, Afzal S, Bhasker M, Finney D. Provider directory solutions report (2012) | HealthIT.gov [Internet]. Office of the National Coordinator for Health Information Technology; 2012 [cited July 31, 2015]. Available from: <http://www.healthit.gov/providers-professionals/implementation-resources/provider-directory-solutions-report-2012>.

[11] The Direct Project overview [Internet] 2010 [cited July 24, 2015]. Available from: <http://directproject.org/content.php?key=overview>.

[12] Indiana health information exchange. DOCS4DOCS [Internet]. n.d. [cited July 5, 2015]. Available from: <http://www.ihie.org/docs4docs>.

[13] National Center for Health Workforce Analysis. Health professions minimum data set [Internet]. Health Resources and Services Administration; n.d. [cited June 20, 2015]. Available from: <http://bhpr.hrsa.gov/healthworkforce/data/minimumdataset/index.html>.

[14] National Council for Palliative Care. Minimum data set [Internet] 2015 [cited July 5, 2015]. Available from: <http://www.ncpc.org.uk/minimum-data-set>.

[15] Health & Social Care Information Centre. Workforce minimum data set (wMDS) [Internet] n.d. [cited July 5, 2015]. <Available from: http://www.hscic.gov.uk/wMDS>.

[16] Rural Health Workforce Australia 2015 [cited July 5, 2015]. Available from: <http://www.rhwa.org.au/site/index.cfm?display=25615>.

[17] Chen C, Baird S, Ssentongo K, Mehtsun S, Olapade-Olaopa EO, Scott J, et al. Physician tracking in sub-Saharan Africa: current initiatives and opportunities. Hum Resour Health 2014;12:21.

[18] Middleton S, Gardner G, Gardner A, Della P, Gibb M, Millar L. The first Australian nurse practitioner census: a protocol to guide standardized collection of information about an emergent professional group. Int J Nurs Pract 2010;16(5):517–24.

[19] ITI Technical Committee. IHE IT Infrastructure (ITI) technical framework supplement: Sharing Value Sets (SVS) [Internet] 2010 [cited July 5, 2015]. Available from: <http://www.ihe.net/Technical_Framework/upload/IHE_ITI_Suppl_SVS_Rev2-1_TI_2010-08-10.pdf>.

[20] HL7. Value sets defined in FHIR—FHIR v0.0.82 [Internet]. 2014 [cited July 31, 2015]. Available from: <http://www.hl7.org/implement/standards/fhir/terminologies-valuesets.html>.

[21] CTS2. About CTS2 [Internet] n.d. [cited July 5, 2015]. Available from: <http://informatics.mayo.edu/cts2/index.php/About>.

[22] Centre for Workforce Intelligence. Horizon 2035: International responses to big picture challenges [Internet] 2014 [cited July 5, 2015]. Available from: <http://www.cfwi.org.uk/publications/horizon-2035-international-responses-to-big-picture-challenges>.

[23] Barnett K, Mercer SW, Norbury M, Watt G, Wyke S, Guthrie B. Epidemiology of multimorbidity and implications for health care, research, and medical education: a cross-sectional study. Lancet Lond Engl 2012;380(9836):37–43.

[24] Health Workforce Australia. Health Workforce 2025—doctors, nurses and midwives, Volumes 1–3 [Internet] 2012 [cited July 5, 2015]. Available from: <https://www.hwa.gov.au/our-work/health-workforce-planning/health-workforce-2025-doctors-nurses-and-midwives>.

[25] OECD. Health at a glance 2013: OECD indicators [Internet]. OECD Publishing; 2013 [cited July 5, 2015]. Available from: http://www.oecd.org/els/health-systems/Health-at-a-Glance-2013.pdf.

[26] World Health Organization. A universal truth: no health without a workforce [Internet] 2014 [cited July 5, 2015]. Available from: <http://www.who.int/workforcealliance/knowledge/resources/GHWA-a_universal_truth_report.pdf>.

[27] World Health Organization. WHO|Global strategy on human resources for health: Workforce 2030 [Internet]. WHO. 2015 [cited July 31, 2015]. Available from: <http://www.who.int/hrh/resources/globstrathrh-2030/en/>.

PART IV

THE VALUE OF HEALTH INFORMATION EXCHANGE

CHAPTER

14

The Evidence Base for Health Information Exchange

William R. Hersh[1,2], *Annette M. Totten*[1], *Karen Eden*[1], *Beth Devine*[1,3], *Paul Gorman*[1,2], *Steven Z. Kassakian*[1], *Susan S. Woods*[1,4], *Monica Daeges*[1], *Miranda Pappas*[1] and *Marian S. McDonagh*[1]

[1]Pacific Northwest Evidence-based Practice Center, Department of Medical Informatics and Clinical Epidemiology, Oregon Health & Science University, Portland, OR [2]Department of Medicine, Oregon Health & Science University, Portland, OR [3]University of Washington Centers for Comparative and Health Systems Effectiveness (CHASE) Alliance, Seattle, WA [4]Veterans Affairs Maine Healthcare System, Augusta, ME

OUTLINE

INTRODUCTION

Over the last decade, there has been substantial growth in the adoption of the electronic health record (EHR) systems in ambulatory and hospital settings across the United States, fueled largely by incentive funding provided by the Health Information Technology for Economic and Clinical Health (HITECH) Act. As a result of HITECH, 94% of nonfederal hospitals [1], 78% of hospital-based physicians [2], 84% of emergency departments, and 73% of hospital outpatient departments in the United States have adopted EHR systems [3]. The motivation to increase the adoption of EHR systems is grounded in evidence that health information technology (HIT) can improve the quality, safety, efficiency, and satisfaction with care, as has been reported in a series of systematic reviews [4–7].

A major challenge to effective use of HIT, however, is that most patients in the United States, especially those with multiple conditions, receive care across a number of settings [8,9]. To enable data to follow patients wherever they receive care, attention has recently focused on health information exchange (HIE), defined as the reliable and interoperable electronic sharing of clinical information among physicians, nurses, pharmacists, other health care providers, and patients across the boundaries of health care institutions, health data repositories, states, and other entities who are not within a single organization or among affiliated providers [10]. The HITECH Act recognized that EHR adoption alone was insufficient to realize the full promise of HIT, allocating $563 million for states or state-designated entities to establish HIE capability among health care providers and hospitals [11]. As a result of HITECH funding, HIE adoption has grown in a parallel though somewhat smaller manner. By 2014, 76% of US hospitals had engaged in some form of HIE [12]. An annual survey of organizations engaged in HIE found 135 in the United States in 2014 [13].

Evaluating the effectiveness of HIE (and HIT generally) has been challenging [14]. HIE is a technology that is intermediate to improving care delivery, allowing clinicians and others' improved access to patient data to inform decisions and facilitate appropriate use of testing and treatment. HIE is not specific to any health issue or diagnosis. HIE implementations have often been supported by one-time start-up funding, without long-term support to sustain the programs long enough for evaluation.

There are three previously published systematic reviews that focus exclusively on HIE [15–17]. One of these reviews is almost a half-decade old [15], another focused only on US-based and clinical-only (ie, not public health) activities [16], and a third assessed only care outcomes and not larger issues of facilitators, barriers, and sustainability [17]. This chapter reports on a systematic review of HIE that updated the previous ones and categorized results based on (1) effectiveness of HIE in improving clinical, economic, population, and intermediate outcomes; (2) use of HIE; (3) usability and facilitators and barriers to use of HIE; and (4) HIE implementation and sustainability. A technical report further describes the methods and includes search strategies and additional information [18].

METHODS

As is done in a typical systematic review, a research librarian conducted electronic database searches identifying relevant articles published between January 1990 and February 2015 in MEDLINE (Ovid), PsycINFO, CINAHL, and the Cochrane Library databases. Searches were peer-reviewed by another librarian and supplemented by references identified from additional sources, including reference lists, table of contents of journals not indexed in databases searched, gray literature sources, and experts. English language studies of HIE that reported on outcomes related to our key questions were included. We included comparative studies of effectiveness and other designs for more qualitative outcomes. Two investigators independently evaluated each study to determine inclusion eligibility. Disagreement was resolved by consensus with a third investigator making the final decision as needed.

Details of included studies were extracted by one investigator and reviewed for accuracy and completeness by a second. Investigators rated the quality (risk of bias) of the individual effectiveness studies and strength of the body of evidence based on preestablished criteria. The strength of evidence consisted of four major categories: high, moderate, low, or insufficient based on the methodological limitations of studies; consistency across studies; precision of estimates; and directness of effect. Ratings were reviewed by a second investigator, and disagreements were resolved by consensus or involvement of a third investigator if necessary.

Data could not be combined in a quantitative meta-analysis because of heterogeneity in the interventions, the outcomes measured, and the way data were reported. Therefore, we combined studies qualitatively based on similarity of the type of HIE, the implementation of the HIE, outcomes measured, and results reported. Where studies were not similar in these areas, we provided results of the individual studies without grouping them.

RESULTS

Out of 5211 potentially relevant citations identified in our literature searches, 850 articles were selected for full-text review and 136 studies were ultimately included. Search and selection results are summarized in Fig. 14.1. Of the 136 studies included, two randomized controlled trials (RCTs) described in three papers and 32 observational and survey studies addressed clinical, economic, population, and intermediate outcomes. Most were conducted in the United States, although eight were from Europe, Canada, Israel, and South Korea. These studies reported clinical or public health process, economic, or population outcomes, while no studies reported harms of HIE. The majority were assessed to be of low risk of bias (ie, good internal validity) but also contained mostly retrospective observational evidence. We identified 58 studies that addressed the use of HIE. The majority were conducted in the United States and were low risk of bias or used study designs that were not amenable to rating. Twenty-two studies were identified that addressed usability and facilitators and barriers to use. Most were assessed to be of moderate risk of bias and were conducted in the United States, Austria, and Australia. A total of 52 studies addressed HIE implementation and sustainability. These studies used varying types of qualitative methods that we did rate for risk of bias or used study designs that were not amenable to rating.

Improving Clinical, Economic, Population, and Intermediate Outcomes

Of 34 studies, 26 reported clinical (intermediate), economic, or population outcomes, while eight were found to report on perceptions of outcomes. No studies evaluated primary clinical outcomes from HIE (eg, mortality and morbidity) nor explicitly assessed harms. We list the study designs and geographic locations in Table 14.1.

The most common study design for assessing outcomes was retrospective cohort, typically with HIE use associated with a specific outcome factor (Table 14.1). The next most common design was survey, which was usually focused on perception of outcomes. Two studies were RCTs, one of a particular directed information exchange (two published papers,

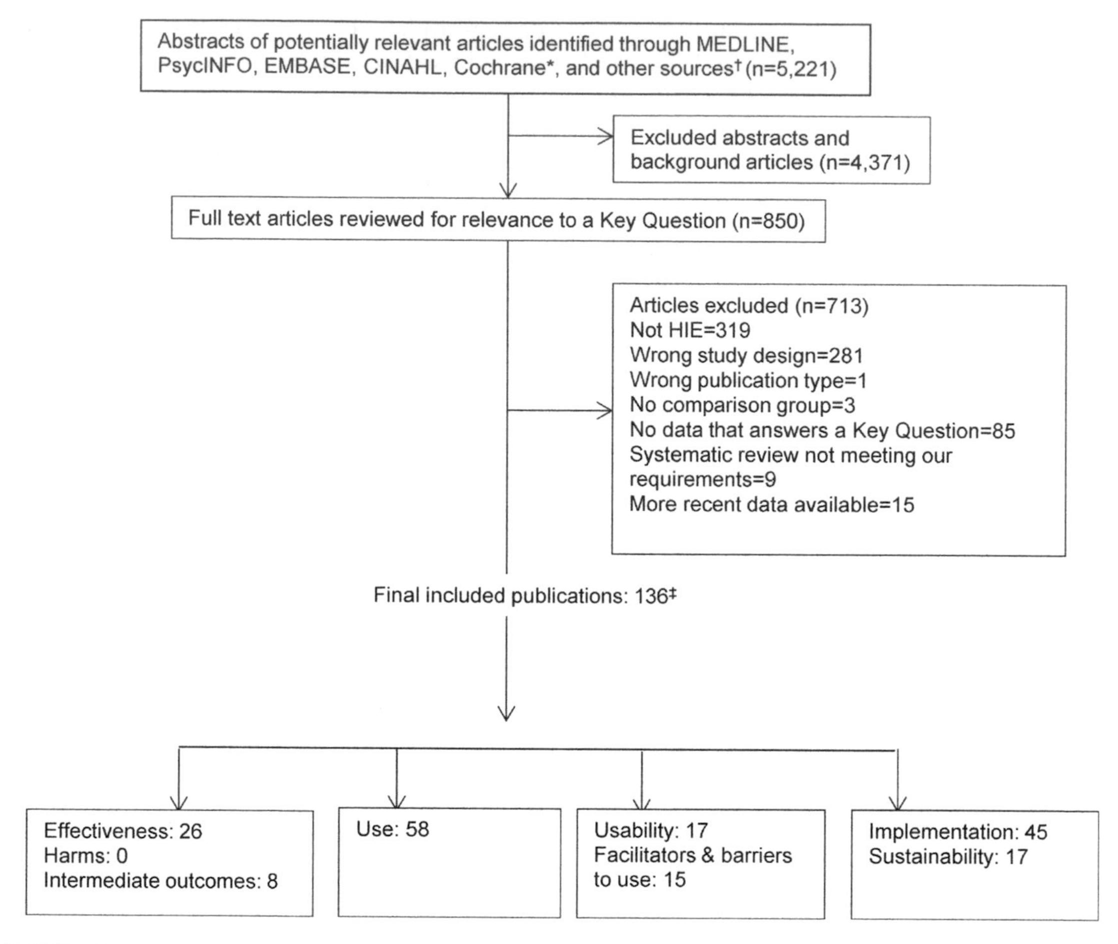

FIGURE 14.1 Results of the literature search. *Cochrane databases include the Cochrane Database of Systematic Reviews, Cochrane Central Register of Controlled Trials, Database of Abstracts of Reviews of Effects, and National Health Sciences Economic Evaluation Database. †Identified from reference lists, hand searching, suggested by experts, and other sources. ‡Publications may address more than one key question, studies may have multiple publications.

one on clinical outcomes and the other on perceptions) and the other of a clinical decision support intervention using data from an HIE implementation. Two studies used cross-sectional analyses of large databases to compare those having access to HIE with those without access. Two other studies used a case series methodology, one of which involved asking clinicians if HIE access avoided undesirable resource use and then calculating the costs saved and the other that retrospectively analyzed data to determine duplicative testing averted. For additional information on study designs, refer to chapter "Measuring the Value of Health Information Exchange" which describes how to evaluate HIE.

The identified studies were performed mostly in the United States, but we identified eight studies from five other countries. Of the 26 US studies, two assessed multiple HIE implementations across the entire United States, one assessed multiple HIE

TABLE 14.1 Study Designs and Locations

Design (Number)	References
Retrospective cohort (18)	19–36
Survey (8)	37–44
Randomized controlled trial (3)	45–47
Cross-sectional (2)	48,49
Case series (2)	50,51
Location (Number)	**References**
Austria (1)	38
Canada (2)	45,47
Finland (2)	27,42
Israel (2)	24,52
South Korea (1)	43
All of United States (2)	44,48
California and Florida	49
Colorado (1)	30
Indiana (3)	25,29,40
Louisiana (1)	28
Massachusetts (1)	41
Minnesota (1)	51
North Carolina (1)	46
New York (6)	26,31,35–37,39
Oklahoma (1)	21
South Carolina (1)	50
Tennessee (3)	20,22,23
Texas (1)	34
Virginia (1)	19
Wisconsin (2)	32,33

implementations in two states (California and Florida), and the remaining 23 studies were conducted in 13 states. Most studies used retrospective designs, usually with an approach examining the association of HIE use with one or more clinical variables. All of these studies focused on the direct effect of HIE, usually in reducing resource use or costs, without determining its larger impact (eg, overall total or proportion of spending in an emergency department (ED) vs the total dollar amounts that HIE appeared to save). None of the studies analyzed individual episodes of care to determine clinical appropriateness of possible changes brought about by HIE use.

The prospective studies also had limitations. The RCTs were focused on highly specific uses of HIE, namely directed exchange of ED reports in one and pharmacotherapy clinical decision support in another. Of note, however, was that neither study showed benefit of HIE. The other prospective study was limited by methodology of physicians self-reporting of resources not utilized when HIE was used, with no follow-up or validation of their decisions or analysis of more holistic views of clinical outcomes or costs.

Most of these studies had reasonable but not strong internal validity. As the HIE intervention was only one of many potential influences on clinical outcome (ie, many more factors go into clinical outcomes than the decision to consult an HIE on a patient), there was possible confounding. As a result, most studies with appropriate retrospective methods are listed as having low or moderate risk of bias.

Due mainly to the study designs and performance or reporting limitations, the lack of ability to combine results, and other factors, the strength of this body of evidence was rated as low, meaning that future studies have the potential to alter these findings in magnitude or direction. In addition, the number of studies and their locations in the United States represent a small fraction of those reporting to be operational, sustainable, or innovating according to the eHealth Initiative Annual Data Exchange Survey, which reported a total of 84 such HIE implementations in 2013 [53] and 106 in 2014 [13]. In other words, while a substantial number of HIE implementations exist in the

United States, only a small number have been subject to evaluation. This low number of studies relative to HIE efforts also makes it difficult to generalize factors about aspects of them, such as location, HIE type, and setting, with results of research.

Improving Resource Use

Most of the studies of HIE effectiveness focused on resource use. We categorized these as follows (Table 14.2): laboratory testing, radiology testing, hospital admissions, hospital readmissions, referrals and consultations, ED costs, public heath reporting, quality of care, and other aspects of HIE. Although the risk of bias in most studies was low, the resulting evidence from them was mostly of low strength due to retrospective designs. This low-strength evidence mostly favored the value of HIE in reducing resource use and costs, especially in the ED, but used a very narrow cost perspective and did not account for how HIE was used or its impact on the overall care of the patient beyond the immediate setting where it was used.

Perceptions

Eight studies evaluated clinician or patient perceptions of outcomes from HIE, with all showing partial or complete perception of HIE leading to improved outcomes. Clinician perceptions of the value of HIE, where studied, were generally positive. How such perceptions translate into improved care is unknown. This body of evidence was rated as low strength.

Factors Associated With Outcomes

To determine whether effectiveness of HIE varied by study type, health care setting, location, or HIE type, we categorized these factors by whether HIE was found to have some beneficial effect or not. As shown in Table 14.3, the preponderance of studies showed that HIE use for different functions, in various settings, and of varying types was mostly positive. While the number of positive versus negative studies was not an indicator of the overall direction of the evidence, we did note that for each "negative" study, there was at least one "positive" one. For "Type of HIE," there was no clear pattern of findings to suggest that one type is clearly better than another, even indirectly. The two RCTs we found were described in three papers. Two of these reported outcomes, one for each RCT, both of which showed no benefit for the HIE intervention [45,46]. A perceptions study of one of the RCTs found impressions of improved patient outcomes and their management [47]. These were in contrast with the observational study designs where almost all found beneficial effects of HIE. For HIE setting, only ambulatory and ED had enough studies to evaluate patterns, with outpatient settings less likely to find beneficial results compared with studies in ED settings, but again based on indirect comparisons only. The sparseness of studies across geographic settings did not allow for identification of patterns, although across most studies in the United States, the findings were positive.

Use of HIE

Fifty-eight studies described either level of use or primary uses of HIE. Many of these were at low risk of bias. Fifteen nationwide surveys conducted in the United States suggested that the proportion of hospitals using HIE has risen substantially in recent years, from 11% (2009) [54] to between 30% and 58% till date [55–57]. Data from the Office of the National Coordinator for Health Information Technology (ONC) from 2014 suggested that more than three-quarters (76%) of nonfederal acute care hospitals electronically exchanged laboratory results, radiology reports, clinical care summaries, and/or medication lists with any outside providers [12]. In ambulatory care settings, 38% of office-based physicians reported exchanging information with other providers or hospitals [58]. Characteristics of higher HIE use were larger

TABLE 14.2 Study Results by Categories

Category (Number)	Results
Laboratory testing (6)	Six studies demonstrated a benefit for HIE in reducing overall tests, although estimates of impact on cost were mixed [20,27,30,32,50,51]. Four of these studies took place in the ED setting, all showing some aspect of reduced testing and cost savings [20,32,50,51]. Two studies were conducted in ambulatory settings, with one showing an increase [27] and the other showing a reduction in the increased overall rate of testing [30].
Radiology testing (9)	Seven studies carried out in the ED setting showing reduced testing [20,22,23,32,49–51]. Two studies were conducted in ambulatory settings, with one showing a decrease [27] and the other showing no change in rate of testing [30].
Hospital admissions (8)	2 studies found a reduction in hospital admissions and lower costs using methods previously described [20,50]. Three other studies also measured some benefit for HIE use in reducing hospital admissions [24,36,52], although three additional studies found no such reduction [33,34,45].
Hospital readmissions (2)	For reducing hospital readmissions, one study showed benefit for HIE [35] but the other did not [48].
Referrals and consultations (2)	Two studies, described previously, assessed HIE for reducing referrals and/or consultations, with conflicting results [27,50].
ED costs (2)	Two studies found reduced overall ED costs per patient when HIE was available [20,32]. Neither study reported overall ED expenditures, making it unknown what proportion of overall ED spending was impacted by HIE.
Public heath reporting (3)	Three studies assessed HIE in public health settings, all of which were conducted in the United States and reported improved automated laboratory reporting [29], improved completeness of reporting for notifiable diseases [25], and improved identification of HIV patients for follow-up care [28].
Quality of care in ambulatory settings (3)	Two retrospective studies found HIE associated with improved quality of care [21,26], while an RCT focused on medication reconciliation found increased ability to detect medication adherence problems but was unable to show improvement in adherence after it was identified and address by providers [46].
Other aspects of HIE (3)	Three studies assessed other aspects of HIE, including reduction in time for processing of social security disability claims [19], increased ability to identify frequent ED users [31], and associated of HIE implementation with improved patient satisfaction scores in hospitals [44].

ED, emergency department; HIE, health information exchange; HIV, human immunodeficiency virus; RCT, randomized controlled trial.

practice size, practice owned by a health system (vs physician owned), and multispecialty (vs single specialty) practice. Hospitals and ambulatory care providers both provided and used data, while laboratory services provided data and community clinics mostly used data [59]. At least 50% of these organizations have reached an advanced stage of use of core functionalities, with many supporting health care reform initiatives and advanced analytics [13,53]. Use varied by type of health care professional, with higher use by nurses and clerks compared with physicians [60,61]. Limited data from residential care settings suggested that use of HIE in this setting is very low (<1%) [62,63], with the consistent pattern of nonprofits having wider use than for-profit entities. An additional 30 studies analyzed the extent to which HIE was

TABLE 14.3 Factors That May Affect Outcomes and Perceptions

	Studies of Outcomes	Studies of Perceptions	Studies Reported as Beneficial	Studies Reported as No Benefit	Total
STUDY TYPE					
Retrospective cohort	20		19	1	20
Randomized controlled trial	2	1	1	2	3
Cross-sectional	2		1	1	2
Case series	2		2		2
Survey[a]		8	8		8
SETTING					
All	1			1	1
Emergency department	13	3	13	3	16
Government	1		1		1
Health management organization	2		2		2
Hospital	1			1	1
Outpatient	5	5	9	1	10
Public health	3		3		3
LOCATION					
United States, multistate	3		2	1	3
Colorado	1		1		1
Indiana	2	1	3		3
Louisiana	1		1		1
Massachusetts	1		1		1
Minnesota	1		1		1
North Carolina	1			1	1
New York	4	2	6		6
Oklahoma	1		1		1
South Carolina	1		1		1
Tennessee	3		3		3
Texas	1			1	1
Virginia	1		1		1
Wisconsin	2		1	1	2
Austria		1	1		1
Canada	1	1	1	1	2
Finland	1	1	1	1	2
Israel	2		2		2
South Korea		1	1		1
HEALTH INFORMATION EXCHANGE TYPE					
Directed	5	5	8	2	10
Query	18	2	19	1	20
Multiple	3	1	3	1	4

[a]*One survey study was also a randomized controlled trial.*

implemented in a state or across a region. These studies evaluated inpatient, outpatient, community clinic, and ED use, but few regions provided data. Results suggested that actual use of HIE is still not well integrated into clinical care, being used in fewer than 10% of visits in both Tennessee [60] and Texas [64], with higher use for ED visits (15%) [61]. Results from nine international or multinational studies suggested the same finding of low to moderate use [65].

Usability and Facilitators and Barriers to Use

Twenty-two cross-sectional multiple site case studies and before–after studies provided descriptive and qualitative data on usability as well as barriers and facilitators to electronically exchanging health data. The main sources of evidence from 17 US studies included survey data from 225 clinician and 174 health professional HIE users, interview transcripts and focus group transcripts of 177 clinician users, and 118 health professional users [37,60,61,66–79]. Five international studies provided survey data that included responses from more than 11,000 clinicians from 31 European countries [38,80–82] and Australia [83]. The most frequent users rated usability higher than infrequent users. Comparison of usability by type of HIE function (directed exchange or push vs query-based or pull) and architecture (eg, whether the query-based system used a centralized or federated model) was difficult as the authors described HIE differently and there was no standard classification. Additionally, users reported barriers to HIE centered on three main themes: lack of critical mass (eg, limited participation in HIE limiting availability of data needed by providers); inefficient workflow; and poorly designed interface.

Implementation and Sustainability

A relatively large number of studies identified in this review assessed factors that impact the implementation (45 studies) and/or sustainability (17 studies) of HIE [19–21,55,66,67, 79,80,84–127]. Adopting and then supporting ongoing HIE are organizational decisions, and the research provides insight into what organizations experience as barriers and facilitators. Implementation and sustainability are linked (ie, organizations consider sustainability potential when deciding whether to implement a new technology), but sustainability has been the subject of fewer studies likely because HIE is still a comparatively new innovation (refer to chapter: Managing the Business of Health Information Exchange: Toward Sustainability). Across these studies the most commonly cited implementation facilitators were general organizational characteristics such as leadership and IT readiness. The most frequently cited barriers to implementation were factors viewed as disincentives including competition, costs, limited return on investment, and concerns about data misuse and privacy. Positive influences identified for sustainability were desire for the expected outcomes from HIE and the selection of HIE functions most likely to have financial benefit. The most frequently cited negative influence was competition that limited the collaboration necessary to support HIE. A major limitation of this body of evidence is that the studies have not been designed to directly compare the relative impact of these factors or to prioritize what should be addressed in order to promote the implementation and sustainability of HIE.

CONCLUSIONS

The findings of this systematic review are summarized in Table 14.4. We conclude that a collection of low-quality evidence on HIE suggests value for reducing duplicative laboratory and radiology test ordering, lowering ED costs, reducing hospital admissions (less so for readmissions), improving public health reporting,

TABLE 14.4 Summary of Evidence

Topic	Number of Included Studies and Its Type	Main Findings	Primary Limitations of the Evidence
Effectiveness	34 20 Retrospective cohort 3 Randomized controlled trial 2 Cross-sectional 2 Case series 8 Survey (1 survey study was an RCT)	Low-quality evidence somewhat supports the value of HIE for reducing duplicative laboratory and radiology test ordering, lowering ED costs, reducing hospital admissions (less so for readmissions), improving public health reporting, increasing ambulatory quality of care, and improving disability claims processing. No evidence of harms was reported.	Studies were from a small number of the functioning HIE implementations, with similarity to unstudied ones unknown, possibly limiting generalizability. Studies looked at limited outcomes compared with the intended scope of the impact of HIE.
Use	58 25 Surveys 13 Audit Logs 9 Retrospective database 7 Mixed methods 2 Focus Groups 1 Time-motion 1 Geocoding	Proportion of hospitals and ambulatory care practices that have adopted HIE is increasing. Currently, proportion of clinicians using HIE and proportion of patients or episodes associated with HIE use are generally low.	While there are relatively high-quality national and regional surveys and reports that are tracking the expansion of HIE among health care organizations, there is not a corresponding comprehensive effort to track changes in rates of use within organizations.
Usability and other factors affecting use	22; 9 Multiple site case studies 11 Cross-sectional 2 Before–after	Three most commonly cited barriers to HIE use were: incomplete patient information (eight studies); inefficient workflow (six studies); poorly designed interface and update features (six studies).	Studies of usability did not relate it to effectiveness and do not permit comparisons across settings or type of HIE. Studies had limitations such as incomplete reporting on sampling, low response rates or selection of a narrow setting or patient population which minimize applicability.
Implementation and sustainability	52 26 Cross-sectional 17 Multiple site case studies 2 Before–after 3 Retrospective cohorts 2 Prospective cohorts 2 Time series	Most facilitators of implementation are characteristics of the HIE or the internal organizational environment. Many barriers to implementation are external, environmental factors. Factors related to sustainability overlap with those identified for implementation.	Studies do not allow comparison of the impact of different barrier and facilitators. The definition and appropriate measure of sustainability are not yet clear.

ED, emergency department; HIE, health information exchange; RCT, randomized controlled trial.

increasing ambulatory quality of care, and improving disability claims processing. The evidence is low-quality, because the retrospective nature of the studies and limited scope of the questions they address reduce their applicability. It is unlikely that additional studies of the kind included in this review will substantially alter the overall conclusion that HIE can reduce laboratory and imaging tests associated with episodes of care without broadening their scope and using more rigorous designs. Though the preponderance of evidence supports positive effects in terms of reduced resource use and improved quality of care, it is entirely possible that focused studies with stronger study designs and more comprehensive assessment of utilization or clinical outcomes might reach a different conclusion.

Comparison With Other Reviews

The present systematic review of HIE can be compared with two other systematic reviews of HIE: one by Rudin et al. [16] and another by Rahurkar et al. [17]. All three systematic reviews used generally similar approaches, with similar definitions of HIE and focus on studies of HIE impact, excluding system descriptions and simple case studies. The three reviews differed, however, in their scope and inclusiveness. Our review was the broadest in scope and the most inclusive in the search for evidence. In addition to patient and population health outcomes, economic, utilization process outcomes, and barriers and facilitators to implementation and use, our review also included studies concerned with use and usability of HIE. We also included studies beyond the United States and those reporting on public health and surveillance as well as exchange of administrative and financial information. The overall result is that we examined a more diverse and more inclusive collection of evidence, especially with respect to usability and use as well as assessing public health settings, although we came to largely similar conclusions. Rahurkar et al. performed a multivariate analysis that found study design was the only characteristic associated with finding a beneficial effect, with the most rigorous studies being less likely to report benefits of HIE [17].

Applicability

One of the concerns of our results is how applicable they might be under "real-world" conditions in health systems, hospitals, and clinics in the United States. One concern has been that the bulk of the evidence about HIT impact has arisen out of a relatively small number of leading HIT centers [4]. These centers have been referred to as such because they are typically large academic medical centers with internally developed HIT systems, implemented incrementally, and refined over a long period of time. In the present review of HIE the concentration of evidence phenomenon is also present, with large numbers of published studies emanating from relatively few areas. Yet this time, it is regional implementation programs rather than academic health centers, such as those in Indiana, New York, and Tennessee, for which we observe a concentration of the evidence. Related to the "HIT leader," concern is the issue of systems evaluated by their developers, also observed in other aspects of HIT [128] such as clinical decision support that tend to achieve more positive outcomes from their evaluation than external evaluators.

Future Research Needs

Given the limited conclusions that can be reached after review of so much published literature on the effects, use, sustainability, and barriers to implementation and use of HIE, what are the implications for future research? Researchers of HIE should work to develop greater focus and clarity about the level at which interventions are operating as well as the types and levels at which outcomes are measured. The outcomes of interest and the factors influencing them may be quite different at different levels of analysis, from specific systems or functionalities of HIE; to individual patients, providers, or episodes of care; to health care units such as the ED, primary care practice, or hospital ward; to institutions such as hospitals; to aggregates such as health systems; or broader regional multiorganization entities or regions.

What types of studies should be performed? RCTs are impractical for technologies with wide-ranging purposes like HIE. Yet, retrospective studies associating HIE versus nonuse for outcomes such as test ordering and hospital admissions limit the conclusions that can be drawn. Research is also challenging because many of the important clinical outcomes that could benefit from HIE have many other potential contributing and confounding factors relating to the patient, his or her clinicians, the quality of care delivered, the EHR system, and other HIT used, the nature of the health care delivery system, the regulatory environment, and many more.

Future studies should be prospective, carried out in mature HIE settings, assessing patients who are likely to benefit from HIE and comparing appropriate outcomes for the use or nonuse of HIE. The prospective collection of data from diverse settings where HIE is used could allow for prospective cohort studies that could identify aspects of HIE associated with beneficial outcomes. This will likely require an effort comparable in scope to national data collection efforts, such as the Patient-Centered Outcomes Research Institute Clinical Data Research Network initiative [129]. Ideally, such an undertaking could be synergistic with these other large-scale efforts.

The full impact of HIE on clinical outcomes and potential harms is insufficiently studied, although evidence provides some support for benefit in reducing use of some specific resources and achieving improvements in quality of care measures. Use of HIE has increased over time and is the highest in hospitals and the lowest in residential care settings. However, use of HIE within organizations that offer it is still low. Barriers to HIE use include incomplete patient information, inefficient workflow, and poorly designed interface and update features, but factors affecting implementation and sustainability remain unclear. To advance our understanding of HIE, future studies need to address comprehensive questions, use more rigorous designs, and be part of a coordinated systematic approach to studying HIE.

Acknowledgments

The authors gratefully acknowledge the following individuals for their contributions to this project: Andrew Hamilton, MLS, MS, for conducting literature searches and Spencer Dandy, BS, for assistance with preparing this manuscript (all are located at the Oregon Health & Science University); and Jon White, MD, Task Order Officer (TOO) at the Agency for Healthcare Research and Quality (AHRQ).

References

[1] Charles D, Gabriel M, Furukawa M. Adoption of electronic health record systems among U.S. non-federal acute care hospitals: 2008–2013. Washington, DC: The Office of the National Coordinator for Health Information Technology; 2014. [March 2, 2014]; Available from: <http://www.healthit.gov/sites/default/files/oncdatabrief16.pdf>.

[2] Hsiao C-J, Hing E. Use and characteristics of electronic health record systems among office-based physician practices: United States, 2001–2013. Hyattsville, MD: National Center for Health Statistics; 2014. [March 3, 2015]; Available from: <http://www.cdc.gov/nchs/data/databriefs/db143.htm>.

[3] Jamoom E, Hing E. Progress with electronic health record adoption among emergency and outpatient departments: United States, 2006–2011. Hyattsville, MD: National Center for Health Statistics; 2015. [March 3, 2015]; Available from: <http://www.cdc.gov/nchs/data/databriefs/db187.htm>.

[4] Chaudhry B, Wang J, Wu S, Maglione M, Mojica W, Roth E, et al. Systematic review: impact of health information technology on quality, efficiency, and costs of medical care. Ann Intern Med 2006;144(10):742–52. Epub May 17, 2006.

[5] Goldzweig CL, Towfigh A, Maglione M, Shekelle PG. Costs and benefits of health information technology: new trends from the literature. Health Aff (Millwood) 2009;28(2):w282–93. Epub January 29, 2009.

[6] Buntin MB, Burke MF, Hoaglin MC, Blumenthal D. The benefits of health information technology: a review of the recent literature shows predominantly positive results. Health Aff (Project Hope) 2011;30(3):464–71. Epub March 09, 2011.

[7] Jones SS, Rudin RS, Perry T, Shekelle PG. Health information technology: an updated systematic review with a focus on meaningful use. Ann Intern Med 2014;160(1):48–54. Epub February 28, 2014.

[8] Bourgeois FC, Olson KL, Mandl KD. Patients treated at multiple acute health care facilities: quantifying information fragmentation. Arch Intern Med 2010;170(22):1989–95. Epub December 15, 2010.

[9] Finnell JT, Overhage JM, Grannis S. All health care is not local: an evaluation of the distribution of emergency department care delivered in Indiana. AMIA Annu Symp Proc 2011;2011:409–16. Epub December 24, 2011.

[10] What is HIE (Health Information Exchange)? Washington, DC: Department of Health and Human Services; 2012 [cited 2014 April 18, 2014]; Available from: <http://www.healthit.gov/providers-professionals/health-information-exchange/what-hie>.

[11] Williams C, Mostashari F, Mertz K, Hogin E, Atwal P. From the office of the national coordinator: the strategy for advancing the exchange of health information [Erratum appears in Health Aff (Millwood). 2012;31(3):886]. Health Aff 2012;31(3):527–36.

[12] Swain M, Charles D, Patel V, Searcy T. Health information exchange among U.S. non-federal acute care hospitals: 2008–2014. Washington DC: The Office of the national Coordinator for Health Information Technology (ONC); 2015. ONC Data Brief No. 24 Contract No.: ONC Data Brief No. 24.

[13] eHealth Initiative. Post HITECH: The landscape of Health Information Exchange. 2014 [updated January 9, 2014]; Available from: <http://www.ehidc.org/resource-center/publications/view_document/461-reports-2014-ehi-data-exchange-survey-key-findings>.

[14] Kern LM, Ancker JS, Abramson E, Patel V, Dhopeshwarkar RV, Kaushal R. Evaluating health information technology in community-based settings: lessons learned. J Am Med Inform Assoc 2011;18(6):749–53. Epub August 03, 2011.

[15] Hincapie A, Warholak T. The impact of health information exchange on health outcomes. Appl Clin Inform 2011;2(4):499–507. Epub January 1, 2011.

[16] Rudin RS, Motala A, Goldzweig CL, Shekelle PG. Usage and effect of health information exchange: a systematic review. Ann Intern Med 2014;161(11):803–11. Epub December 2, 2014.

[17] Rahurkar S, Vest JR, Menachemi N. Despite the spread of health information exchange, there is little evidence of its impact on cost, use, and quality of care. Health Aff. (Project Hope) 2015;34(3):477–83. Epub March 4, 2015.

[18] Hersh W, Totten A, Eden K, Devine B, Gorman P, Kassakian S, et al. Health Information Exchange. Rockville, MD: Agency for Healthcare Research and Quality; 2015.

[19] Feldman SS, Horan TA. Collaboration in electronic medical evidence development: a case study of the Social Security Administration's MEGAHIT System. Int J Med Inf 2011;80(8):e127–40.

[20] Frisse ME, Johnson KB, Nian H, Davison CL, Gadd CS, Unertl KM, et al. The financial impact of health information exchange on emergency department care. J Am Med Inform Assoc 2012;19(3):328–33.

[21] Nagykaldi ZJ, Yeaman B, Jones M, Mold JW, Scheid DC. HIE-i-health information exchange with intelligence. J Ambulatory Care Manage 2014;37(1):20–31.

[22] Bailey JE, Wan JY, Mabry LM, Landy SH, Pope RA, Waters TM, et al. Does health information exchange reduce unnecessary neuroimaging and improve quality of headache care in the emergency department? J Gen Intern Med 2013;28(2):176–83.

[23] Bailey JE, Pope RA, Elliott EC, Wan JY, Waters TM, Frisse ME. Health information exchange reduces repeated diagnostic imaging for back pain. Ann Emerg Med 2013;62(1):16–24.

[24] Ben-Assuli O, Shabtai I, Leshno M. The impact of EHR and HIE on reducing avoidable admissions: controlling main differential diagnoses. BMC Med Inform Decis Mak 2013;13:49.

[25] Dixon BE, McGowan JJ, Grannis SJ. Electronic laboratory data quality and the value of a health information exchange to support public health reporting processes. AMIA Annu Symp Proc 2011;2011:322–30.

[26] Kern LM, Barrón Y, Dhopeshwarkar RV, Kaushal R. Health information exchange and ambulatory quality of care. Appl Clin Inform 2012;3(2):197–209.

[27] Mäenpää T, Asikainen P, Gissler M, Siponen K, Maass M, Saranto K, et al. Outcomes assessment of the regional health information exchange: a five-year follow-up study. Methods Inf Med 2011;50(4):308–18.

[28] Magnus M, Herwehe J, Gruber D, Wilbright W, Shepard E, Abrams A, et al. Improved HIV-related outcomes associated with implementation of a novel public health information exchange. Int J Med Inf 2012;81(10):e30–8.

[29] Overhage JM, Grannis S, McDonald CJ. A comparison of the completeness and timeliness of automated electronic laboratory reporting and spontaneous reporting of notifiable conditions. Am J Public Health 2008;98(2):344–50.

[30] Ross SE, Radcliff TA, Leblanc WG, Dickinson LM, Libby AM, Nease Jr. DE. Effects of health information exchange adoption on ambulatory testing rates. J Am Med Inform Assoc 2013;20(6):1137–42.

[31] Shapiro JS, Johnson SA, Angiollilo J, Fleischman W, Onyile A, Kuperman G. Health information exchange improves identification of frequent emergency department users. Health Aff 2013;32(12):2193–8.

[32] Tzeel A, Lawnicki V, Pemble KR. The business case for payer support of a community-based health information exchange: a humana pilot evaluating its effectiveness in cost control for plan members seeking emergency department care. Am Health Drug Benefits 2011;4(4):207–15.

[33] Tzeel A, Lawnicki V, Pemble KR. "Hidden" value: how indirect benefits of health information exchange further promote sustainability. Am Health Drug Benefits 2012;5(6):333–40.

[34] Vest JR. Health information exchange and healthcare utilization. J Med Syst 2009;33(3):223–31.

[35] Vest JR, Kern LM, Silver MD, Kaushal R. The potential for community-based health information exchange systems to reduce hospital readmissions. J Am Med Inform Assoc 2014;22(2):435–42. Epub August 8, 2014.

[36] Vest JR, Kern LM, Campion Jr. TR, Silver MD, Kaushal R. Association between use of a health information exchange system and hospital admissions. Appl Clin Inform 2014;5(1):219–31. Epub April 16, 2014.

[37] Campion Jr. TR, Ancker JS, Edwards AM, Patel VN, Kaushal R, Investigators H Push and pull: physician usage of and satisfaction with health information exchange. AMIA Annu Symp Proc 2012;2012:77–84.

[38] Machan C, Ammenwerth E, Schabetsberger T. Evaluation of the electronic transmission of medical findings from hospitals to practitioners by triangulation. Methods Inf Med 2006;45(2):225–33. Epub March 16, 2006.

[39] Altman R, Shapiro JS, Moore T, Kuperman GJ. Notifications of hospital events to outpatient clinicians using health information exchange: a post-implementation survey. Inform Prim Care 2012;20(4):249–55.

[40] Chang KC, Overhage JM, Hui SL, Were MC. Enhancing laboratory report contents to improve outpatient management of test results. J Am Med Inform Assoc 2010;17(1):99–103.

[41] Kaushal R, Dhopeshwarkar R, Gottlieb L, Jordan H. User experiences with pharmacy benefit manager data at the point of care. J Eval Clin Pract 2010;16(6):1076–80.

[42] Maass MC, Asikainen P, Mäenpää T, Wanne O, Suominen T. Usefulness of a regional health care information system in primary care. A case study. Comput Methods Programs Biomed 2008;91(2):175–81.

[43] Park H, Lee S-I, Kim Y, Heo E-Y, Lee J, Park JH, et al. Patients' perceptions of a health information exchange: a pilot program in South Korea. Int J Med Inf 2013;82(2):98–107.

[44] Vest JR, Miller TR. The association between health information exchange and measures of patient satisfaction. Appl Clin Inform 2011;2(4):447–59. Epub January 1, 2011.

[45] Lang E, Afilalo M, Vandal AC, Boivin JF, Xue X, Colacone A, et al. Impact of an electronic link between the emergency department and family physicians: a randomized controlled trial. CMAJ 2006;174(3):313–8. Epub January 10, 2006.

[46] Willis JM, Edwards R, Anstrom KJ, Johnson FS, Del Fiol G, Kawamoto K, et al. Decision support for evidence-based pharmacotherapy detects adherence problems but does not impact medication use. Stud Health Technol Inform 2013;183:116–25. Epub February 8, 2013.

[47] Afilalo M, Lang E, Léger R, Xue X, Colacone A, Soucy N, et al. Impact of a standardized communication system on continuity of care between family physicians and the emergency department. CJEM 2007;9(2):79–86. Epub March 30, 2007.

[48] Jones SS, Friedberg MW, Schneider EC. Health information exchange, Health Information Technology use, and hospital readmission rates. AMIA Annu Symp Proc 2011;2011:644–53.

[49] Lammers EJ, Adler-Milstein J, Kocher KE. Does health information exchange reduce redundant imaging? Evidence from emergency departments. Med Care 2014;52(3):227–34.

[50] Carr CM, Gilman CS, Krywko DM, Moore HE, Walker BJ, Saef SH. Observational study and estimate of cost savings from use of a health information exchange in an academic emergency department. J Emerg Med 2014;46(2):250–6.

[51] Winden TJ, Boland LL, Frey NG, Satterlee PA, Hokanson JS. Care everywhere, a point-to-point HIE tool: utilization and impact on patient care in the ED. Appl Clin Inform 2014;5(2):388–401. Epub July 16, 2014.

[52] Ben-Assuli O, Shabtai I, Leshno M. Using electronic health record systems to optimize admission decisions: the creatinine case study. Health Informatics J 2015;21(1):73–88. Epub April 3, 2014.

[53] eHealth initiative. Result from survey on Health Data Exchange 2013. The challenge to connect. 2013 [March 3, 2015]; Available from: <http://www.ehidc.org/resource-center/reports/view_document/458-survey-results-results-from-survey-on-data-exchange-2013-data-exchange>.

[54] Adler-Milstein J, Bates DW, Jha AK. U.S. regional health information organizations: progress and challenges. Health Aff 2009;28(2):483–92.

[55] Adler-Milstein J, Jha AK. Health information exchange among U.S. hospitals: who's in, who's out, and why? Healthcare 2014;2(1):26–32.

[56] Audet A-M, Squires D, Doty MM. Where are we on the diffusion curve? Trends and drivers of primary care physicians' use of health information technology. Health Serv Res 2014;49(1 Pt 2):347–60.

[57] Furukawa MF, Patel V, Charles D, Swain M, Mostashari F. Hospital electronic health information exchange grew substantially in 2008–12. Health Aff 2013;32(8):1346–54.

[58] Furukawa MF, King J, Patel V, Hsiao C-J, Adler-Milstein J, Jha AK. Despite substantial progress in EHR adoption, health information exchange and patient engagement remain low in office settings. Health Aff 2014:1–8.

[59] Adler-Milstein J, McAfee AP, Bates DW, Jha AK. The state of regional health information organizations: current activities and financing. Health Aff 2008;27(1):w60–9.

[60] Johnson KB, Gadd CS, Aronsky D, Yang K, Tang L, Estrin V, et al. The midsouth eHealth alliance: use and impact in the first year. AMIA Annu Symp Proc 2008:333–7.

[61] Johnson KB, Unertl KM, Chen Q, Lorenzi NM, Nian H, Bailey J, et al. Health information exchange usage in emergency departments and clinics: the who, what, and why. J Am Med Inform Assoc 2011;18(5):690–7.

[62] Caffrey C, Park-Lee E. Use of electronic health records in residential care communities. NCHS Data Brief 2013;128:1–8.

[63] Hamann DJ, Bezboruah KC. Utilization of technology by long-term care providers: comparisons between for-profit and nonprofit institutions. J Aging Health 2013;25(4):535–54.

[64] Vest JR, Zhao H, Jaspserson J, Gamm LD, Ohsfeldt RL. Factors motivating and affecting health information exchange usage. J Am Med Inform Assoc 2011;18(2):143–9.

[65] Schoen C, Osborn R, Squires D, Doty M, Rasmussen P, Pierson R, et al. A survey of primary care doctors in ten countries shows progress in use of health information technology, less in other areas. Health Aff (Project Hope) 2012;31(12):2805–16. Epub November 17, 2012.

[66] Bouhaddou O, Bennett J, Cromwell T, Nixon G, Teal J, Davis M, et al. The Department of Veterans Affairs, Department of Defense, and Kaiser permanente nationwide health information network exchange in San Diego: patient selection, consent, and identity matching. AMIA Annu Symp Proc 2011;2011:135–43.

[67] Byrne CM, Mercincavage LM, Bouhaddou O, Bennett JR, Pan EC, Botts NE, et al. The Department of Veterans Affairs' (VA) implementation of the Virtual Lifetime Electronic Record (VLER): findings and lessons learned from Health Information Exchange at 12 sites. Int J Med Inf 2014;83(8):537–47.

[68] Kierkegaard P, Kaushal R, Vest JR. How could health information exchange better meet the needs of care practitioners? Appl Clin Inform 2014;5(4):861–77.

[69] Myers JJ, Koester KA, Chakravarty D, Pearson C, Maiorana A, Shade SB, et al. Perceptions regarding the ease of use and usefulness of health information exchange systems among medical providers, case managers and non-clinical staff members working in HIV care and community settings. Int J Med Inf 2012;81(10):e21–9.

[70] Ozkaynak M, Brennan PF. Revisiting sociotechnical systems in a case of unreported use of health information exchange system in three hospital emergency departments. J Eval Clin Pract 2013;19(2):370–3.

[71] Thorn SA, Carter MA, Bailey JE. Emergency physicians' perspectives on their use of health information exchange. Ann Emerg Med 2014;63(3):329–37.

[72] Unertl KM, Johnson KB, Lorenzi NM. Health information exchange technology on the front lines of healthcare: workflow factors and patterns of use. J Am Med Inform Assoc 2012;19(3):392–400.

[73] Finnell JT, Overhage JM. Emergency medical services: the frontier in health information exchange. AMIA Annu Symp Proc 2010;2010:222–6. Epub February 25, 2011.

[74] Gadd CS, Ho Y-X, Cala CM, Blakemore D, Chen Q, Frisse ME, et al. User perspectives on the usability of a regional health information exchange. J Am Med Inform Assoc 2011;18(5):711–6.

[75] Hincapie AL, Warholak TL, Murcko AC, Slack M, Malone DC. Physicians' opinions of a health information exchange. J Am Med Inform Assoc 2011;18(1):60–5.

[76] McCullough JM, Zimmerman FJ, Bell DS, Rodriguez HP. Electronic health information exchange in underserved settings: examining initiatives in small physician practices & community health centers. BMC Health Serv Res 2014;14:415. Epub September 23, 2014.

[77] Rudin R, Volk L, Simon S, Bates D. What affects clinicians' usage of health information exchange? Appl Clin Inform 2011;2(3):250–62. Epub December 20, 2011.

[78] Yeager VA, Walker D, Cole E, Mora AM, Diana ML. Factors related to health information exchange participation and use. J Med Syst 2014;38(8).

[79] Messer LC, Parnell H, Huffaker R, Wooldredge R, Wilkin A. The development of a health information exchange to enhance care and improve patient outcomes among HIV+ individuals in rural North Carolina. Int J Med Inf 2012;81(10):e46–55.

[80] Codagnone C, Lupiañez-Villanueva F. Benchmarking deployment of eHealth among general practitioners (2013)—final report. Luxembourg: European Commission; 2014.

[81] Hyppönen H, Reponen J, Lääveri T, Kaipio J. User experiences with different regional health information exchange systems in Finland. Int J Med Inf 2014;83(1):1–18.
[82] Nohr C, Kristensen M, Andersen SK, Vingtoft S, Lippert S, Berstein K, et al. Shared experience in 13 local Danish EPR projects: the Danish EPR Observatory. Stud Health Technol Inform 2001;84(Pt 1): 670–4. Epub October 18, 2001.
[83] Massy-Westropp M, Giles LC, Law D, Phillips PA, Crotty M. Connecting hospital and community care: the acceptability of a regional data linkage scheme. Aust Health Rev 2005;29(1):12–16.
[84] Adjerid I, Padman R. Impact of health disclosure laws on health information exchanges. AMIA Annu Symp Proc 2011;2011:48–56.
[85] Adler-Milstein J, Bates DW, Jha AK. A survey of health information exchange organizations in the United States: implications for meaningful use. Ann Intern Med 2011;154(10):666–71. Epub May 18, 2011.
[86] Adler-Milstein J, Bates DW, Jha AK. Operational health information exchanges show substantial growth, but long-term funding remains a concern. Health Aff (Project Hope) 2013;32(8):1486–92. Epub July 11, 2013.
[87] Agency for Healthcare Research and Quality. Evolution of state Health Information Exchange/A Study of vision, strategy, and progress. 2006 [11/20/2014]; Available from: <http://www.avalerehealth.net/research/docs/State_based_Health_Information_Exchange_Final_Report.pdf>.
[88] Dixon B, Miller T, Overhage M. Barriers to achieving the last mile in health information exchange: a survey of small hospitals and physician practices. J Healthc Inf Manag 2013;27(4):55–8.
[89] Dobalian A, Claver ML, Pevnick JM, Stutman HR, Tomines A, Fu Jr. P. Organizational challenges in developing one of the Nationwide Health Information Network trial implementation awardees. J Med Syst 2012;36(2):933–40.
[90] Dullabh P, Hovey L. Large scale health information exchange: implementation exp eriences from five states. Stud Health Technol Inform 2013;192:613–7.
[91] Dullabh P, Ubri P, Hovey L. The state HIE program four years later: key findings on grantees' experiences from a six-state review. Washington, DC: Office of the National Coordinator for Health Information Technology; 2014.
[92] Fairbrother G, Trudnak T, Christopher R, Mansour M, Mandel K. Cincinnati Beacon community program highlights challenges and opportunities on the path to care transformation. Health Aff 2014;33(5):871–7.
[93] Feldman SS, Schooley LB, Bhavsar PG. Health information exchange implementation: lessons learned and critical success factors from a case study. JMIR Med Inform 2014;2(2):e19.
[94] Foldy S. Inventory of electronic health information exchange in Wisconsin, 2006. WMJ 2007;106(3):120–5.
[95] Fontaine P, Zink T, Boyle RG, Kralewski J. Health information exchange: participation by Minnesota primary care practices. Arch Intern Med 2010;170(7):622–9.
[96] Genes N, Shapiro J, Vaidya S, Kuperman G. Adoption of health information exchange by emergency physicians at three urban academic medical centers. Appl Clin Inform 2011;2(3):263–9. Epub January 1, 2011.
[97] Goldwater J, Jardim J, Khan T, Chan K. Emphasizing public health within a health information exchange: an evaluation of the district of Columbia's health information exchange program. EGEMS (Wash DC) 2014;2(3):1090. Available from: http://dx.doi.org/10.13063/2327-9214.1090.
[98] Grossman JM, Kushner KL, November EA. Creating sustainable local health information exchanges: can barriers to stakeholder participation be overcome? Res Briefs 2008;2:1–12.
[99] Herwehe J, Wilbright W, Abrams A, Bergson S, Foxhood J, Kaiser M, et al. Implementation of an innovative, integrated electronic medical record (EMR) and public health information exchange for HIV/AIDS. J Am Med Inform Assoc 2012;19(3):448–52.
[100] Hessler BJ, Soper P, Bondy J, Hanes P, Davidson A. Assessing the relationship between health information exchanges and public health agencies. J Public Health Manag Pract 2009;15(5):416–24.
[101] Kern LM, Barrón Y, Abramson EL, Patel V, Kaushal R. HEAL NY: promoting interoperable health information technology in New York State. Health Aff 2009;28(2):493–504.
[102] Kern LM, Wilcox A, Shapiro J, Dhopeshwarkar RV, Kaushal R. Which components of health information technology will drive financial value? Am J Manag Care 2012;18(8):438–45.
[103] Kern LM, Wilcox AB, Shapiro J, Yoon-Flannery K, Abramson E, Barrón Y, et al. Community-based health information technology alliances: potential predictors of early sustainability. Am J Manag Care 2011;17(4):290–5.
[104] Lobach DF, Kawamoto K, Anstrom KJ, Kooy KR, Eisenstein EL, Silvey GM, et al. Proactive population health management in the context of a regional health information exchange using standards-based decision support. AMIA Annu Symp Proc 2007: 473–7.

[105] McCarthy DB, Propp K, Cohen A, Sabharwal R, Schachter AA, Rein AL. Learning from health information exchange technical architecture and implementation in seven beacon communities. EGEMS (Wash DC) 2014;2(1):6.

[106] McGowan JJ, Jordan C, Sims T, Overhage JM. Rural RHIOs: common issues in the development of two state-wide health information networks. AMIA Annu Symp Proc 2007:528–32.

[107] Merrill JA, Deegan M, Wilson RV, Kaushal R, Fredericks K. A system dynamics evaluation model: implementation of health information exchange for public health reporting. J Am Med Inform Assoc 2013;20(e1):e131–8.

[108] Miller AR, Tucker C. Health information exchange, system size and information silos. J Health Econ 2014;33:28–42.

[109] Miller RH. Satisfying patient–consumer principles for health information exchange: evidence from California case studies. Health Aff 2012;31(3):537–47.

[110] Morris G, Afzal S, Bhasker M, Finney D. Query-based exchange: key factors influencing success and failure. Office of the National Coordinator for Health Information Technology; 2012.

[111] Nykänen P, Karimaa E. Success and failure factors in the regional health information system design process—results from a constructive evaluation study. Methods Inf Med (Washington, DC) 2006;45(1):85–9. Epub February 17, 2006.

[112] Overhage JM, Evans L, Marchibroda J. Communities' readiness for health information exchange: the National Landscape in 2004. J Am Med Inform Assoc 2005;12(2):107–12.

[113] Pagliari C, Gilmour M, Sullivan F. Electronic clinical communications implementation (ECCI) in Scotland: a mixed-methods programme evaluation. J Eval Clin Pract 2004;10(1):11–20. Epub 21 January, 2004.

[114] Phillips AB, Wilson RV, Kaushal R, Merrill JA, Investigators H Implementing health information exchange for public health reporting: a comparison of decision and risk management of three regional health information organizations in New York state. J Am Med Inform Assoc 2014;21(e1):e173–7.

[115] Pirnejad H, Bal R, Berg M. Building an inter-organizational communication network and challenges for preserving interoperability. Int J Med Inf 2008;77(12):818–27.

[116] Pouloudi A. Information technology for collaborative advantage in healthcare revisited. Inf Manage 1999;35(6):345–56.

[117] Ross SE, Schilling LM, Fernald DH, Davidson AJ, West DR. Health information exchange in small-to-medium sized family medicine practices: motivators, barriers, and potential facilitators of adoption. Int J Med Inf 2010;79(2):123–9.

[118] Rudin RS, Simon SR, Volk LA, Tripathi M, Bates D. Understanding the decisions and values of stakeholders in health information exchanges: experiences from Massachusetts. Am J Public Health 2009;99(5):950–5.

[119] Saff E, Lanway C, Chenyek A, Morgan D. The Bay Area HIE. A case study in connecting stakeholders. J Healthc Inf Manag 2010;24(1):25–30.

[120] Schabetsberger T, Ammenwerth E, Andreatta S, Gratl G, Haux R, Lechleitner G, et al. From a paper-based transmission of discharge summaries to electronic communication in health care regions. Int J Med Inf 2006;75(3–4):209–15.

[121] Sicotte C, Paré G. Success in health information exchange projects: solving the implementation puzzle. Soc Sci Med 2010;70(8):1159–65.

[122] Silvester BV, Carr SJ. A shared electronic health record: lessons from the coalface. Med J Aust 2009;190(11 Suppl):S113–6.

[123] Steward WT, Koester KA, Collins SP, Maiorana A, Myers JJ. The essential role of reconfiguration capabilities in the implementation of HIV-related health information exchanges. Int J Med Inf 2012;81(10):e10–20.

[124] Tripathi M, Delano D, Lund B, Rudolph L. Engaging patients for health information exchange. Health Aff 2009;28(2):435–43.

[125] Unertl MK, Johnson BK, Gadd SC, Lorenzi MN. Bridging organizational divides in health care: an ecological view of health information exchange. JMIR Med Inform 2013;1(1):e3.

[126] Vest JR. More than just a question of technology: factors related to hospitals' adoption and implementation of health information exchange. Int J Med Inf 2010;79(12):797–806.

[127] Vest JR, Issel LM. Factors related to public health data sharing between local and state health departments. Health Serv Res 2014;49(1 Pt 2):373–91.

[128] Roshanov PS, Fernandes N, Wilczynski JM, Hemens BJ, You JJ, Handler SM, et al. Features of effective computerised clinical decision support systems: meta-regression of 162 randomised trials. BMJ 2013;346:f657. Epub February 16, 2013.

[129] Fleurence RL, Curtis LH, Califf RM, Platt R, Selby JV, Brown JS. Launching PCORnet, a national patient-centered clinical research network. J Am Med Inform Assoc 2014 amiajnl-2014-002747.

CHAPTER

15

Measuring the Value of Health Information Exchange

Brian E. Dixon[1] *and Caitlin M. Cusack*[2]

[1]Indiana University Richard M. Fairbanks School of Public Health; and the Center for Biomedical Informatics, Regenstrief Institute, Inc., Indianapolis, IN [2]Insight Informatics, Manchester, NH

OUTLINE

LEARNING OBJECTIVES

At the end of this chapter, the reader should be able to

- Define evaluation in the context of health information exchange.
- Compare and contrast the various categories of evaluation.

- List and describe the domains of evaluation commonly examined in health information exchange.
- Discuss the importance of developing an evaluation plan.
- Identify the various roles recommended for inclusion as part of the evaluation team.
- Outline important considerations for the design of an evaluation plan.
- State the key sections or components of an evaluation plan.
- Describe why dissemination is an important aspect of evaluation.
- Prepare an evaluation plan to measure some aspect of health information exchange.

INTRODUCTION

Given the dearth of evidence on the effective use of health information exchange (HIE) to improve outcomes for patients or populations as described in the chapter "The Evidence Base for Health Information Exchange," there is a clear need to evaluate the implementation, use, and impact of HIE by those investing in it within a community, state, or nation. While literature reviews and journal articles argue for comparative studies and research agendas, the evidence base for HIE will not be developed by research scientists alone. Demonstrating HIE's effectiveness in reducing costs, improving outcomes, and creating more efficient care delivery systems will come from a combination of scientific research and practice-based evaluation. This chapter describes strategies and methods for evaluating HIE, principally from the perspective of a health system or other entity engaged in the implementation and use of HIE. The chapter begins with a review of the various types of evaluation, including research. Then the chapter outlines a strategy and the methods for the evaluation of HIE. Finally, the chapter provides guidance for how to disseminate outcomes from HIE development, implementation, adoption, and use. Only by evaluating HIE and sharing lessons will the evidence base for HIE be strengthened. It is incumbent upon all of us in both academia and practice to further develop the evidence base if we desire HIE to be sustainable.

THE SPECTRUM OF EVALUATION

Evaluation seeks to examine the "worth, merit, or significance" [1] of an object (eg, program, HIE, device). Many organizations routinely conduct evaluations to determine whether their business operations, internal initiatives, or external partnerships are effective. Efforts found to be effective are sustained or expanded, and ineffective efforts are either improved or terminated. These activities are often labeled as quality improvement projects, lean manufacturing, six sigma, or operations research. Research, therefore, is just one type of evaluation performed to determine whether an information system, program, or process is meritorious.

Despite the fact many health care organizations routinely evaluate their clinical or administrative operations, health care leaders often equate evaluation of HIE with research and therefore entrust it to academics. A decade ago, the US Agency for Healthcare Research and Quality (AHRQ) awarded grants to over 100 health systems across America to implement health information technology (health IT) [2]. The list of grantees included a number of organizations seeking to deploy HIE in their local community or across their state [3,4]. Each grantee organization was asked to complete an evaluation as a component of their project. While projects led by academic research organizations submitted evaluation plans in a timely fashion, projects led by health systems and community organizations struggled to develop their evaluation plans [5]. In a series of meetings with grantees, AHRQ learned that practice-based organizations viewed evaluation as synonymous with scientific research and therefore struggled to come up with what they perceived as "rigorous research" of their HIE efforts.

Many in health care associate the term "research" with a randomized controlled trial (RCT) in which subjects are randomly assigned to either receive a new medication (drug) or a placebo (an inert substance also referred to as a sugar pill). While RCTs are considered the hallmark of scientific research for demonstrating the effectiveness of a new medication, therapy, or health delivery process, they are not the only form of scientific research performed in health care. Nor are they the only kind of evaluation that can support the implementation and adoption of new technologies in health care. In fact, RCTs are very challenging to do in the domain of health IT and HIE, because it is often either unethical to deny HIE benefits to some people in a community or impractical to partially implement HIE in a health system. Moreover, RCTs are costly and lengthy as they require significant human resources to coordinate the implementation of HIE into carefully selected, controlled environments. Therefore the health system must utilize an array of evaluation methods beyond RCTs to study HIE and other information technologies [5,6]. Evaluations of HIE can be grouped into the following categories: formative evaluation, summative evaluation, and scientific research.

Formative Evaluation

Formative evaluation takes place before or during implementation with the aim of improving the design and performance of the technology being implemented [6]. Evaluations of this type are sometimes referred to as "playing smallball," a baseball analogy that suggests the goal of a formative evaluation is not to hit a Grand Slam but to simply make a base hit [7]. For HIE, formative evaluations tend to be focused on a singular aspect of the exchange, and thus can be carried out by a relatively small team overseen by a project manager or program director. For example, the project director may wish to ensure that health care organization leaders are on board with the formation of an HIE effort in the community, or the creation of a new HIE service. A stakeholder analysis would facilitate systematic collection of feedback from the health care leaders useful to decision-making at the local HIE while simultaneously providing insights useful to other HIEs that could be shared in the form of a whitepaper or professional conference presentation.

Formative evaluation can occur during multiple phases of HIE development as summarized in Table 15.1. Several existing HIE efforts have used formative evaluation to assess readiness for HIE adoption [8,9], the design of HIE services [10,11], or the early adoption of HIE in an organization or geographic region [12,13]. Qualitative methods, those that focus on open-ended questions and emergent discovery of knowledge, lend themselves well to this form of evaluation.

Summative Evaluation

Summative evaluation, which can be referred to as ex-post evaluation (meaning after the event), typically occurs after implementation, and focuses on the impact of a given technology. Most often this form of evaluation is used to measure whether or not a technology such as HIE achieved its desired aims or goals. For example, a summative evaluation might measure the impact of HIE on specialty care referrals from primary care clinicians. The focus of summative evaluation is on outcomes, however, and

TABLE 15.1 The Stages of HIE in Which Formative Evaluation Can Be Used to Gather Insight, Lessons, and Evidence

	Formation	Development	Implementation
Purpose of the evaluation	To understand or clarify the need for HIE.	To understand user needs or rationale for design decisions.	To ensure that HIE activities are being delivered efficiently and effectively.
Examples	Review of available literature to convince stakeholders of the need for HIE.	Conduct a focus group to gather ideas on the design of services offered by the HIE.	Review project team materials to assess whether the implementation is on schedule and within budget.
	Analyze the readiness of organizations in the community to engage in HIE.	Interview IT staff at HIE member organizations to gather input on the design of the HIE architecture.	Observe clinical users to assess access to and early adoption of HIE services and applications.
	Observe clinicians' request and use of information from outside providers or organizations to identify potential workflow, improvements given in HIE.	Survey health care organizations to assess market interest and customer price points.	Assess the quality of data transmitted from source systems (eg, laboratory information system).

Includes examples of formative evaluation methods for assessing specific aspects of HIE.

not process. So the emphasis in an e-referral project would be on care coordination, including timeliness of follow up by specialists and primary care physicians' satisfaction with the service, instead of simply counting the number of e-referrals sent by primary care doctors. In other words, summative evaluation measures the value of HIE with respect to clinical decision-making, health care delivery, as well as patient and population outcomes. This kind of evaluation can also be used to measure HIE usage, such as measuring how many patients' records in the HIE are accessed or under what conditions emergency department clinicians access the HIE. The results of summative evaluations can be shared in the form of reports or peer-reviewed journal articles in addition to conference presentations. Summative evaluations often use quantitative methods, although qualitative methods are used in some cases.

Real world examples of summative evaluations performed in HIE include the following:

- Measuring the impact of HIE on repeated diagnostic imaging and related costs in emergency back pain evaluation [14].
- Barriers to usage of HIE in interorganizational patient transfers [15].
- Assessment of the association between HIE system usage and 30-day same-cause hospital readmissions [16].
- Assessment of HIE impact on surveillance of the H1N1 influenza outbreak in a local health jurisdiction [17].

Scientific Research

Scientific research aims at producing generalizable knowledge using replicable methods to measure the impact of HIE on some outcome. While summative evaluation also measures outcomes, scientific research attempts to control for various extraneous factors such as organizational, behavioral, or policy factors. By controlling for these extraneous factors, scientists seek to find out whether and how much HIE influenced the outcome beyond policy changes (eg, Meaningful Use) or a charismatic HIE champion. Furthermore, scientific research can examine patterns and trends beyond a single HIE implementation. For example, a cross-sectional study might survey hospitals about their adoption and usage of HIE to infer trends across a state, region, or nation. Scientific research also includes RCTs as well as large observational studies of patient populations, provider organizations that participate in HIE, and HIE initiatives themselves. Quantitative, qualitative, and mixed methods studies are all used in scientific research.

Real world examples of scientific research performed in HIE include the following:

- An examination of lessons and challenges from 12 sites within the US Department of Veterans Affairs (VA) that implemented HIE with non-VA providers [18].
- A national survey in the United States of ambulatory care providers to identify how many and which types of practices participate in HIE activities [19].
- A national, 5-year study in Finland looking at the impact of HIE on the volume of laboratory tests, radiology examinations, appointments, emergency visits, and referrals [20].
- A study in South Korea which examined the impact of HIE on physicians' access to past clinical information as well as reductions in diagnostic test utilization and health care costs [21].

Domains of Evaluation

No matter the type, evaluation examines one or more aspects of HIE. Prior work developed a framework [22] that defines five broad domains in which evaluation of HIE can occur (see Table 15.2). Each domain is broad, encompassing a range of possible questions that a health system, HIE initiative, policymaker, or research scientist might wish to ask. While the Value domain focuses on the impact of HIE on outcomes, the other domains support evaluation questions that address the impact of HIE or its components (eg, technical aspects, a certain type of data) on patients, providers, organizations, usage, or adoption. This framework is useful for thinking about the kinds of questions certain stakeholders might ask about the development, implementation, or use of HIE.

DEVELOPING AN EVALUATION PLAN

To effectively evaluate an aspect of an operational HIE initiative or the development of HIE for a specific use case, one must have a plan. The plan outlines the goals of both the HIE project as well as the evaluation; it specifies what is to be measured, how it is to be measured, and by whom; it considers costs, personnel, and timelines; and it serves as an overall guide for the team conducting the evaluation. Although aspects of the evaluation will likely evolve and change during execution of the plan, it is critical to the success of an evaluation to begin with a well-constructed plan.

The following sections of the chapter outline the various components of an evaluation plan. One can think of the section headers as a checklist of elements that could be embodied in a document shared amongst a team as well as stakeholders, such as the people or organization funding the evaluation. The content in these sections is derived from the authors' many years of evaluating HIE as well as from their work with AHRQ grantees seeking to do the same. A corollary document that those interested in HIE evaluation might find valuable is the "Guide to Evaluating Health Information Exchange Projects" published by AHRQ [23].

The Evaluation Team

One of the first tasks to evaluating HIE is putting together the right team. Just as HIE development and implementation teams involve multiple individuals with different

TABLE 15.2 Domains of Evaluation for HIE

Domain	Description	Evaluation Question Examples
Technology	Evaluations in this domain focus on the technical aspects of HIE, including performance of the software, hardware, and architectural choices made by the HIE. This domain also allows for comparison of technical designs, maintenance costs, and system usability.	What is the accuracy of the master person index? Which text mining methods can best identify active medications in a hospital discharge summary? Which data encryption tools perform well in a federated HIE network of mental health clinics?
Data	Evaluations in this domain focus on the data captured, stored, and managed by the HIE. This can include the quality of the data from various sources as well as which data are accessed under what conditions by certain types of user groups.	Which sources of data are most accessed by primary care clinicians? How complete and timely are immunization records sent by emergency departments? Under what conditions do clinicians click on discharge summaries that are more than 5 years old?
Implementation	Evaluations in this domain focus on the facets of design, use, and implementation of HIE in a health system or community. They can range from measuring adoption by certain providers to the cost of interface development to the challenges of mapping local terminologies to a reference terminology.	What is the average total cost associated with implementing an interface to emergency department information systems for syndromic surveillance? Which providers tend to use the HIE and under what conditions? How many full-time equivalents are needed to staff the help desk at HIEs of various sizes and maturity levels?
Policy	Evaluations in this domain focus on the influence of local, state, and national policies on the adoption and use of HIE. Evaluations can examine stakeholder engagement as well as aspects of privacy. They can also include measuring the degree to which use is mandated by hospital administration.	Does HIE adoption vary based on the size and governance structure of a hospital? What is the impact of Stage 3 Meaningful Use on the adoption of HIE among physician practices with less than five providers? Would a change in privacy policy impact the adoption and use of HIE among patients in Indiana?
Value	Evaluations in this domain focus on the impact of HIE on clinical and population outcomes. They can further measure the effect of HIE on health care costs, utilization, and access.	Does HIE between VA and non-VA providers improve access to care for Veterans? What is the impact of HIE within an accountable care organization on rehospitalizations? Can HIE between primary care and specialty providers improve the coordination of care?

Adapted from Ref. [22].
Includes evaluation questions representative of each domain.

expertise, so does the evaluation team. The evaluation team can be led by someone from the implementation team, or it could be a consultant hired to conduct the evaluation. While the exact composition of the evaluation team will vary depending on the goals of the evaluation, one should consider including experts in the following areas: evaluation methodology, health care operations, technical implementation, clinical care, and project management. In addition, having someone who represents the patient or consumer viewpoint could be helpful. Each of these areas is considered below.

Evaluation Methodology

The benefits of working with an expert in evaluation methodology when conducting an evaluation are obvious. For HIE evaluation, it is best to identify someone who is experienced in health services or public health evaluations. These individuals can be recruited from academic organizations, or they may be employed by a consulting firm. Experts in evaluation methodology may advise on what to measure, how to measure the outcomes of interest, and the process for conducting the evaluation. Furthermore, they may assist in the analysis and interpretation of results. Experts can further provide oversight of evaluation activities, human subjects' protection, and confidentiality of evaluation data including compliance with the Health Insurance Portability and Accountability Act of 1996 (HIPAA).

Health Care Operations

Experts in this area are individuals with detailed understanding of the administrative and business side of health care organizations. They can be particularly helpful when measuring impact of HIE on health care workflows. Such an expert can communicate with organizational staff and administrators before and during the evaluation, represent their needs to the evaluation team, and help determine what health care organizations and stakeholders need to collect or extract from administrative systems as part of the evaluation. In addition, health care operations expertise can help determine the validity of measures for financial assessments of HIE costs and savings, such as reduced utilization of services.

Technical Implementation

Experts in this area are individuals who are familiar with health IT systems and HIE transactions. They can help the evaluation team determine what is feasible to extract from electronic health record (EHR) systems, clinical data warehouses, or other components of the HIE in order to measure system performance, HIE usage, volume of transactions, or impact on patient and population outcomes. Technical experts are often familiar with health IT data standards as well as how data are entered and stored in systems. They can further assist the evaluation team in managing the data it will ultimately collect for analysis.

Clinical Care

Experts in clinical care are current or former practicing clinicians who understand clinical decision-making processes as well as workflow. They can inform study designs that aim at measuring the impact of HIE on patient outcomes as well as diagnosis, treatment plans, or care coordination. Clinical expertise is especially important to evaluation efforts that seek to measure adherence to clinical guidelines, clinical performance, patient safety, or quality of care. Sometimes it is possible to recruit a senior clinician with administrative experience who can inform both clinical and operations aspects of an evaluation. In other instances, this role may be filled by a clinician champion involved in the implementation of HIE within a health system or community.

Project Management

Experts in project management are important not only for implementation of HIE but also its evaluation. Evaluations can involve complex data collection from multiple EHR systems or organizations, and efforts to obtain consent from study participants as well as schedule observations of workflow require coordination. An experienced project manager can support execution of the evaluation plan by coordinating team activities while helping to ensure the evaluation is completed on time and within budget.

Patient (Consumer) Representation

Patients and their caregivers can provide useful insights into the type of metrics or study questions that would be most beneficial to other patients and caregivers. If the evaluation seeks to measure patient satisfaction, quality of life, or patient reported outcomes, consider adding one or more patient representatives to the evaluation team. Ideally, patient representatives should be familiar with the health care consumer experience and able to share first-hand experiences of being a patient or caregiver.

Defining Goals, Objectives, and Stakeholders

To measure the impact of HIE, one must first define the impact(s) to be measured. Planning an evaluation therefore begins by defining the goals and objectives of the HIE, and it requires defining the stakeholders who care about whether the HIE is successful or fails.

First, identify key stakeholders who care about the success of HIE. These stakeholders might be those who are funding the implementation of HIE, or they may be the participants in HIE. Health systems are often stakeholders in HIE as are clinicians. However, there may be other groups that stand to benefit if HIE is successful, or lose if HIE fails. It is these stakeholders who will be interested in the results of the evaluation, and their perspective matters to the evaluation plan.

Next, enumerate the goals and objectives of HIE, usually within a particular use case. For example, a community may wish to improve the exchange of immunization records to enhance the ability of the health system to both measure vaccine coverage and forecast vaccines for a particular patient population (eg, children, the elderly). Such goals and objectives would likely suggest an evaluation plan that would seek to measure a change in documented vaccine administration records, as well as accurate vaccine forecasts generated for the patient population of interest. The objectives of an evaluation plan (eg, what it seeks to measure) stem from the goals and objectives of HIE mediated by stakeholders. Table 15.3 provides

TABLE 15.3 Example Alignment of HIE Goals and Objectives Mediated by Stakeholder Groups for the Use Case of Electronic Laboratory Reporting

Goal and Objective of the Health Information Exchange	Stakeholder Groups and Their Interests	Evaluation Plan Objectives (Measures)
Goal: To improve the completeness and timeliness of disease reporting by successfully transmitting laboratory results electronically to public health authorities in the State of Indiana. *Objective*: To exchange at least 80% of laboratory results from private hospital and independent laboratories electronically within 18 months.	Public health department receiving complete lists of cases faster. Health systems—cutting costs for paper and time to fax results to health department. Providers—reducing costs and time for faxing lab results to health authorities.	Measure change at the health department in the number and percent of fax-based laboratory reports to electronically delivered laboratory reports. Measure change in time (# days) between when the laboratory test was performed and when it was reported to a public health department. Measure change in time (# minutes) clinic and laboratory staff spend handling laboratory reports. Measure change in number of laboratory reports received from stakeholders per unique disease case (redundant reporting).

an example showing the alignment between the goals and objectives of a project to electronically report laboratory results to public health authorities mediated by the interests of stakeholder groups.

Identifying Potential Measures

Once the stakeholders, goals, and objectives are known, the evaluation team can then identify potential measures. Eventually the evaluation project will measure some change as a result of the HIE. This might be a change in patient attitudes or knowledge, provider attitudes or knowledge, efficiency of care processes, or clinical or population outcomes. Although measurement is an action (verb), evaluations use measures (nouns) or variables to indicate whether a change has occurred. Measures can be clinical or process indicators such as blood pressure versus the number of days to schedule an appointment. A successful evaluation is one that selects feasible measures, or measures that are readily available and can be objectively collected for analysis.

The first step in selecting measures for a given evaluation is to generate a list of candidate measures. There are two methods for generating the list: (1) perform a literature review and (2) brainstorm possible measures. While either method can generate a list of candidate measures, it is recommended that both methods be used, because they complement one another and can ensure that a comprehensive list of candidate measures is generated.

A literature review is a process to identify relevant material from both peer-reviewed and gray literature (information that falls outside the mainstream of published journals and monographs), reading through the material, and analyzing the information in the material. Librarians in hospitals, academic medical centers, or the public library are excellent resources to consult when conducting a literature review. They can assist in designing a broad but specific search. Furthermore, they can help identify relevant sources of gray literature that may not appear in an online search.

The second method involves gathering the evaluation team plus key stakeholders to brainstorm measures of interest. Brainstorming is a group exercise designed to generate ideas through open and constructive discussion. Health care executives and clinical leaders are familiar with a wide range of indicators they review on a regular basis: indicators they might want to see affected by HIE. Evaluation experts will also be familiar with commonly used indicators in prior evaluations. Discussion should center on the goals and objectives of the HIE use case as well as the evaluation. Candidate measures should be related to the evaluation target.

The group should solicit ideas from all attendees, and emphasize that "no idea is a bad idea." Keep in mind that this list will be further reviewed, discussed, and paired down. Therefore it is best to start with a large list since many measures will be eliminated when the evaluation plan is finalized.

Designing the Evaluation

Now that the team has a list of possible measures, it is time to design the evaluation. The evaluation team must decide upon the study design and methods. The study design, whether formative, summative, or scientific research, should be informed by the stage of HIE development and purpose of the evaluation, as discussed at the beginning of the chapter. The study methods should be informed by the study design.

Study methods produce the data and are grouped into three categories: quantitative, qualitative, and mixed. In general, quantitative methods produce numbers that describe what has changed; while qualitative methods produce information that describes why or how a change occurred. Mixed methods use a combination of quantitative and qualitative methods to produce a more comprehensive understanding of an outcome. Table 15.4 summarizes and compares study methods as well as example data they produce.

An example of a mixed methods study evaluating HIE is the AHRQ-funded "Improving Population Health through Enhanced Targeted Regional Decision Support" project [24], which aims to use a community-based HIE to electronically prepopulate provider-submitted notifiable condition case reporting forms with available clinical, lab, and patient data. The evaluation-specific objectives of this project are to assess the implementation of the reporting form intervention at the clinic level to:

1. Identify barriers and facilitators to implementation, adoption, and utilization of the prepopulated reporting form;
2. Measure impacts of the tool on workflow, provider awareness, and end-user satisfaction; and
3. Describe the contextual factors that impact the effectiveness of the intervention within heterogeneous clinical settings and the HIE.

To evaluate the intervention, the study is using a concurrent mixed methods design, in which the quantitative and qualitative methods occur in parallel both pre- and postimplementation to enable comparison. Because the study is scientific research, the study will also collect data from control clinics, which are peers of the intervention sites but are not adopting the HIE intervention until a later date (presumably when the study team demonstrates value of the intervention).

In each phase of the study, the evaluation team will use closed-ended surveys (quantitative),

TABLE 15.4 Comparison of Study Methods and the Data They Produce

Study Methods	Examples of Methods	Examples of Data Produced
Quantitative	Surveys/questionnaires	• Likert scale values 1–5 based on respondents' answer selection. • Demographics of the subjects. • Ordinal data based on respondents' multiple choice answers.
	Analysis of administrative datasets such as diagnosis codes or user access logs	• Count of each ICD-10 code recorded for patients in the emergency department. • List of clinical users and the date/time they accessed the HIE portal or viewer.
	Analysis of clinical datasets such as laboratory results or postsurgical outcomes	• Count of HbA1c tests performed for patients with diabetes. • Average value of HbA1c test results. • List of patients with a 30-day readmission following a surgical procedure.
Qualitative	Observations	• Long lists of activities performed by clinicians during the observation period. • After synthesis, patterns of activities or decision-making processes during a shift.
	Interviews	• Pages of transcribed questions and answers from the people interviewed. • Video or audio of the interviews; notes taken by the study team.
	Focus groups	• Pages of transcribed discussion among small groups of people. • Video or audio of the sessions. • Notes from the focus group leader and observers.
	Document review	• Copies of notices of privacy practice from clinics. • Notes taken during implementation team meetings over an 18-month period.

time-series data (eg, quantitative reporting rates by physicians over time), data quality measures (eg, quantitative completeness of data, quantitative timeliness of reports), interviews with clinical as well as public health staff (qualitative), and open-ended survey questions (qualitative) as methods to collect data on the intervention from the perspective of both clinical and public health. The main components of the evaluation plan, including data sources, are summarized in Table 15.5.

Data Sources

The next step in the process is identifying the sources of the data to support evaluation of the potential measures for the target study design. Data are everywhere in the health system as well as in health information systems. The challenge is defining how the data are to be captured or extracted so they can be used in the evaluation. Furthermore, the team needs to consider where the extracted data will be stored for use during the analysis phase. There are likely to be many data of interest, but only a limited set of data that can be feasibly captured from health services or extracted from existing systems.

Given the proposed study design and list of candidate measures, the team should systematically identify the sources and extraction methods for the data that will be used for each proposed measure. Potential sources include: laboratory information system, radiology information system, emergency department information system, billing system, registration system, disease registry, pharmacy orders, medication administration systems, personal health record system, and nursing documentation. Other systems to consider: enterprise clinical data warehouse; interface engines that move data between information systems; edge servers that queue incoming or outgoing messages or documents; or the client registry. Some of these systems will be readily available to the HIE or health system, while others (eg, disease registry, immunization information system) might be available through a partner, such as the public health authority, insurance company, or independent laboratory.

Each system will likely have a different process by which the team can extract, transform, and load (ETL) data into a study database that will enable analysis. This is where having technical expertise on the evaluation team will be vital. Moreover, extracting data from information systems managed by partners may require coordination and discussions with their technical staff. External data sources may also require executing a data use agreement or business associate agreement, a task that can be handled by the project manager with review and input from legal counsel and project director. Keep in mind that legal agreements can take weeks to months to negotiate and finalize.

A final consideration is how the data captured by the evaluation team (eg, interview data) or extracted from an information system (eg, laboratory results) will be analyzed. Qualitative data usually require multiple iterations in which the raw notes or documents are synthesized into themes and patterns. Quantitative data often need manipulation prior to their use in an analysis. For example, laboratory test result data are often quite complex—especially microbiology results. Some results might have a numeric value and a reference range, allowing the team to easily assess whether the value falls inside or out of the range and is therefore indicative of disease or a given health status. Yet many results are reported as cryptic values of "present" or "suspected" while they are sent to public health lab for confirmation, leaving the final result determination up to the evaluation team when analyzing the data. Moreover, many patients with a given disease, such as diabetes, may not have a formal, documented diagnostic code for the disease. Therefore the team may need to derive a formula for determining, based on available

TABLE 15.5 Evaluation Details for an Community-Based HIE Study to Test the Impact of an Intervention on Public Health Reporting Processes Described in Ref. [24]

Evaluation Construct	Data Collected	Method	Pre	Post	Analysis
Reporting rates	Number of reports submitted by primary care providers to public health departments—collect from control and intervention sites	C	X	X	ITS
Completeness	Completed/missing provider report data fields	C	X	X	ITS
	Comparison of completeness	C	X	X	PPC
	Provider perceptions of completeness of prepopulated forms	S/I	X	X	QUAL/DESC
Accuracy	Inaccurate provider report data fields	C	X	X	ITS
	Comparison of accuracy	C	X	X	PPC
	Provider perceptions of accuracy of intervention	S/I	X	X	QUAL/DESC
Timeliness	Time between data when lab test performed and when the result was reported to public health	C	X	X	ITS
	Comparison of timeliness	C	X	X	PPC
	Provider perceptions of timeliness of intervention	S/I	X	X	QUAL/DESC
Burden	Volume and duration of phone and fax communications by public health staff with staff at the control and intervention clinics	C	X	X	ITS
	Provider perceptions regarding reporting burden	S/I	X	X	QUAL/DESC
Data quality	Provider perceptions regarding quality of data in prepopulated reporting forms (intervention)	S/I	X	X	QUAL/DESC
Benefits & utility	Provider perceived benefits & utility of intervention	S/I	X	X	QUAL/DESC
Adoption & use	Provider perceived barriers & facilitators to adopting & using prepopulated report forms	S/I	X	X	QUAL/DESC
	Level of acceptance & satisfaction with intervention	S/I	X	X	QUAL/DESC
	Provider perceived ease of operations	S/I	X	X	QUAL/DESC
	Provider acceptability of interface	S/I	X	X	QUAL/DESC
Workflow	Public health workflow observations	O	X	X	DESC
	Provider reported impact of intervention on work & information flows	S/I	X	X	QUAL/DESC
Context	Clinic demographics	S/I	X	X	DESC

C, census of public health report forms & data fields; DESC, descriptive statistics; ITS, interrupted time-series; FG, focus groups; I, semi-structured interviews; PPC, pre-post comparison; O, observations; Pre, before implementation; Post, post pre-populated report form implementation; QUAL, qualitative data analysis; S, clinician surveys.

data, whether a given patient has a particular disease or outcome. The need to transform data prior to analysis should be considered when discussing how best to capture data for a given measure.

Assessing Feasibility of Evaluation Measures

Reaching this step in the planning process is not an easy task. However, by systematically thinking through the study design, evaluation methods, potential measures, data sources, and data extraction methods, the team will be well aware of the challenges, complexities, and effort that may be required to measure everything on the list thus far. This awareness will be useful during this step: assessing feasibility of the candidate evaluation measures.

In this step, the team discusses the candidate measures, the sources of the data for those measures, and the relevant ETL methods, in the context of the study design and evaluation methods. To guide the discussion, we suggest asking the team to collectively place each candidate measure in one of the quadrants within a 3 × 3 decision matrix (Fig. 15.1). The measures should be considered with respect to two aspects: (1) their importance to stakeholders and (2) their feasibility to capture. Measures that are both important to stakeholders and feasible to obtain for analysis should be prioritized in the evaluation plan. Quadrants 1–3 are marked in green (light gray in the print version) to suggest that, after discussion, the measures placed in them should be retained for the final evaluation plan. The measures in quadrants 4 and 5 should be further discussed and kept in the plan as time and resources permit. Measures that are not feasible, meaning that their capture or extraction would come at a large expense or significant time, should be eliminated. The goal is to help the team prioritize the measures that will best meet stakeholder needs given the budget, time, and people available to perform the evaluation.

Finalizing the Plan

With a completed decision matrix, the team is ready to finalize the evaluation plan. At this stage, the output from each section above can be combined into a single document. The document should be drafted by the team, internally reviewed, and potentially reviewed by external experts or advisors. Once fully drafted, the plan can be presented to a funder for review, or it can be shared with a Board for advice and consent. Once approved by stakeholders, the team will be ready to execute the plan.

		Feasibility		
		1: Feasible	2: Feasible With moderate effort	3: Not Feasible
Importance	1. Very Important	(1)	(2)	
	2. Moderate Important	(3)	(4)	
	3. Not Important	(5)		

FIGURE 15.1 A decision matrix to guide the selection of important and feasible measures for use in the final evaluation plan. *Source: Adapted from Ref. [25].*

BOX 15.1

SAMPLE EVALUATION PLAN OUTLINE

1. Overview of the HIE project or organization
2. Goals and objectives of the HIE project or use case for evaluation
3. Questions or objectives of the evaluation
4. Evaluation measures
   a. First measure—quantitative or qualitative?
      i. Description of measure
      ii. Timeframe for measurement
      iii. Study design/method
      iv. Data collection plan
         - Data source and description
         - Data extraction methods, including the name of any specific database field name where the data are stored
      v. Analysis plan
         - Data coding methods
            - Quantitative data: How should the data be calculated or transformed prior to analysis?
            - Qualitative data: Which themes is the team trying to find in the unstructured notes/documents?
         - Data analysis methods
         - Power calculations or sample size considerations
         - Tools or software to support the analysis
   b. Repeat the above for each subsequent measure...
5. Budget considerations
6. Conclusion

The information in Box 15.1 is a sample outline for the various sections to be included in the evaluation plan document. Each final measure should be fully described, although the exact elements and sections included in the plan may vary depending on the study design.

DISSEMINATION OF FINDINGS

Evaluating the impact of an HIE project or intervention remains incomplete until the results or lessons from the evaluation are shared. Disseminating findings is what builds the evidence base for HIE, and provides closure to the evaluation. Stakeholders interested in, or whom may have funded, the evaluation will want to see a report or presentation. There are benefits to disseminating the findings more broadly to peers (eg, other organizations that may be HIE initiatives or health systems) as well as the biomedical science community. Presentations at professional or scientific conferences can improve the reputation of the evaluation team members as well as the organization for which they work. Publication of the results in a peer-reviewed journal also enhances stature of individuals and organizations. These dissemination methods enable others in the HIE and health IT communities to learn from the experiences of implementing or using HIE.

Strategies for Success

Although dissemination beyond the local environment may be challenging, it is feasible as many audiences are interested in the outcomes from and barriers to HIE. Results from the evaluation plus a well-documented

BOX 15.2

DISSEMINATION RESOURCES

Statement on Reporting of Evaluation Studies in Health Informatics (STARE_HI) [26,27]

These are guidelines created by the International Medical Informatics Association (IMIA) to help individuals structure a document that reports the findings from an evaluation. The advice in STARE-HI can guide the evaluation team in drafting an article for submission to a peer-reviewed journal.

Just Plain Data Analysis [28]

This resource offers suggestions for how to present numerical evidence from evaluations for use in policymaking contexts. The advice can guide evaluation team members in presenting their findings to conference attendees, Board members, and the general public.

How to Write a Paper or Conference Abstract [29]

This is a blog post by an academic on how to craft a successful abstract. The guidance in this post provides a blueprint for evaluation teams to succinctly state their findings useful in many contexts, including peer-reviewed article submissions, professional conference abstract submissions, and communicating with stakeholders.

evaluation plan provide sufficient inputs into developing an abstract, article, or manuscript for submission to a professional conference or journal. The resources in Box 15.2 provide further advice and guidance on disseminating findings from HIE evaluations.

EMERGING TRENDS

A Growing Evidence Base

Finishing the analysis and writing up the findings for publication in a peer-reviewed journal can take time, especially when the evaluation team members include practicing clinicians, HIE leaders, and health care executives. Moreover, the peer-review process usually requires at least 1 year before a submitted article is first published online. This can delay the development of the HIE evidence base.

Many of the HIE initiatives funded by the Office of the National Coordinator for Health Information Technology (ONC) are beginning to publish their findings and lessons in the peer-reviewed literature. It is expected that more findings and evidence from these efforts will emerge in the literature over the next 2–3 years. This evidence will be important as the ONC funding represents a significant investment in HIE infrastructure across the United States.

Return-on-Investment

Despite a growing evidence base, there is continued need for evaluation. This is especially true for results of return-on-investment (ROI) analyses, which continues to represent a minority of the available evidence. Health systems, accountable care organizations, and policymakers are all keen to understand whether HIE can result in reduced health care costs either by improving the efficiency of health services or through savings afforded by better outcomes that coincide with lower utilization. Where possible, evaluation teams should consider adding economic expertise to facilitate conduct of ROI as a component of HIE evaluation. Funders of HIE evaluations are encouraged to support ROI analyses to advance this segment of the evidence base.

Meaningful Use and Beyond

At time of writing, ONC and the Centers for Medicaid and Medicare Services (CMS) were reviewing comments submitted on proposed regulations for Stage 3 of the Meaningful Use program. The proposed regulations would take effect as early as 2017, and many of the criteria seek to advance the development, implementation, and use of HIE. Increased adoption and use of HIE provides an opportunity to further evaluate its implementation and impact. Therefore as health systems engage in HIE for Stage 3 Meaningful Use, government agencies, private foundations, and health systems are encouraged to invest in the evaluation of HIE. Lessons from this next phase of HIE adoption and use will help to guide not only the continued refinement of HIE services but also the development of the Learning Health System, Accountable Care Organizations, and other health system reforms necessary to achieve the Triple Aim of improving the health of populations, as well as the quality of and satisfaction with care delivery, while reducing the per capita cost of health care.

SUMMARY

The evaluation of HIE remains a need for a health system in the middle of reform. Despite growth in the adoption and use of HIE, the evidence base supporting its business case, as well as best practices, is limited. More work is necessary to measure the impact of HIE on clinical as well as population outcomes, in addition to the business of health care delivery. Readers are encouraged to not only contribute to the development and implementation of HIE but also its evaluation.

QUESTIONS FOR DISCUSSION

1. Under what circumstances might summative evaluation be considered research? How about vice versa? Is one better than the other?
2. Which study designs and methods lend themselves best to evaluations on a "shoestring budget"?
3. What are the ethical implications of conducting an evaluation of HIE in a community setting?
4. How might the evaluation plan for a low-to-middle income country differ from an evaluation plan in the United States?
5. Who are potential funders of HIE evaluation in the United States? Internationally?
6. Why should health systems or accountable care organizations fund evaluation of HIE? Isn't research funding best left to government?

References

[1] Scriven M. Minimalist theory: the least theory that practice requires. Am J Eval 1998;19(1):57–70.

[2] AHRQ. HHS awards $139 million to drive adoption of health information technology. Rockville, MD: Agency for Healthcare Research and Quality; [updated October 13, 2004; August 3, 2009]. Available from: <http://www.ahrq.gov/news/press/pr2004/hhshitpr.htm>.

[3] Nocella KC, Horowitz KJ, Young JJ. Against all odds: designing and implementing a grassroots, community-designed RHIO in a rural region. J Healthc Inf Manag 2008;22(2):34–41. PubMed PMID: 19266993. Epub March 10, 2009. eng.

[4] Agency for Healthcare Research and Quality. State and Regional Demonstration Projects. Rockville, MD: Agency for Healthcare Research and Quality; 2009 [updated December 2014; cited June 24, 2015]. Available from: <http://healthit.ahrq.gov/ahrq-funded-projects/state-and-regional-demonstration-projects>.

[5] Poon EG, Cusack CM, McGowan JJ. Evaluating healthcare information technology outside of academia: observations from the national resource center for healthcare information technology at the Agency for Healthcare Research and Quality. J Am Med Inform Assoc 2009;16(5):631–6. PubMed PMID: 19567800. PMCID: 2744713. Epub July 2, 2009. eng.

[6] McGowan JJ, Cusack CM, Poon EG. Formative evaluation: a critical component in EHR implementation. J Am Med Inform Assoc 2008;15(3):297–301. PubMed PMID: 18308984. Epub March 1, 2008. eng.
[7] Johnson KB, Gadd C. Playing smallball: approaches to evaluating pilot health information exchange systems. J Biomed Inform 2007;40(Suppl. 6):S21–6. PubMed PMID: 17931981. Epub October 13, 2007. eng.
[8] Dixon BE, Miller T, Overhage JM. Assessing HIE stakeholder readiness for consumer access: lessons learned from the NHIN trial implementations. J Healthc Inf Manag 2009;23(3):20–5. PubMed PMID: 19663160. Epub August 12, 2009. eng.
[9] Overhage JM, Evans L, Marchibroda J. Communities' readiness for health information exchange: the National Landscape in 2004. J Am Med Inform Assoc 2005;12(2):107–12. PubMed PMID: 15561785. Epub November 25, 2004. eng.
[10] Revere D, Dixon BE, Hills R, Williams JL, Grannis SJ. Leveraging health information exchange to improve population health reporting processes: lessons in using a collaborative-participatory design process. eGEMs (Generating Evidence & Methods to improve patient outcomes) [Internet]. 2014;2(3):[Article p. 12]. Available from: <http://repository.academyhealth.org/egems/vol2/iss3/12/>.
[11] Reeder B, Revere D, Hills RA, Baseman JG, Lober WB. Public health practice within a health information exchange: information needs and barriers to disease surveillance. Online J Public Health Inform 2012;4:3.
[12] Abramson EL, McGinnis S, Edwards A, Maniccia DM, Moore J, Kaushal R. Electronic health record adoption and health information exchange among hospitals in New York State. J Eval Clin Pract 2012;18(6):1156–62. PubMed PMID: 21914089. Epub September 15, 2011. eng.
[13] Vest J. Health information exchange: the determinants of usage and the impact on utilization [3397326]. Texas, TX: The Texas A&M University System Health Science Center; 2010.
[14] Bailey JE, Pope RA, Elliott EC, Wan JY, Waters TM, Frisse ME. Health information exchange reduces repeated diagnostic imaging for back pain. Ann Emerg Med 2013;62(1):16–24. PubMed PMID: 23465552. Epub March 8, 2013. eng.
[15] Richardson JE, Malhotra S, Kaushal R. A case report in health information exchange for inter-organizational patient transfers. Appl Clin Inform 2014;5(3):642–50. PubMed PMID: 25298805. PMCID: 4187082. Epub October 10, 2014. eng.
[16] Vest JR, Kern LM, Silver MD, Kaushal R. The potential for community-based health information exchange systems to reduce hospital readmissions. J Am Med Inform Assoc 2014 PubMed PMID: 25100447. Epub August 8, 2014. Eng.
[17] Shapiro JS, Genes N, Kuperman G, Chason K, Richardson LD. Health information exchange, biosurveillance efforts, and emergency department crowding during the spring 2009 H1N1 outbreak in New York City. Ann Emerg Med 2010;55(3):274–9. PubMed PMID: 20079955. Epub January 19, 2010. eng.
[18] Byrne CM, Mercincavage LM, Bouhaddou O, Bennett JR, Pan EC, Botts NE, et al. The Department of Veterans Affairs' (VA) implementation of the Virtual Lifetime Electronic Record (VLER): findings and lessons learned from Health Information Exchange at 12 sites. Int J Med Inform 2014;83(8):537–47. PubMed PMID: 24845146. Epub May 23, 2014. eng.
[19] Furukawa MF, King J, Patel V, Hsiao CJ, Adler-Milstein J, Jha AK. Despite substantial progress in EHR adoption, health information exchange and patient engagement remain low in office settings. Health Aff 2014;33(9):1672–9. PubMed PMID: 25104827. Epub August 12, 2014. eng.
[20] Maenpaa T, Asikainen P, Gissler M, Siponen K, Maass M, Saranto K, et al. The utilization rate of the regional health information exchange: how it impacts on health care delivery outcomes. J Public Health Manag Pract 2012;18(3):215–23. PubMed PMID: 22473113. Epub April 5, 2012. eng.
[21] Park H, Lee SI, Hwang H, Kim Y, Heo EY, Kim JW, et al. Can a health information exchange save healthcare costs? Evidence from a pilot program in South Korea. Int J Med Inform 2015 PubMed PMID: 26048738. Epub June 7, 2015. Eng.
[22] Dixon BE, Zafar A, Overhage JM. A framework for evaluating the costs, effort, and value of nationwide health information exchange. J Am Med Inform Assoc 2010;17(3):295–301. PubMed PMID: 20442147. PMCID: 2995720. Epub May 6, 2010. eng.
[23] Pan E, Byrne CM, Damico D, Crimmins M. Guide to Evaluating Health Information Exchange Projects. Rockville, MD: Agency for Healthcare Research and Quality; 2014 [cited June 26, 2015]. Prepared for the Agency for Healthcare Research and Quality under Contract No. 290200900023-I. Available from: <http://healthit.ahrq.gov/health-it-tools-and-resources/guide-evaluating-health-information-exchange-projects>.
[24] Dixon BE, Grannis SJ, Revere D. Measuring the impact of a health information exchange intervention on provider-based notifiable disease reporting using mixed methods: a study protocol. BMC Med Inform Decis Mak 2013;13(1):121. PubMed PMID: 24171799. PMCID: 3819468. Epub November 1, 2013. Eng.
[25] Cusack CM, Byrne CM, Hook JM, McGowan J, Poon E, Zafar A. Health Information Technology Evaluation Toolkit: 2009 Update. (Prepared for the AHRQ National Resource Center for Health Information Technology under Contract No 290-04-0016) AHRQ

Publication No 09-0083-EF. Rockville, MD: Agency for Healthcare Research and Quality; 2009.

[26] Brender J, Talmon J, de Keizer N, Nykanen P, Rigby M, Ammenwerth E. STARE-HI—Statement on Reporting of Evaluation Studies in Health Informatics: explanation and elaboration. Appl Clin Inform 2013;4(3):331–58. PubMed PMID: 24155788. PMCID: 3799207. Epub October 25, 2013. eng.

[27] Talmon J, Ammenwerth E, Brender J, de Keizer N, Nykanen P, Rigby M. STARE-HI—Statement on reporting of evaluation studies in Health Informatics. Int J Med Inform 2009;78(1):1–9. PubMed PMID: 18930696. Epub October 22, 2008. eng.

[28] Klass G. Just plain data analysis: finding, presenting, and interpreting social science data., 2nd ed. New York, NY: Rowman and Littlefield Publishers; 2012.

[29] Kelsky K. How to write a paper or conference proposal abstract; 2011 [cited June 30, 2015]. Available from: <http://theprofessorisin.com/2011/07/12/how-tosday-how-to-write-a-paper-abstract/>.

PART V

THE FUTURE OF HEALTH INFORMATION EXCHANGE

CHAPTER

16

Future Directions in Health Information Exchange

Julia Adler-Milstein[1] *and Brian E. Dixon*[2]

[1]School of Information, University of Michigan, Ann Arbor, MI [2]Indiana University Richard M. Fairbanks School of Public Health; and the Center for Biomedical Informatics, Regenstrief Institute, Inc., Indianapolis, IN

OUTLINE

LEARNING OBJECTIVES

By the end of the chapter, the reader should be able to:

- Identify current challenges facing health information exchange (HIE) adoption and use.
- Describe the strategies underway to address current HIE challenges.
- List opportunities for researchers and for practitioners to address current HIE challenges.
- Describe future trends likely to shape and be shaped by HIE.

INTRODUCTION

Health information exchange (HIE) is defined as the electronic transfer of health-related information across diverse and often competing health care organizations [1]. As noted in the chapter "What Is Health Information Exchange?", the term HIE is used as both a *verb* and a *noun*. While some chapters have used it as a noun, in this chapter, we consider HIE principally as a verb, emphasizing the electronic exchange of data or information among various stakeholders within a nation or health care system.

There are many motivations for pursuing HIE. For clinicians, optimal clinical decision-making requires access to prior health information about the patient, regardless of where it was generated. When such information is unavailable, care decisions are less safe, less effective, and can result in duplicative utilization. For administrators, HIE can also result in operational efficiencies; there are tangible cost savings associated with shifting from manual approaches to sharing information to electronic approaches, particularly for the exchange of images. For public health authorities, HIE enables more reliable and less costly reporting of key information related to immunizations, communicable disease cases, and early detection of emerging threats to health.

While there is widespread agreement on the potential value from HIE, there is less clarity around the optimal approach to enabling HIE. The United States has pursued HIE with limited top-down regulation, allowing multiple approaches to HIE to develop and coexist as discussed in many chapters as well as the case studies in this book. Today, HIE efforts that limit which participants can share information (private and vendor-facilitated efforts) exist in the market alongside HIE efforts that take a more open approach to participation (government-facilitated and community-based efforts). Furthermore, current efforts to enable HIE tend to focus on distinct HIE use cases—some efforts target the exchange of specific types of information (eg, lab results) or documents (eg, summary of care records) while others attempt to create a comprehensive longitudinal patient record. While this heterogeneity allows tailoring of the HIE approach to the needs of the participants involved in the effort, this approach also leaves gaps, and the reality is that we have yet to achieve the ultimate goal of ensuring that information is readily available electronically when needed across the full spectrum of care delivery.

In this chapter, we examine the key near-term challenges facing HIE development, implementation, and use. These challenges present opportunities for HIE research and development, which we highlight and discuss. Finally, we examine long-term trends that are anticipated to shape the direction of HIE in the future.

KEY CHALLENGES FACING HIE AND ASSOCIATED OPPORTUNITIES FOR RESEARCH AND PRACTICE

Throughout the book, we describe challenges to pursuing HIE within an enterprise as well as within and across nations. Here we recap and expand upon key challenges facing HIE. We highlight the opportunities created for professionals as well as researchers across the wide spectrum of health sciences, health services research, health informatics, and health information management to help the field address the challenges facing broad uptake of HIE.

Adoption and Use of Standards

As described in the chapters "Syntactic Interoperability and the Role of Standards" and "Standardizing Health Care Data Across an Enterprise," standards enable interoperability between health information systems. Yet, implementation and adoption of standards is challenging. First, doing so requires organizations to harmonize workflow and business processes to support standardized capture of data and information as they are generated in health care delivery. Second, it can require EHR systems to be designed to standardize data and information as they are captured, stored, and exchanged. While HIE infrastructures support term mapping and harmonization across disparate EHR systems, mapping processes and changes to workflow require significant investment of time and/or money by health systems. This can be a major challenge for HIE in countries or communities that lack access to sufficient financial or human resources necessary for data and process standardization.

The meaningful use (MU) incentive program for EHR adoption in the United States is driving adoption of standards required for Certified EHR Technologies (CEHRT), including HIE components. While past research found limited adoption of standards, even after stage 1 MU [2], the second and third stages of MU are likely to increase the adoption of standards among commercial CEHRT. Each successive evolution of the MU program has expanded the number and types of standards called for to support the CEHRT functionalities implemented by health care systems. For example, stage 3 of MU proposes exploration and use of the emerging Health Level 7 FHIR (Fast Healthcare Interoperability Resources) standard, which is already being implemented and tested by EHR vendors and health systems [3,4]. Therefore as health systems in the United States implement CERHT to meet MU criteria, in the background, their technology infrastructures will likely support a greater variety of standard transactions and message formats. While this progress will not immediately solve the data entry and workflow aspects of standardization, it provides an opportunity for health systems to think critically about information capture, processing, storage, and exchange.

As health systems in the United States expand their capacity to support standards-based transactions and message content, HIE specialists (see chapter "Health Information Exchange as a Profession") and researchers have an opportunity to advance the adoption and utilization of standards towards ubiquitous interoperability. Professionals in health systems should leverage the availability of new standards in CEHRT to improve the methods by which data are entered (captured) and shared among health care workers. Workflows might be altered to support expanded use of *Write Once Read Many (WORM)* approaches across health care delivery tasks. For example, documentation of health services might be distributed across a team involving a medical assistant, nurse, and physician; so there is less burden on the physician to enter comprehensive structured information about a patient's symptoms, medications, and care plan. Similarly, CEHRT might be configured to automatically retrieve elements from a patient's medical history from outside care providers to reduce the burden of manual data entry on clinical care team staff.

Outside the United States, many nations are developing or advancing their national eHealth strategies [5,6]. These strategies often call for use of interoperability standards to enable HIE across national health systems as recommended by the World Health Organization and the International Telecommunications Union [7]. While each nation is in a different stage of development or implementation, most strive to lay a strong foundation for incorporating the use of standards. Like in the United States, as other countries implement eHealth technologies, they should, in parallel, develop an infrastructure capable of standards-based transactions and messages. Therefore all nations should think about how data and transactions can be standardized to enable WORM approaches that will support secondary use across clinical and population health use cases. HIE specialists have an opportunity to raise the issue with health authorities while working with local health facilities to adopt standards-based approaches to data entry, storage, management, and exchange.

Researchers not only have an opportunity to measure the adoption and utilization of standards following the implementation of CEHRT but they also have an opportunity to design and evaluate new models for care delivery using integrated HIE technologies. Once available within implemented CERHT, standard transactions and messages could be used for purposes other than those intended by policymakers who developed stages 2 and 3 of the MU incentive program. For example, standards implemented to enable patients to view, download, and transmit their personal health information could be leveraged by HIE networks to enhance how patients interact with their health data. Instead of maintaining three separate patient portal accounts associated with individual providers, patients might be able to unify their ability to view and monitor their health via HIE. Researchers have the opportunity to envision and develop novel technologies that may one day support a wider array of HIE functionalities and systems for use by patients, providers, and public health authorities.

Patient Identification and Matching

Within a single HIE effort, multiple stakeholders typically provide patient data, creating the challenge of patient identification, and matching. This problem also exists when multiple HIE networks seek to connect to each other (ie, a "network-of-networks" approach). In countries without a unique patient identifier, those who provide data need to rely on the fields available across data sources, and a key challenge is data quality within those fields (see chapter "Client Registries: Identifying and Linking Patients"). While the adoption and use of standards may improve how data are captured, standards alone will not alleviate all data entry errors and omissions. Thus there remains a challenge of properly trained human resources responsible for capturing patient identifiers and attributes (eg, date of birth, sex, and address). Because health data are generated and captured across a diverse array of settings, including devices worn by the patient, it is imperative that each device, software application, or EHR system focus on improving how it captures and maintains information used to determine patient identity. Addressing this challenge is an important near-term priority for health systems that wish to accurately develop solutions for measuring, monitoring, and changing population health, as well as HIE efforts across health systems.

While in the near-term solutions like complex matching algorithms used within a client registry (discussed in chapter "Client Registries: Identifying and Linking Patients") will continue to be necessary to sort through messiness of real-world patient identity information captured and exchanged by myriad EHR technologies used across varied provider organizations, two emerging trends may help alleviate inconsistency in patient identification. First, the emergence of voluntary universal health care identifiers (VUHIDs) coinciding with the move towards patient-centered care may leapfrog traditional approaches to patient matching. Second, growing comfort and accuracy of biometric identification may play an important role in improving patient identification.

Health systems around the world are embracing a move towards patient-centered care, where the patient or citizen is conceived to be not only a major actor in their health care but also a significant driver of their individual health and well-being. VUHIDs support patient-centered care, because they enable patients to govern the creation and use of a health-centric identifier. Because patients both request and provide the VUHID, they control which entities within the health system can track their health information over time. Increasing awareness and use of VUHIDs will simplify patient-matching algorithms because they are unique to health care and alleviate the need to rely on less discriminating individual attributes.

Similarly biometrics may significantly contribute to improving the ability of HIE networks to identity and match patients across data sources. Current biometric measurements and analysis have weaknesses. Yet, biometric technologies are rapidly improving. Furthermore, their popularity with mobile device users as well as their depiction in popular media may help to acculturate consumers to biometrics as a normal method of identification.

Health systems and researchers have many opportunities to improve patient identification and matching. Health system leaders, potentially in partnership with researchers, could begin to incorporate VUHIDs and biometrics into patient registration processes within clinics, hospitals, and emergency departments. Their introduction and use could be tested and evaluated. Results will provide valuable lessons for expanding their use or improving their design and effectiveness.

Researchers further have ample opportunities to improve existing patient identification techniques. Algorithms for uniquely identifying patients across larger and more complex networks of health information systems are needed. Existing techniques have limitations that could be improved. Furthermore, research is necessary to examine how best to improve existing techniques and algorithms when VUHIDs and biometric data are available for broader use.

Governance of HIE

Governance is arguably one of the most important and challenging aspects of HIE. Governance creates a framework for trust among those organizations participating in the sharing of protected health information within and across diverse and evolving networks (see chapter "Engaging and Sustaining Stakeholders: Towards Governance"). Yet, governance itself is ever-shifting due to organizational policies and priorities as well as changes in local, state, national, and regional policies affecting health systems and health information. Keeping on top of changing governance needs, stakeholder desires, and legal obstacles is a challenge for HIE efforts of any size or scope.

In the near-term, two specific challenges facing the governance of HIE are receiving substantial attention. First, many HIE efforts face challenges in the interpretation of national policies such as the Health Insurance Portability and Accountability Act (HIPAA). Privacy officers, information technology professionals, and clinical staff in hospitals and health systems can have different interpretations of the restrictions in the law, informing their peers and HIE networks that certain data cannot be shared or used for certain use cases. For example, when HIPAA was first implemented, some in the health sector felt that HIPAA precluded giving the patient his or her own information. With respect to HIE, some health systems have expressed concerns about sharing free text documents (eg, clinical notes) because they are difficult to deidentify. In some cases, fear of sharing data may be justified. Yet in other cases, it demonstrates confusion in the law or general lack of awareness of the details provided in both the law and subsequent administrative rules established by the US Department of Health and Human Services (HHS). Either way, misinterpretation of HIPAA guidelines can interfere with agreement on appropriate HIE governance.

Another challenge facing HIE governance is the complex and challenging set of laws that exist across the various states within the United States. Varying state laws, which can be more restrictive than HIPAA, are difficult to navigate for HIE efforts that serve medical trading areas that span more than one state [8]. While certain use cases might be deemed acceptable in one state under its laws and within the framework of HIPAA, a neighboring state may possess a law that prohibits implementation of the same use cases. Thus far, the federal government has not taken direct steps to solve these issues even though they are well-documented and discussed.

As HIE efforts continue to scale within and across states, governing bodies and HIE leaders must confront these governance challenges. Yet, clear resolution may not always be achievable. Cultivating a diverse set of governing body representatives to include legal as well as policy experts will likely be essential to structuring HIE networks to confront these challenges as they emerge. Broad representation should help HIEs not only resolve ambiguity in existing laws but also identify potential solutions to explore with policymakers and health system leaders. United efforts across regional and national HIE efforts may lead to changes in federal law or new guidance from HHS to eliminate roadblocks to legitimate HIE use cases that have the potential to improve clinical as well as population outcomes.

Using Policy to Drive HIE

Beyond specific challenges impeding HIE, there is a broader challenge of how to create a stronger imperative for HIE development and growth using policy tools. HIE is viewed as a high-priority policy target because of the substantial public value expected to be generated from broad electronic exchange of health data and the slow pace of HIE adoption led by the private sector. In the United States, the MU criteria serve as an influential driver of how health care delivery organizations implement and use EHR systems, including the extent to which they engage in HIE. Because these criteria coordinate with federal EHR certification standards, they dictate what HIE capabilities CEHRT must be able to support. Today, most doctors and hospitals are beginning to pursue stage 2 MU, and the core HIE-related criterion is that for 10% of care transitions, providers must electronically transmit a summary of care record. EHR vendors have to certify that there systems can support, at a minimum, a basic electronic transport approach known as Direct, which is akin to secure email. The 10% threshold for the proportion of care transitions for which a summary care record must be sent electronically was set low, because it is not clear the extent to which providers have the ability to engage in HIE with the other providers to which they transition their patients. For example, if a hospital is the first in its market to achieve stage 2 MU and all other hospitals are still working on stage 1 MU, this would leave few trading partners for that hospital to send summary of care records electronically.

Proposed stage 3 MU criteria seek to increase this threshold to 50% and also offer an alternative measure that is likely more appropriate for providers who more regularly receive patients from other settings. In the proposed transitions-of-care measure, for more than 40% of transitions or referrals received in which the provider has never before encountered the patient, providers must incorporate into the CEHRT an electronic summary of care document from a source other than the provider's own EHR system. Stage 3 MU also newly introduces the concept of open application programming interfaces that would more readily allow information to be pulled from a given EHR, and while this criterion is targeted to support patient access to information, the functionality could support other third parties seeking to facilitate HIE across providers.

Because stage 3 MU is not slated to begin until 2018 (though some organizations could choose to begin in 2017), it remains to be seen whether these new thresholds and criteria will drive broad-based HIE and connectivity between providers. Beyond specific MU criteria, policy efforts seek to ensure that providers have the ability to find (ie, query), send, receive, and integrate information across settings. This broad set of HIE capabilities should serve as the basis for enabling a variety of HIE use cases. Ultimately, HIE is seen as key to enabling a Learning Health System (discussed in the long-term trends section below).

Perhaps the most difficult challenge in the effort to use policy as a driver of HIE is knowing where government involvement is most helpful, where it is likely to be ineffective, and where it may actually slow HIE progress. To date, MU and associated certification criteria have largely set a low bar, hoping that MU will help catalyze broader market-driven HIE, rather than being the sole driving force behind HIE. Federal policy efforts have also targeted complementary areas, such as standards, patient identification and matching, governance, data privacy/security, and creating stronger financial incentives for care coordination through delivery and payment reform.

Whether current policies are pushing HIE development and expansion efforts in the right direction at the right pace is critical to assess. Thus, for researchers, there is substantial opportunity to study where HIE progress is not occurring. There are still many challenges simply measuring HIE and interoperability, given the various dimensions and use cases. Thus, investment in HIE measurement, particularly measures that can feasibly be collected at a national level, is needed. Once we have the ability to characterize HIE progress, an assessment of the upstream enablers and barriers is needed, along with an assessment of how policy efforts are influencing enablers and barriers. Research opportunities will also arise from the need to assess whether HIE is translating into improved care.

While determining that more HIE activity occurring is important, if that information exchange is not resulting in safer, more effective, and more efficient care, we will not have achieved the policy objectives. Two recent HIE evidence reviews [9,10], in addition to chapter "The Evidence Base for Health Information Exchange," point to the need for more studies on HIE impact, and in particular, understanding the conditions under which HIE results in health care process improvement and/or clinical as well as population outcomes.

For professionals, policy efforts to promote HIE are creating new requirements to which provider organizations must respond. Simply keeping up with the requirements—upgrading EHRs and meeting new MU criteria—can feel like a full-time job. Yet the key is ensuring that meeting the criteria results in improved care and this can require new workflows and other strategies in order for HIE capabilities to translate into information available to providers at the point-of-care. In particular, as the volume of HIE activity increases, it will be critical to identify strategies to ensure that providers are not simply overloaded with information; this will likely require a combination of new workflows and new analytic tools that sort through newly available information and identify the relevant subset. More HIE activity also creates newly available data for analytics and performance measurement, and these can be used as broader levers for measuring and improving performance.

Sustainability of HIE Efforts

HIE MU criteria have served as one important driver of demand for HIE capabilities, and, increasingly, demand for HIE is driven by other policy efforts (such as new payment models that shift the risk to providers for the cost and quality of care; see Case Study 4). As providers seek to engage in HIE, they have a variety of options as described in the chapter "What Is Health Information Exchange?" and the options that make sense to pursue depend on the type of data they want to exchange and the partners with which they want to exchange. Today's HIE ecosystem consists of varied types of HIE efforts. Some are large and national in scale, for example, the SureScripts network facilitates electronic transmission of prescriptions for the majority of providers and Epic System's CareEverywhere network allows sharing of a broad set of clinical data across all Epic clients. Other HIE efforts focus on enabling exchange at the community or state level across different EHR vendor platforms. All of these efforts face the challenge of sustainability—how to generate revenue to offset the cost of HIE and associated organizational infrastructure (see chapter "Managing the Business of Health Information Exchange: Toward Sustainability").

HIE sustainability is a challenge because the benefits of HIE can be diffuse; they come in the form of improved access to information that can translate into higher-quality, lower-cost care while in parallel supporting research, surveillance, quality reporting, and population health management. Yet the costs largely fall on those that generate data, primarily provider organizations. Thus, an ongoing issue, particularly for community-oriented HIE efforts, is how to build a sustainable business model in which those who benefit from HIE are the entities that pay for it to occur. While some states view HIE as a public good and fund HIE efforts in their state using public financing models, this remains the exception and most HIE efforts have to establish a business model without heavily relying on public funding. National surveys of HIE efforts suggest that identifying a sustainable business model has been, and continues to be, the most commonly cited challenge to the development of HIE efforts [11,12].

One of the stakeholders thought to benefit from HIE is those who pay for care (ie, health insurers), who accrue the benefits of better care, and in particular, less redundant care that should result from information exchange. Payers are therefore viewed as an important stakeholder in ensuring HIE sustainability. A recent study examined payer perspectives on HIE and their decision-making on whether or not to support HIE efforts [13]. Key findings included the fact that current approaches to HIE diverge from those that generate clear value to payers—specifically, because there are many different HIE efforts, it is rare that a given effort heavily overlaps with the covered lives of a given payer and it is therefore difficult for a payer to justify investment in any given HIE effort. In addition, HIE efforts have not developed to support specific payer HIE use cases and so this further decreases the tangible value from HIE support realized by payers that would justify their investment. Thus, unless they cater more directly to payer needs, HIE efforts are likely to continue to struggle to engage payers, which makes identifying a sustainable business model difficult.

This leaves open the question of the extent to which current HIE efforts will be able to identify sustainable business models, particularly as one-time funding for HIE included in the HITECH Act is spent, and which business models work for different types of networks. A particular concern is that community-oriented HIE efforts will struggle, while enterprise and EHR vendor exchange efforts, which face fewer sustainability challenges, will not. These concerns were recently heightened by a congressional request to investigate the practice of information blocking. Information blocking occurs when persons or entities knowingly and unreasonably interfere with the exchange or use of electronic health information [14].

Certain business, technical, and organizational practices by provider organizations and

EHR vendors are perceived to interfere with the exchange of electronic health information. These practices may include:

1. contract terms, policies, or other business or organizational practices that restrict individuals' access to their electronic health information or restrict the exchange or use of that information for treatment and other permitted purposes,
2. charging prices or fees (such as for data exchange, portability, and interfaces) that make exchanging and using electronic health information cost prohibitive,
3. developing or implementing health IT in nonstandard ways that are likely to substantially increase the costs, complexity, or burden of sharing electronic health information, especially when relevant federal interoperability standards, and
4. developing or implementing health IT in ways that are likely to "lock in" users or electronic health information; lead to fraud, waste, or abuse; or impede innovations and advancements in HIE and health IT-enabled care delivery.

To the extent that information blocking is occurring, in combination with the challenges to identifying a sustainable business model for HIE efforts, the result could be that most of the HIE efforts that survive are those that fall along the lines of provider enterprises or EHR vendor user communities. This will limit the extent to which patient information can flow freely, regardless of where patients choose to seek care, and therefore limit the extent to which we will achieve the overarching goal of HIE.

For researchers, continuing to identify sustainable business models for HIE efforts, and the impact of varied market forces and policies on which HIE efforts are sustainable, is critical. Specifically on the topic of information blocking, we know little about the different forms it takes, where it is occurring, and what approaches may be effective to counter it. For practitioners, the diverse and evolving HIE ecosystem can make it difficult to know where to invest limited resources or even what options are available to engage in HIE. Gaining a clear understanding of the costs and benefits of various options is likely the best place to start.

KEY HEALTH CARE TRENDS LIKELY TO IMPACT LONG-TERM HIE FOCUS

As described above, HIE is an active and vibrant field facing a number of key challenges. Despite specific challenges, we believe that HIE implementation and use will continue to expand in nations across the globe. Fundamentally HIE is a necessary, even if not always sufficient, component to improving health care practice, services, and outcomes. In this section, we describe key trends within health care that are likely to both shape and benefit from HIE.

Care Coordination and Team-Based Care

A major focus of HIE is to enable access to patient information where and when it is needed regardless of its source. A key driver of HIE is the fact that today providers often lack information from prior settings in which their patients received care. While closing information gaps is helpful, it is not clear that HIE will be sufficient to truly achieve coordinated care.

Care coordination is a term associated with the coordinated distribution of health services for a given patient or consumer. Many health systems and countries are implementing team-based care models in which a broad set of providers work together to coordinate their delivery of health services. For example, recall the example of Bob, the patient with diabetes from the chapter "Client Registries: Identifying and Linking Patients." Bob visits multiple providers for various aspects of his management of diabetes, including his primary care provider

(PCP), endocrinologist, podiatrist, and ophthalmologist. Ensuring that Bob receives the most appropriate care and management for his diabetes can often fall solely on the PCP. In a coordinated care scenario, all of Bob's providers would communicate with each other and work off a shared coordinated care plan for Bob. HIE could be used simply to make information about Bob's past care available to all of the providers involved in his care. While this is a necessary step towards enabling care coordination, it is not sufficient, because a given set of patient data does not reveal the clinical thinking that went into the generation of that data (ie, why a particular drug was selected or a particular test ordered) or the envisioned long-term care plan for Bob who will manage diabetes for the rest of his life. Thus, as HIE matures, its focus will likely shift from simply making data more broadly available to enabling care coordination and shared care planning.

Today, we are beginning to operationalize what coordinated care looks like across a team of providers, particularly during key care transitions—such as post-hospitalization—as well as key health events—such as a new diagnosis. Several of these common workflows are becoming standardized through efforts like Integrating the Healthcare Enterprise (IHE) in which technical standards and HIE transactions are designed to support each scenario (see chapter "Syntactic Interoperability and the Role of Standards"). Yet, these efforts are only a few years old and are rapidly evolving. Once such efforts mature, the associated enabling tools can be implemented, such as dynamic shared care plans, and more advanced HIE capabilities can come to the fore.

Patient-Centered Care

Ultimately, effective shared care planning needs to extend to include the patient and their caregivers, and care will evolve to be truly patient-centered. When this occurs, patients will meaningfully engage with their health information and care planning. Today, patients are being given increasing access to their health data. They are also being asked to increasingly participate in decisions about their care. Models of care such as patient-centered medical homes and patient-aligned care teams advocate for active patient engagement in combination with care coordination enabled by EHR systems as well as HIE [15,16].

While patient access to data is an important step, it is still several steps removed from patient-centered care. What broader patient data access allows, however, is the development of new tools and technologies to help patients understand and engage with the data. As these emerge, HIE will shift from a largely provider-centric activity to one that is patient-centric. Specifically, we will move from the current state in which patients can electronically access and download certain static pieces of their record, such as lab test results, to a state in which data can automatically flow to one or more tools of the patients' choice and members of the patients' designated care team. This might include the use of independent health record banks [17,18] or personal health record systems [19,20]. Yet patient-centered approaches will likely offer the opportunity for patients to interact with other key sources of their health data, ranging from sensors to family members to the environment. Patient-centered HIE will further offer the opportunity for patients to access, input and monitor the social determinants of health [21–23] including economic, housing, transportation, and recreation facilities in their communities that contribute to their overall health and well-being. Access to and interaction with a broader set of data and information is likely to help patients adhere to care plans and support health-promoting behaviors.

Population Health Management

Historically, health care in the United States has predominately been delivered using a fee-for-service model in which providers are incentivized to focus on each distinct encounter, diagnosis, or procedure regardless of the broader population health implications. This model has contributed to rising health care costs with marginal improvement in population health.

In the last decade, there has been a growing movement in the United States to move away from a fee-for-service basis towards value-based care that operationalizes a "Triple Aim" framework described by the Institute for Healthcare Improvement [24], which seeks to:

1. improve the patient experience of care (including quality and satisfaction);
2. improve the health of populations (and not just patients under care); and
3. reduce the per-capita cost of care.

Efforts to make health systems in the United States "accountable" for achieving the Triple Aim include the Affordable Care Act of 2010 as well as the Veterans Access, Choice, and Accountability Act of 2014 [25]. Unlike prior regulations that metaphorically locked patients into a particular network of providers, the newer laws enable patients to seek care where they desire but designate a specific provider organization to be accountable for their health and well-being. At the organizational level, accountable care providers are responsible for populations of patients and must therefore have access to information on their designated populations, regardless of source, which necessitates broader adoption and use of HIE [26].

The implementation of accountable value-based care is in its infancy. The management of population health continues to evolve as do EHR and HIE tools to support it. Early applications of HIE tend to focus on gathering insurance claims data to measure health care consumption and costs. While useful, these approaches are limited. Future efforts to fully implement population health will likely necessitate new capabilities to access clinical information and more powerful visualization tools to aggregate and analyze population-level data made up of both claims and EHR data. These needs will drive new HIE services and capabilities, including tools to quickly assess multiple types of data across multiple dimensions of health care outcomes for subpopulations. More on population health management and its intersection with HIE can be found in Case Study 4.

Learning Health System

As HIE matures, another key use is the ability to access large sets of electronic data to facilitate more rapid learning about health and health care, and then apply new knowledge when and where it is needed. This cycle of continuous learning is termed the Learning Health System (LHS), and such a system requires HIE capabilities as the foundation [27]. Today, a nationwide LHS is a vision articulated for the future by many influential stakeholders such as the Institute of Medicine [28] and the Office of the National Coordinator for Health IT (in their 10-year interoperability roadmap) [29].

A growing number of learning health networks and learning health infrastructures exist today. Examples include:

- The HMO Research Network, a public, nonproprietary, research-focused data model implemented at 17 health care systems across the United States focused on supporting the generation on new knowledge through research [30].
- Observational Health Data Sciences and Informatics (OHDSI), a multistakeholder, interdisciplinary collaborative that designs and implements open-source tools to

conduct large-scale analytics on over one billion patients to generate evidence about all aspects of health care [31,32].

- PopMedNet, a distributed health data network that advances the secondary use of electronic health information by creating standardized and reusable data sources in multiple sites, as well as tools to use them [33].

These early initiatives serve as examples for what is hoped can be brought to scale at a national level. As such networks mature and others are implemented, they will not only utilize HIE models and services but also define new HIE capabilities for conducting large-scale observational studies efficiently to rapidly inform health care practice.

Cross-Country Learning

While much of the discussion has focused on the future of HIE efforts in the United States, many countries are at a similar stage in the evolution of their HIE implementation and use. This creates a valuable opportunity for cross-country learning as nations are likely to encounter similar challenges. To date, cross-country learning has been hampered by a lack of common terminology for health information and communications technologies (ICTs). For example, the term HIE has different meanings across countries, making it very difficult to determine which policies and approaches could serve as models. Until definitional issues as well as variations in approach to measurement are resolved, we cannot know for certain which countries are successful in the varied domains of HIE.

In response, an international effort, led by the Organisation for Economic Co-operation and Development (OECD) is underway to develop benchmark measures of health ICTs that can be applied by countries to track their progress [34]. In this effort, the domain of HIE was defined as the process of electronically transferring, or aggregating and enabling access to, patient health information and data across provider organizations. Exchange may take place between different types of entities, for example, e-transfer of patient data between ambulatory care providers or e-transfer of data at the regional level. Specific HIE measures focus on three HIE functions: (1) secure messaging between professionals; (2) ordering and reporting of medications and laboratory tests with result receipt; and (3) patient referrals. The first set of comparative data from more than 10 countries that piloted the OECD model survey is expected to be reported shortly after the release of this book and will enable countries to more readily identify models from which they could learn.

CONCLUSION

While hard to know for certain, HIE appears to be in its teenage years. Much of the formative, developmental work has been accomplished and we now understand the key dimensions of HIE in detail. In some parts of the health care system, HIE is robust. However, many key challenges remain to be addressed and, until they are, HIE will not mature sufficiently to deliver on the substantial benefits it promises.

Today, there are large holes in needed connectivity, and uncertainty around how best to fill those holes—particularly using policy levers to address issues related to standards, patient matching, governance, and a sustainable business model. Encouragingly, efforts are underway to ensure that, as HIE matures, it can serve as the foundation for driving major changes in healthcare—from realizing the vision of person-centered care to powering an LHS. And these changes are poised to impact not just the US health care system but also health care systems across the globe. The motivation and the vision for what HIE can and should be are coming into focus—ensuring that HIE drives sustainable change to health systems, processes, and outcomes—as is the fact that much hard work remains to achieving this. HIE is a journey, not a destination; and the road ahead is long.

References

[1] Dixon BE, Zafar A, Overhage JM. A framework for evaluating the costs, effort, and value of nationwide health information exchange. J Am Med Inform Assoc 2010;17(3):295–301. Epub May 6, 2010.

[2] Dixon BE, Vreeman DJ, Grannis SJ. The long road to semantic interoperability in support of public health: experiences from two states. J Biomed Inform 2014;49:3–8. Epub April 1, 2014.

[3] Kasthurirathne SN, Mamlin B, Grieve G, Biondich P. Towards standardized patient data exchange: integrating a FHIR based API for the open medical record system. Stud Health Technol Inform 2015;216:932. Epub August 12, 2015.

[4] Alterovitz G, Warner J, Zhang P, Chen Y, Ullman-Cullere M, Kreda D, et al. SMART on FHIR genomics: facilitating standardized clinico-genomic apps. J Am Med Inform Assoc 2015;0:1–6. http://dx.doi.org/10.1093/jamia/ocv045. Epub July 23, 2015.

[5] Oluoch T, Muturi D, Kiriinya R, Waruru A, Lanyo K, Nguni R, et al. Do interoperable national information systems enhance availability of data to assess the effect of scale-up of HIV services on health workforce deployment in resource-limited countries? Stud Health Technol Inform 2015;216:677–81. Epub August 12, 2015.

[6] Alander T, Scandurra I. Experiences of healthcare professionals to the Introduction in Sweden of a Public eHealth Service: patients' online access to their electronic health records. Stud Health Technol Inform 2015;216:153–7. Epub August 12, 2015.

[7] World Health Organization National eHealth strategy toolkit. Geneva, Switzerland: World Health Organization and International Telecommunication Union; 2012.

[8] Dimitropoulos L.L., Loft J. Health information privacy and security collaboration. Rockville, MD: Agency for Healthcare Research and Quality; 2014 [cited August 20, 2015]; Available from: <https://healthit.ahrq.gov/ahrq-funded-projects/privacy-and-security-project>.

[9] Rudin RS, Motala A, Goldzweig CL, Shekelle PG. Usage and effect of health information exchange: a systematic review. Ann Intern Med 2014;161(11):803–11.

[10] Rahurkar S, Vest JR, Menachemi N. Despite the spread of health information exchange, There is little evidence of its impact on cost, use, and quality of care. Health Aff 2015;34(3):477–83.

[11] Adler-Milstein J, Bates DW, Jha AK. U.S. Regional health information organizations: progress and challenges. Health Aff 2009;28(2):483–92.

[12] Adler-Milstein J, Bates DW, Jha AK. Operational health information exchanges show substantial growth, but long-term funding remains a concern. Health Aff (Millwood) 2013;32(8):1486–92. Epub July 11, 2013.

[13] Cross DA, Lin SC, Adler-Milstein J. Assessing payer perspectives on health information exchange. J Am Med Inform Assoc 2015;0:1–7. http://dx.doi.org/10.1093/jamia/ocv072.

[14] Office of the National Coordinator for Health Information Technology. Report on Health Information Blocking. Washington, DC: US Department of Health and Human Services; 2015 [cited August 27, 2015]; Available from: <http://www.healthit.gov/sites/default/files/reports/info_blocking_040915.pdf>.

[15] Stange KC, Nutting PA, Miller WL, Jaen CR, Crabtree BF, Flocke SA, et al. Defining and measuring the patient-centered medical home. J Gen Intern Med 2010;25(6):601–12. Epub May 15, 2010.

[16] Piette JD, Holtz B, Beard AJ, Blaum C, Greenstone CL, Krein SL, et al. Improving chronic illness care for veterans within the framework of the patient-centered medical home: experiences from the Ann Arbor patient-aligned care team laboratory. Behav Med Pract Policy Res 2011;1(4):615–23.

[17] Yasnoff WA, Shortliffe EH. Lessons learned from a health record bank start-up. Methods Inf Med 2014;53(2):66–72. Epub January 31, 2014.

[18] Cimino JJ, Frisse ME, Halamka J, Sweeney L, Yasnoff W. Consumer-mediated health information exchanges: the 2012 ACMI debate. J Biomed Inform 2014;48:5–15. Epub February 25, 2014.

[19] Nazi KM. The personal health record paradox: health care professionals' perspectives and the information ecology of personal health record systems in organizational and clinical settings. J Med Internet Res 2013;15(4):e70. Epub April 6, 2013.

[20] Tang PC, Ash JS, Bates DW, Overhage JM, Sands DZ. Personal health records: definitions, benefits, and strategies for overcoming barriers to adoption. J Am Med Inform Assoc 2006;13(2):121–6. Epub December 17, 2005.

[21] Hripcsak G, Forrest CB, Brennan PF, Stead WW. Informatics to support the IOM social and behavioral domains and measures. J Am Med Inform Assoc 2015;22:921–4. http://dx.doi.org/10.1093/jamia/ocv035. Epub April 29, 2015.

[22] Bazemore AW, Cottrell EK, Gold R, Hughes LS, Phillips RL, Angier H, et al. Community vital signs:

incorporating geocoded social determinants into electronic records to promote patient and population health. J Am Med Inform Assoc 2015 Epub July 16, 2015.
[23] Comer KF, Grannis S, Dixon BE, Bodenhamer DJ, Wiehe SE. Incorporating geospatial capacity within clinical data systems to address social determinants of health. Public Health Rep 2011;126(Suppl. 3):54–61. Epub August 13, 2011.
[24] Berwick DM, Nolan TW, Whittington J. The triple aim: care, health, and cost. Health Aff (Millwood) 2008;27(3):759–69. Epub May 14, 2008.
[25] Veterans access, choice, and accountability act of 2014, Congress, 113th Session (2014).
[26] Dixon BE, Haggstrom DA, Weiner M. Implications for informatics given expanding access to care for Veterans and other populations. J Am Med Inform Assoc 2015;22(4):917–20. Epub April 3, 2015.
[27] Institute of Medicine Digital infrastructure for the learning health system: the foundation for continuous improvement in health and health care: workshop series summary. Washington, DC: The National Academies Press; 2011.
[28] Olsen L, Aisner D, McGinnis JM, editors. The learning healthcare system: workshop summary (IOM roundtable on evidence-based medicine). Washington, DC: The National Academies Press; 2007.
[29] ONC. Connecting health and care for the nation: a shared nationwide interoperability roadmap. In: Services DoHaH, editor. Washington DC: 2015.
[30] Ross TR, Ng D, Brown JS, Pardee R, Hornbrook MC, Hart G, et al. The HMO research network virtual data warehouse: a public data model to support collaboration. EGEMS 2014;2(1):1049.
[31] Hripcsak G, Duke JD, Shah NH, Reich CG, Huser V, Schuemie MJ, et al. Observational Health Data Sciences and Informatics (OHDSI): opportunities for observational researchers. Stud Health Technol Inform 2015;216:574–8. Epub August 12, 2015.
[32] Boyce RD, Ryan PB, Noren GN, Schuemie MJ, Reich C, Duke J, et al. Bridging islands of information to establish an integrated knowledge base of drugs and health outcomes of interest. Drug Saf 2014;37(8):557–67. Epub July 6, 2014.
[33] PopMedNet. Available from: <http://www.popmednet.org>.
[34] Adler-Milstein J, Ronchi E, Cohen GR, Winn LA, Jha AK. Benchmarking health IT among OECD countries: better data for better policy. J Am Med Inform Assoc 2014;21(1):111–6. Epub June 1, 2013.

PART VI

CASE STUDIES IN HEALTH INFORMATION EXCHANGE

CASESTUDY

1

The Indiana Health Information Exchange

J. Marc Overhage

Cerner Corporation, Kansas City, MO

OUTLINE

MAJOR THEMES

Major themes that should be evident in this case study include the ongoing goal to sustainably create value for the citizens of Indiana by improving the quality and efficiency of health care. This goal was achieved through persistence, systematically building on successes and pragmatism.

INTRODUCTION

When we began to create what would become the Indiana Health Information Exchange (IHIE), efforts to create Community Health Information Networks (CHINs) and Community Health Management Information Systems had, with a very few exceptions, failed. Initially these efforts focused primarily on administrative transactions and depended on relatively expensive and early technologies. By the mid-1990s, investigators at the Regenstrief Institute, who had created an enterprise medical record system referred to as the Regenstrief Medical Record System, started to evolve the system to serve the needs of faculty and resident physicians of the Indiana University School of Medicine who routinely practiced across the county, Veterans Administrations, University Hospitals, and patients who received care across these facilities all located on a single campus—clinical not administrative functions were most important for this work.

Rapid evolution of the Internet in combination with Regenstrief Institute investigators leadership and experience with health care IT standards stimulated a technological evolution creating an opportunity to develop a low-cost scalable approach to health information exchange (HIE).

Finally, while IHIE grew out of a research initiative, early emphasis on sustainability and practicality has ensured that broad adoption, long-term growth, and economic viability would be key drivers for the project.

These guiding principles served as the foundation for the 2004 incorporation of the IHIE as a not-for-profit supporting organization with the initial goals of:

- making Central Indiana a national leader in the use of electronic health information to deliver superior health care and to lower the cost of that care;
- developing and implementing an HIE that enables hospitals, physicians, laboratories, pharmacies, and other health services providers to deliver faster, more accurate, safer, higher quality and less redundant medical care to patients in Central Indiana;
- benefiting the work of medical and public health researchers by making available the unique databases that will be developed through the HIE, which will, in turn, benefit hospitals, payers, pharmacy benefits managers, employers, public health agencies, drug companies, and ultimately patients; and
- facilitating the development and adoption of new health-related technologies, which is likely to result in new job opportunities in the Central Indiana economy.

BACKGROUND OR CONTEXT

In the mid-1990s, investigators at the Regenstrief Institute, an international leader in developing and evaluating health information technology, with funding from the Agency for Healthcare Research and Quality and the National Library of Medicine, engaged central Indiana stakeholders including health systems, public health departments, physicians, businesses, payers, and philanthropies to build on previous work to create the Indiana Network for Patient Care (INPC) [1].

Since 1994, the INPC system has evolved and expanded while maintaining its original focus and priorities. INPC first facilitated data exchange within a single hospital system. While developing the INPC, we focused on solving the problems of clinicians who had incomplete patient data. Patients were often seen by physicians in an emergency care setting, for example, without critical data about their condition and treatment being made available to the medical staff. The INPC was developed in collaboration with 27 data sharing partners; including representation from hospitals, practices, community health clinics, and homeless care sites. Initial features included a secure wide-area network, a clinical data repository, and software to enable a cross-institutional combined view of an individual's medical results.

A series of grants from federal agencies (including the Agency for Healthcare Research and Quality, National Library of Medicine, National Cancer Institute, and Office of the National Coordinator for Health Information

Technology) and private foundations (Regenstrief Foundation, Markle Foundation, and Fairbanks Foundation) allowed us to build the core technological infrastructure and operate the exchange [2–6] while studying the core problems such as patient identify management, privacy and confidentiality, data normalization, and assessing the value created through the exchange of health information [7, 8].

In 2003, Indianapolis business community leaders commissioned a report from Battelle to identify priority focus areas for business development. The report indicated that life sciences should be a priority. In response, a new organization named BioCrossroads (www.biocrossroads.com) convened work groups which determined that health IT should be developed in Indiana. Based on these recommendations, BioCrossroads commissioned the Boston Consulting Group to conduct a study on the most effective way to develop and implement health IT in the community.

There were three major early challenges which could have scuttled the IHIE project. First, hospital CIOs asked whether IHIE competes with the individual hospital IT strategies to link physician offices. This was resolved by recognizing that the EHR systems in the hospitals addressed institutional workflows and that participation in the city-wide network could reduce their operating costs.

Second, hospital CFOs asserted, "I do not see any significant ROI and recommend to CEO's not to proceed." Fortunately a return on investment analysis showed that the economies of scale created hard returns as a result of lower costs for delivering clinical results to ambulatory provider practices, in addition to the likely intangible returns. Based on these results the health system CEOs vision that INPC is the infrastructure for future health care initiatives and cost savings carried the day.

Finally, the inevitable question of who would capitalize the project came to the fore. Fortunately the Regenstrief Institute's development of the INPC coincided with overcoming the other challenges. So in 2004, Indianapolis civic leaders created IHIE to provide technical support and help develop a sustainable business model for the INPC. This blending of research and commercial perspectives proved to be a successful formula for community HIE.

The HIE landscape has changed in many ways over the last 15 years. By the time the HITECH act passed, the INPC had had over a decade of experience building community trust, assessing needs, and responding to issues such as privacy and security. Current efforts to foster interoperability will not have the luxury of developing at this pace and must demonstrate value early in the implementation process. The high costs of building infrastructure may make it difficult for HIEs to demonstrate their value to stakeholders at inception, and delaying value creation can slow the HIE's momentum. Emerging interoperability efforts do, however, have the advantage of existing data nomenclature standards such as LOINC and RxNorm, technical solutions for patient matching, and commercial products for HIE.

CASE STUDY MAIN CONTENT

Organization

IHIE is the service provider that works to expand the reach of currently available services, providing customer support, business development, technical resources, and physician liaisons. IHIE also is responsible for identifying potential sources of capital and assessing the feasibility of potential use cases, with emphasis on identifying the value of participation for different stakeholders. Initially the Regenstrief Institute was responsible for the INPC's technical direction, implementation, and operations, including application and technical support. Over time, IHIE has taken on more of the operations responsibility and expanded the technology partners.

The stakeholders in IHIE were aligned across a number of categories including external environment, organizational environment, consensus about goals, consensus about means, unique local aspects of the market, consensus about roles, the potential value that IHIE could bring, and consensus around behavioral expectations [9].

IHIE is a nonprofit 501(c)3 supporting organization. It operates through a variety of governance structures that facilitate efficient consultation with the diverse set of stakeholders. The major stakeholder structure is a Board of Directors which consists of 16 organizations representing the hospital networks, public agencies, medical societies, physicians, consumers, and researchers. The hardest work was establishing trusted organizational models, consensus on goals and requirements, and crafting participation agreements that met the legal, clinical, and ownership requirements of each party. We have advisory groups that provide guidance and expertise to assist with future development. Membership is multidisciplinary including representation encompassing technical, clinical, customer service, and users.

The INPC Management Committee, which operates separately from the Board, evaluates each proposed use of the system, such as adding a data type to the exchange, for its appropriateness. They evaluate aspects of the change such as how many patients are affected, what organizations need to be involved, how to implement the new service, and how much it will cost. This approach has been in place since IHIE's inception. By understanding the stakeholders' objectives and developing the exchange to support those objectives, we achieved a degree of social alignment primarily through a complex and somewhat organic communication process.

Community Engagement

Regenstrief and IHIE engage clinicians and health plans by contacting them to present their business case. For example, the potential savings offered by Quality Health First (QHF) or through various accountable care models is one of the major reasons payers have engaged. Because of the community priority on life sciences and health IT, many potential participants have existing collegial relationships which facilitate willingness to participate. Other factors that facilitate interest in participation are INPC's cost-effective solution for results delivery and increasing interest and investment in health IT across Indiana. INPC notes that its relationships have been built over a long time. They use the services of BioCrossroads to help facilitate discussions among stakeholders. Early on, candidates for participation are often unaware of HIE in the state, and a long period of education and communication was required to engage them. Of course, awareness is higher now but deep engagement still requires considerable time and effort. For example, members of the nursing home industry were in discussions with INPC for 5 years prior to the first long-term care facility signing a participation agreement in spring 2010.

As of July 2015, 106 hospitals, two long-term care groups, laboratories, imaging centers, and pharmacies, are connected to INPC with approximately 4 billion structured observations (Fig. 1) on over 24.8 million registrations (11.4 million unique patients). As evident in Fig. 2, participation and scale have grown from a focus in Indianapolis and central Indiana to statewide participants. Over 22,000 physicians use the HIE. Indiana Medicaid shares administrative data, including prescription records. Nearly all Indiana Emergency Departments are connected to capture real-time chief complaint data for biosurveillance and outbreak detection. The Indiana State Department of Health and the Marion County Health Department share childhood immunization information, public health laboratory results, and tumor registry data.

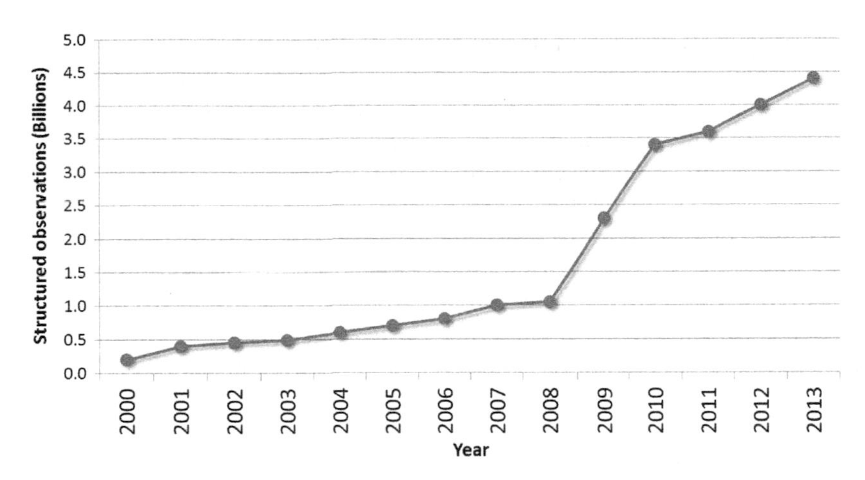

FIGURE 1 Growth in the number of structured observations captured and stored in the INPC data repository between 2000–2013.

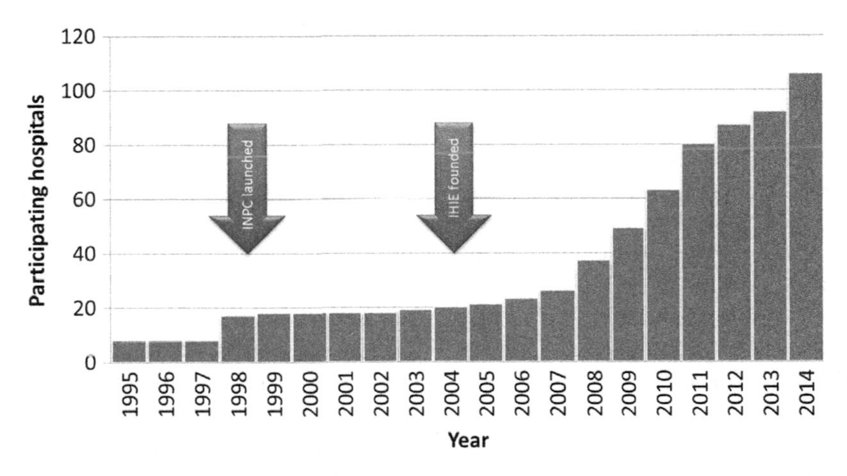

FIGURE 2 Timeline showing the growth in hospital participation over time while indicating both when the INPC evolved from a research project to an operational HIE and the launch of the Indiana Health Information Exchange corporation.

A key factor in engaging participants is what services IHIE offers. IHIE has to be cautious in choosing what services to implement in what order since each service needs to be financially self-sustaining; sources of participant engagement, sources of capital to create the service, technological capabilities, and business models have to be in alignment. By alignment we mean creating an architectural, operational, and business approach that distributes value across all stakeholders rather than about funding. According to a 2006 report by the Deloitte Center for Health Solutions, while "financing and ROI issues often receive a disproportionate share of stakeholder attention, successful HIEs keep their purpose and mission at the forefront." IHIE has kept its focus on value and facilitating the business need to share patient data in order to improve quality, safety, and efficiency [10].

HIE can be expected to improve efficiency and reduce cost growth. However, if their primary purpose becomes cost control, they will likely fail as did the CHINs of the 1990s [11]. IHIE has explored implementing more than 30 value-added services that rely on using normalized data. These include syndromic surveillance, EMT access, and INPC access at mass sporting events (eg, Indianapolis Motor Speedway).

Not all services proved successful. For example, early on IHIE had discussions with pharmacy benefit managers and payers about an incremental approach to e-prescribing. The initial step for this approach was to support delivery of a printed medication history synthesizing data from multiple medication sources. A combination of factors resulted in our choice of not to pursue this service because by time the technical challenges had been overcome and a business model evolved, e-prescribing had begun to rapidly expand. We were essentially too late. More recently, an image exchange service never gained enough participants to be sustainable due to a combination of chance events and competing priorities that limited marketing and sales efforts.

Financial Model

Operation of the exchange has been self-sustaining since 2011. Its operational costs are covered through its "bundled" subscription fees (including clinical messaging and clinical repository services). Initially, IHIE charged per transaction (clinical message delivered). However, large aggregated transaction fees served to discourage utilization among large providers and IHIE transitioned to a membership fee model based upon adjusted patient days. IHIE continually works to identify ways to leverage data, such as electronic lab reporting, multidrug resistant organism surveillance, and determining disability eligibility for the Social Security Administration.

Organizations providing HIE face the challenge of any multiparty network service [12]. To survive, they must reach a critical mass of users. Expanding the number of users and uses allows IHIE to distribute the core costs of data capture, normalization, and storage. Cost distribution supports sustainability. Some value-added services become less expensive and more technologically feasible as more organizations share the costs of an HIE infrastructure. The cost of standardizing a given kind of data source is relatively independent of the volume of data produced; any organization supporting interoperability must focus their resources on the high-volume data producers in order to reach critical mass. In most communities, these will be the large health systems.

IHIE creates value primarily by extracting data out of silos within participant organizations, and establishing trust in the community allowing the data to be aggregated and accessible by providers and other stakeholders who need information to improve patient and population health. The INPC's architecture is designed to support and facilitate data use and reuse. To some, the term reuse, or secondary use, has a negative connotation. However, the reality is that in health care, nearly every use is a reuse beyond the primary reason for collecting the data (eg, documentation or billing). Therefore, some prefer to use the term "continuous use" of data rather than reuse. Regardless of what term is used, data and information are valuable for a range of purposes in health care and therefore HIEs, like IHIE, create value when they can make data and information available in a wide range of contexts for use.

HIE operation, like most service businesses, is labor intensive. Building and maintaining interfaces to and from data sources as well as the initial and ongoing semantic normalization of data from different sources (ie, "mapping") makes up roughly half of ongoing expenses.

The training and support of new and existing customers makes up another quarter. The remaining quarter is divided, in decreasing portions, among software, database setup and maintenance, project management, data center and hardware, and professional services.

The business model created for access to the INPC clinical data repository relies on health systems paying a fee scaled by their size, and this access will, in return, improve the quality, safety, and efficiency of care they provide.

IHIE's sustainability strategy is based on principles key to HIE being a self-sustaining endeavor:

- HIE is a business
- Leverage high-cost, high-value assets
- No loss leaders
- Independent, local sustainability
- HIEs are natural monopolies
- There is an optimal size for an HIE—the need for scale
- Avoid grants for operational cost—HIE services must be able to generate revenue equal to or in excess of expenses

For more information about these principles, refer to chapter "Managing the Business of Health Information Exchange: Toward Sustainability."

Technical Approach

To facilitate participation and engagement, INPC strives to keep its technical architecture simple. The INPC system stores data in a federated model, with all data physically residing in a central location [6]. Data are logically separated, however, by source institution, even though they operate in the same software system. Messages from many source systems flow into one centralized facility, where IHIE implements routines to standardize the HL7 messages, map local observations, and report codes to a universal standard (eg, reference terminology as described in chapter "Standardizing Health Care Data Across an Enterprise"), and link multiple patient and physician identifiers for one individual to a global identifier (eg, client registry as described in chapter "Client Registries: Identifying and Linking Patients").

The INPC system matches patients within and across institutions, creating a longitudinal patient-centric record (eg, shared health record as described in chapter "Shared Longitudinal Health Records for Clinical and Population Health"). The current patient-matching infrastructure requires a patient identifier or medical record number assigned by a known registration authority to be associated with results or observations about the patient. A deterministic matching algorithm links multiple records for one patient, enabling a view of the patient's data; no matter its source.

Different data services require different standardization efforts. On the one hand, report delivery services such as DOCS4DOCS require a relatively small (a few person-weeks) effort per data source, most of which is consumed by standardizing the local provider codes used to identify report recipients. For other use cases, INPC maps local laboratory, radiology, and/or drug codes to national terminology standards.

Mapping to a common code system, or reference terminology, allows the INPC to consolidate patient data for use in decision support, public health, and research. The INPC's perspective is that data can only be leveraged for use and reuse if represented in a standard format. Therefore, supporting use of Logical Observation Identifiers and Name Codes (LOINC) and RxNorm were central to INPC's early work. Regenstrief developed, maintains, and supports LOINC for laboratory observations. The National Library of Medicine (NLM) developed RxNorm as standard nomenclature for medications. The INPC maps all institution laboratory codes to LOINC.

The use of CCDs, or continuity of care documents, to provide data has increased gradually. Currently more than 100,000 CCDs per month are received from 55 hospitals, yet this still represents a minority of all data exchanged. IHIE delivers copies of the CCDs to providers through the DOCS4DOCS system and retains a copy with the intent to eventually parse them into discrete data. IHIE can also deliver CCDs in response to queries such as those originated by EPIC's Care Everywhere system. In addition, as part of the Veterans' Administration, VLER project IHIE exchanges CCDs with VA facilities across the country. Unfortunately, providers are still dissatisfied with the content and workflow associated with CCDs as a medium for HIE [13].

Over the last decade, we made a number of significant enhancements to the underlying technical infrastructure of the INPC. First, we completely redeveloped the software, moving from a locally developed hierarchical database to a commercial relational database (Oracle), and reimplemented the code in JAVA to create a contemporary, service-oriented architecture. Second, we fully virtualized the system and migrated it from the public hospital's data center, where the exchange had been hosted since its inception to a contemporary hardware and storage environment in a commercial data center. This move increased reliability, performance, and security. One of the most important technical infrastructure efforts we undertook was to create and refine an improved process for interfacing participants. The process for "onboarding" new organizations had proven to be a rate-limiting step in the network's growth. It is also a challenge for other HIEs, as well as public health departments seeking to onboard providers for meaningful use.

Our approach to onboarding included establishing a project management office, monthly status tracking, dedicated interface engineers, and detailed process maps. While this approach certainly improved the process, we were still not satisfied with the rate of progress and continue to explore new ways to improve our interfacing capability. We also established a master provider index (eg, health worker registry as described in chapter "Health Worker Registries: Managing the Health Care Workforce") with matching during the project. This functionality allows us to link all data for a provider even though different provider identifiers might be used. For example, a prescription record from Surescripts might be identified by a DEA number while a laboratory result is identified by the local laboratory ID for that provider. This capability was used to facilitate access to the clinical data repository across provider organizations to aggregate data for clinical data reporting and other similar functions.

A related technological improvement was the creation of a provider attribution system. This system utilizes a predictive model that uses data about the transactions passing through the exchange to identify providers who can be considered accountable for the patient's care. This attribution is used, for example, to select the patients used for provider quality reporting. It is also used as the basis for an access control method, which allows a patient's primary provider to access their record.

Privacy and Confidentiality

The INPC system contains and discloses highly confidential information that is protected by both federal and state law. As a result, the agreement contains stringent confidentiality provisions. All information stored on and received through the INPC network must be kept confidential pursuant to all applicable laws, as well as each participant's own internal rules and regulations relating to the confidentiality of patient health information. The terms and conditions agreement that govern INPC members' participation in the INPC incorporate recent changes to HIPAA under HITECH as well as a reporting process for serious breaches of confidentiality. The agreement allows the use of the repository data for prescribed treatment, public health and research, and purposes with oversight by the INPC Management Committee. Only authorized INPC member users associated with a given institution are given INPC access to the records of patients according to the agreed-upon "trigger and access window rules" based on the approved uses. It permits research on deidentified data extracts but prohibits research that compares institutions or providers, even if deidentified, unless specifically approved by the involved parties.

Because the INPC pool of patients is so large and inclusive, rules are applied that go beyond Health Insurance Portability and Accountability Act (HIPAA) requirements and constrain clinicians' access to a stingy subset of the total INPC population at any given point in time.

We based our first rule on "proximity" between patient and provider. The INPC knows when a patient has checked into a given facility, because it receives all check-in messages. It uses the aforementioned check-in information to give physicians working within each facility access to the INPC records of patients who are also there. We have been using this proximity-based approach in Indianapolis emergency departments for years. We are now implementing the same approach for physicians and patients in a given hospital.

We based our second rule on institutional privileging. This rule allows providers who have staff privileges at two or more INPC institutions to access the INPC data from all of their institutions at once, so they can look at a patient's data as one record. In the combined view, individual results are footnoted with their institutional source to clarify the data's origin. Physicians already have the right to look at the medical record data in each hospital by virtue of their staff privileges; the INPC makes access easier and the data more digestible.

Services

IHIE offers three basic services: DOCS4DOCS, the INPC Clinical Repository and Results Viewer, and Accountable Care Organization (ACO) services. An important turning point in INPC's evolution was developing the DOCS4DOCS report delivery system. When INPC first began exchanging data, they used a "pull" model offering a comprehensive view of patients' records at the point of care. In 2003, INPC learned that clinicians would not always look up data and wanted a "push" model. Regenstrief responded by developing DOCS4DOCS, a clinical messaging service which sends text reports such as laboratory, radiology, transcriptions, and cardiology from source systems at hospitals and delivers the information to affiliated providers. DOCS4DOCS provides three methods for physicians to receive or access clinical information from participating organizations:

- *Secure Inbox*—the DOCS4DOCS portal is a secure, web-based "inbox."
- *Direct EHR Integration*—clinical messages can be delivered directly to an ambulatory provider's EHR via an HL7 interface.
- *Fax*—messages can be delivered to physician practices via fax upon request.

DOCS4DOCS uses HL7 interfaces to receive laboratory/transcription/radiology results, discharge summaries, operative notes, EKGs, and other clinical messages from participating data sources. Users can choose which reports are delivered to their inbox, for example, inpatient versus outpatient, preliminary versus final, and report forwarding to other physicians involved in the patient's care. Data sources can "override" these options when delivery is dictated by regulation for example. Data senders, such as hospitals and laboratories, must pay to deliver results to clinicians. DOCS4DOCS offers data delivery at a lower cost than alternatives, providing a value proposition to data senders. As a result, they are invested in the system at a business level. This approach to getting data to users consistently and reliably has driven growth and is the basis of IHIE's sustainability planning.

The INPC Clinical Repository and Results Viewer is a statewide health repository system that securely aggregates individual patient health information from multiple sources into a single virtual patient medical record which provides views of a clinical abstract and results of the most accurate up-to-date information available for a patient, regardless of treatment location. The INPC Clinical Repository is organized by patient and segregated by originating institution, aggregating data in real-time to ensure current patient information including the following:

- Emergency department visit data (free-text chief complaint)
- Registration records (demographics)
- Radiology reports
- Discharge summaries
- Operative notes
- Pathology reports
- Medication records
- EKG reports
- Laboratory data
- Inpatient and outpatient hospital encounter data demographics
- Coded diagnoses and procedures for hospital admissions and emergency department visits
- Ambulatory encounter (visit) data.

IHIE's most recent services focus on support for accountable care organizations starting with alerting ACOs to patient care events like admissions or emergency department encounters which build on previous research efforts [14]. The ACOs use these alerts to track where care has been delivered, to support the management of care transitions and follow-up to ensure care has been delivered as needed. In one case study, these alerts and subsequent ACO interventions reduced the number of non-urgent emergency department visits by 53% with a corresponding increase in primary care physician office visits by 68% which, based on the local costs for an emergency department visit versus an office visit, saved the health plan between $2.1 and $4.1 million during the 6-month trial period [15].

Another service, QHF was offered from 2008 until 2013, however we were unable to meet participant needs to scale beyond the State of Indiana. QHF provided patient-level data for two purposes. First, it provides guidance on an individual patient's needs, such as whether they are due for a screening test. Second, it provided monthly reports on physician performance quality by utilizing aggregated clinical and claims data. QHF was developed by physicians, hospital networks, health insurers, Regenstrief Institute, Employers' Forum of Indiana, Indiana State Medical Association, Indiana Department of Health, and Indianapolis Medical Society. This program provided physicians with a disease management, preventive care, and reporting service that delivered patient-specific and population-based reports, alerts, and reminders based upon needs or incentives of participating providers or payers. This program combined clinical data, medical and drug claims, and point-of-care data to monitor patients' health and wellness (eg, cholesterol, diabetes, and asthma) including Physician Quality Reporting Initiative reporting. Physicians were able to compare their individual results to the physician community as a whole. There was no charge to physicians, and no technology or software required for participation in QHF. Payers provided participating physicians with financial incentives for performance improvement and funded QHF on a patient per month basis. This provided the physicians with information about the care they were providing to their patients and provided payers with data about the quality of care physicians were providing across all patients that a physician cares for.

In addition to the services that IHIE provides, the INPC data infrastructure supports other important services including public health and biomedical research.

Because the INPC provides data flows from so many sources including laboratories and emergency department encounters that are of particular interest to public health, investigators from the Regenstrief Institute with the support of local and state public health agencies have created systems [16] that support both electronic laboratory reporting [17–19] and syndromic surveillance [20,21]. In addition, the INPC has been leveraged to support infection control efforts by including data across institutions to support infection control; Regenstrief investigators demonstrated significant improvements in the management of MRSA and VRE [22,23–25].

The INPC also serves biomedical research. Clinical researchers at the IU School of Medicine have long used the INPC repositories to estimate the number and demographic characteristics of patients with particular diseases for research planning and grant writing. Under institutional review board–approved rules, they use the data to verify that study candidates qualify before inviting them into a study and to collect information about outcomes of patients in active studies. The data are also used for epidemiologic studies, a great example of which is the one that discovered the associations between erythromycin and pyloric stenosis among newborns. [26] Research administration at the Indiana University School of Medicine estimates that more than 2000 of their human subjects research studies use data from the INPC repository at any given time. The heavy utilization of the system for research is unique among HIEs, in part as a result of the INPC's legacy as a research effort.

We believe that a variety of different services built on a common technology, and operations base is the best vehicle for HIE sustainability. The model we created was predicated on the principle that sustained funding would require that funders would need to achieve sustained value. The initial service provided was result delivery through the DOCS4DOCS service. Organizations that produced health information paid to have those results delivered to providers. In addition to supporting the costs of interfacing, developing and maintaining relationships with physician practices, and some administrative overhead, the service raised the importance to the participating organizations of maintaining the integrity of the interfaces.

SUMMARY

While we have some strong lessons to share in general from the IHIE experience including:

- do not make it complicated
- "free" the data—get it out of the silos and establish trust in your community
- aggregate the data and do something with it
- do not boil the ocean
- data reuse is the killer application

We most want to emphasize that some of the most difficult and valuable work required to develop an HIE is engagement, operationalization of data sources, and the network externalities created. No matter what interoperability technology or approach is adopted, the data created, stored, and managed in various health care IT systems need to be freed and normalized; and this work is largely "trench warfare." In addition to freeing the data, there must be trust, collaboration, and connectivity between providers.

DISCUSSION QUESTIONS

1. Interoperability can only be achieved when provider organizations do the work necessary to participate. Do provider organizations have the necessary incentives to do that work?
2. Private health information exchanges seem to be growing at a faster pace than public health information exchanges. Public

exchanges should arguably offer more value to patients and lower costs to provider organizations. Why the discrepancy?

3. The INPC, originated as a research project, was initially funded by grants and one of the ongoing value propositions is research use of the data. Is research necessarily critical to success of a health information exchange?
4. Establishing and operating a health information exchange requires a variety of investments including computing and network infrastructure, software systems of various types, legal and operational costs. Would you agree that data capture and normalization is the largest investment required?
5. Computing infrastructure, networking technology, software and clinical information standards will continue to evolve rapidly and investments in the technology will depreciate relatively rapidly. What are the core assets of an HIE if not these things?

References

[1] Overhage JM, Tierney WM, McDonald CJ. Design and implementation of the Indianapolis network for patient care and research. Bull Med Libr Assoc 1995;83(1):48.

[2] Biondich PG, Grannis SJ. The Indiana network for patient care: an integrated clinical information system informed by over thirty years of experience. J Public Health Manag Pract 2004;10:S81–6.

[3] McGowan JJ, Overhage JM, Barnes M, McDonald CJ. Indianapolis I3: the third generation integrated advanced information management systems. J Med Libr Assoc 2004;92(2):179.

[4] McDonald CJ, Overhage JM, Barnes M, Schadow G, Blevins L, Dexter PR, et al. The Indiana network for patient care: a working local health information infrastructure. Health Aff 2005;24(5):1214–20.

[5] Overhage JM. Health information exchange:'lex parsimoniae'. Health Aff 2007;26(5):w595–7.

[6] Zafar A, Dixon BE. Pulling back the covers: technical lessons of a real-world health information exchange. Stud Health Technol Inform 2007;129(Pt 1):488–92.

[7] Overhage JM, Dexter PR, Perkins SM, Cordell WH, McGoff J, McGrath R, et al. A randomized, controlled trial of clinical information shared from another institution. Ann Emerg Med 2002;39(1):14–23.

[8] Finnell JT, Overhage JM, Dexter PR, Perkins SM, Lane KA, McDonald CJ. Community clinical data exchange for emergency medicine patients. AMIA Annu Symp Proc 2003;2003:235–8. American Medical Informatics Association.

[9] West DM, Friedman A. [Internet]. Health information exchange and megachange, Governance Studies at Brookings [cited July 21, 2015] http://www.brookings.edu/research/papers/2012/02/08-health-info-exchange-friedman-west.

[10] Deloitte Center for Health Solutions [Internet]. Health information exchange (HIE) business models: the path to sustainable financial success [cited July 21, 2015] http://www.providersedge.com/ehdocs/ehr_articles/Health_Info_Exchange_Business_Models.pdf.

[11] John A. Hartford Foundation, Benton International, community health management information system: functional specifications. New York: Hartford Foundation; 1991.

[12] Economides N, Himmelberg C. Critical mass and network evolution in telecommunications Brock GW, editor. Toward a competitive telecommunications industry, selected papers from the 1994 telecommunications policy research conference. Mahwah, NJ: Lawrence Erlbaum; 1995.

[13] Byrne CM, Mercincavage LM, Bouhaddou O, Bennett JR, Pan EC, Botts NE, et al. The Department of Veterans Affairs' (VA) implementation of the Virtual Lifetime Electronic Record (VLER): findings and lessons learned from health information exchange at 12 sites. Int J Med Inform 2014;83(8):537–47.

[14] Anand V, Sheley ME, Xu S, Downs SM. Real time alert system: a disease management system leveraging health information exchange. Online J Public Health Inform 2012;4(3).

[15] Indiana Health Information Exchange [Internet]. Indiana: Indiana Health Information Exchange; ADT alerts for reducing ED admissions: a case study [cited July 12, 2015] http://mpcms.blob.core.windows.net/bd985247-f489-435f-a7b4-49df92ec868e//4f798bc8-4c8f-4dce-b145-cab48f3d8787/ihie-adtalerts-casestudy.pdf

[16] Dixon BE, Grannis SJ. Public health informatics infrastructure Public health informatics and information systems. London: Springer; 2014.69.88.

[17] Overhage JM, Grannis S, McDonald CJ. A comparison of the completeness and timeliness of automated electronic laboratory reporting and spontaneous reporting of notifiable conditions. Am J Public Health 2008;98(2):344.

[18] Dixon BE, McGowan JJ, Grannis SJ. Electronic laboratory data quality and the value of a health information

exchange to support public health reporting processes AMIA Annu Symp Proc, 20112011322. American Medical Informatics Association.

[19] Fidahussein M, Friedlin J, Grannis S. Practical challenges in the secondary use of real-world data: the notifiable condition detector AMIA Annu Symp Proc, 20112011402. American Medical Informatics Association.

[20] Mandl KD, Overhage JM, Wagner MM, Lober WB, Sebastiani P, Mostashari F, et al. Implementing syndromic surveillance: a practical guide informed by the early experience. J Am Med Inform Assoc 2004;11(2):141–50.

[21] Grannis S, Wade M, Gibson J, Overhage JM. The Indiana public health emergency surveillance system: Ongoing progress, early findings, and future directions AMIA Annu Symp Proc, 20062006304. American Medical Informatics Association.

[22] Dixon BE, Jones JF, Grannis SJ. Infection preventionists' awareness of and engagement in health information exchange to improve public health surveillance. Am J Infect Control 2013;41(9):787–92.

[23] Kho AN, Doebbeling BN, Cashy JP, Rosenman MB, Dexter PR, Shepherd DC, et al. A regional informatics platform for coordinated antibiotic-resistant infection tracking, alerting, and prevention. Clin Infect Dis 2013;57(2):254–62.

[24] Kho AN, Lemmon L, Commiskey M, Wilson SJ, McDonald CJ. Use of a regional health information exchange to detect crossover of patients with MRSA between urban hospitals. J Am Med Inform Assoc 2008;15(2):212–6.

[25] Rosenman MB, Szucs KA, Finnell SME, Khokhar S, Egg J, Lemmon L, et al. Nascent regional system for alerting infection preventionists about patients with multidrug-resistant gram-negative bacteria: implementation and initial results. Infect Control Hosp Epidemiol 2014;35(S3):S40–7.

[26] Mahon BE, Rosenman MB, Kleiman MB. Maternal and infant use of erythromycin and other macrolide antibiotics as risk factors for infantile hypertrophic pyloric stenosis. J Pediatr 2001;139(3):380–4.

CASESTUDY

2

Using Health Information Exchange to Support Public Health Activities in Western New York: A Case Study

Saira N. Haque, Robert Bailey and Barbara Massoudi
RTI International Center for the Advancement of Health IT, Research Triangle Park, NC

OUTLINE

MAJOR THEMES

- Implementation of a clinical or health information exchange system/component
- Business case for health information exchange/business plan/sustainability
- Use of health information exchange for population health
- Public funding

INTRODUCTION

This case study outlines an expanded use of HEALTHeLINK, the western New York health information exchange (HIE), for population health. Chapter "What is Health Information Exchange?" outlines different types of HIEs: community based, government facilitated, private, and vendor based. HEALTHeLINK was initially developed by payers and providers for administrative data exchange that expanded to become a community-based HIE to also include clinical data. HEALTHeLINK is governed by health care providers, insurers, and other western New York community health organizations. Using a publicly funded grant program, HEALTHeLINK expanded its role to support public health in several ways: reporting to public health agencies, providing public health alerts, and supporting clinical care and public health services. Specific activities in these areas include identification, investigation, treatment, and tracking of sexually transmitted infections, HIV, tuberculosis (TB), possible rabies exposures, HIV-positive patients, and hepatitis patients. In addition, HEALTHeLINK facilitated provision of public health services including quality control and investigations. Thus, less effort is needed for administrative duties, freeing resources for service provision to vulnerable populations. These innovations in routine public health work have allowed public health professionals to save money through time savings, avoided medical treatment and associated indirect costs, and improved health outcomes.

BACKGROUND

HEALTHeLINK is an HIE network that connects data sources and enables querying and data sharing. HEALTHeLINK connects clinical data from all 26 hospitals in an eight-county western New York region as well as eight radiology providers, three independent laboratories, four home health care agencies, four long-term care facilities, three medication history sources, and the Veterans Health Administration [1].

HEALTHeLINK serves the western region of New York state. The major metropolitan area in the region is Buffalo-Niagara [2]. The HIE serves western New York's eight rural and urban counties: Allegany, Cattaraugus, Chautauqua, Erie, Genesee, Niagara, Orleans, and Wyoming [3]. The total population is approximately 1.5 million people. Out of those, approximately 42% have consented to participate in the HIE [4]. The median income is slightly below that of the rest of the state, and the median age is higher.

Socioeconomic disparity is high, which means that public health concerns relative to poverty rates persist in the region. In addition, approximately 30% of the adult population is obese, as well as almost 20% of children. Health concerns in the area include cardiovascular disease, diabetes mellitus, behavioral health, asthma, HIV/AIDS, perinatal care, palliative care, and renal care. The region is characterized by high rates of health disparities, particularly among minority and elderly populations [4].

The HIE was established by a consortium of partners representing hospitals and payers. It has since expanded to include other clinical providers, long-term and postacute care, laboratory services, public health, and pharmacy. To expand the HIE, HEALTHeLINK, and its community partners applied for, and subsequently received, Beacon Community Cooperative Agreement Program funding. This 3-year grant from the Office of the National Coordinator for Health Information Technology supported expansion of HIE infrastructure to include community-based health initiatives [5]. The Beacon Community funding was used to strengthen HEALTHeLINK by connecting additional partners and data sources and develop new functionality to increase HEALTHeLINK's value to users, including the New York State Department of Health (NYSDOH) and the Erie County Department of Health (ECDOH).

Several partners comprise the Western New York Beacon Community (WNY Beacon). They include HEALTHeLINK itself (the HIE for western New York), the P^2 Collaborative of Western New York (the New York eHealth Collaborative regional extension agent, a nonprofit dedicated to improving health in western New York), and 40 community partners. HEALTHeLINK is governed by health care providers, insurers, and representatives from the western New York community, including the Catholic Health System, the Erie County Medical Center, HealthNow New York, the Independent Health Association, Kaleida Health, the Roswell Park Cancer Institute, Univera Healthcare, and the Health Care Efficiency and Affordability Law for New Yorkers Capital Grant Program from New York State (known as HEAL NY).

Although HEALTHeLINK's most noted aim for expansion when seeking Beacon Community funding was to address the region's high rate of diabetes, expansion had public health impacts. Public health officials leveraged the local HIE infrastructure to streamline and improve the effectiveness of communicable disease epidemiologic investigations. The processes developed have allowed public health staff to overcome traditional challenges such as delayed reporting, incomplete information, and resource limitations to acquire more of the demographic and clinical information they need more quickly and with less effort than what the case was previously. They use this information to identify significant clinical or behavioral risk factors, complete surveillance reports, and intervene with patients and contacts more effectively when needed.

HEALTHeLINK does not generate or "push" reports or alerts about public health events. Instead, these come from the Electronic Clinical Laboratory Reporting System (ECLRS), via fax or telephone from clinical laboratories and providers. Once NYSDOH identifies an issue in ECLRS or another one of its databases, it accesses HEALTHeLINK to acquire additional clinical and demographic data. Investigators from ECDOH receive these reports and access HEALTHeLINK to fill in missing clinical data and retrieve demographic and contact information that can aid their investigations [6].

HIE and Public Health

Public health activities rely heavily on information sharing and analysis. Improving access to information can support public health services such as surveillance and monitoring immunization coverage [7].

The Health Information Technology for Economic and Clinical Health Act has provided incentives for providers to implement electronic health records (EHRs). The inclusion of public health-oriented Meaningful Use objectives has led to greater inclusion of information relevant for public health agencies in EHR implementations [8]. Because of funding constraints, public health organizations have been creative in taking advantage of existing resources and infrastructure to access information.

Public health–specific information exchange activities include the BioSense Platform [9] and the Public Health Information Network [10]. In addition to efforts specifically focused on health information technology (IT), some community-based funding initiatives include information exchange such as the Centers for Medicare & Medicaid Services–funded Health Care Innovation Awards [11].

New York state developed a program to help support regional health information organizations (RHIOs) [12], which are described in "Case Study 3." This program has helped to provide infrastructure to overcome barriers to HIE including structures, formats, and vocabularies [13].

These efforts focus on various aspects of public health and information exchange. The following sections discuss ways in which information exchange can support public health.

Uses of HIE in Public Health

Public and population health activities rely on information sharing among health care providers [14]. Facilitating information availability supports HIE to improve public health

BOX 1

USES OF HEALTH INFORMATION EXCHANGE IN PUBLIC HEALTH

Catastrophic events

- Mass-casualty events
- Disaster medical response

Reporting to public health agencies

- Reporting of laboratory diagnoses
- Nonmandatory reporting of laboratory data
- Nonmandatory reporting of clinical data
- Reporting of physician-based diagnoses
- Immunization
- Surveillance

Public health alerting

- Public health alerting—patient level
- Public health alerting—population level

Clinical care

- Clinical care in public health clinics

Public health services

- Public health investigation
- Quality measurement

activities [14,15]. A discussion of several ways in which information exchange can be used to support public health based on Shapiro et al. [15] and the Meaningful Use criteria is shown in Box 1.

Catastrophic Events

HIE is necessary and helpful in catastrophic events, such as mass-casualty events (including natural disasters) or disaster medical response. The response to those events encompasses disaster medical response. In these conditions, exchanging health information is vital to facilitating communication among providers and with the public.

The Southeast Regional HIT-HIE Collaboration (SERCH) project on HIE in Disaster Preparedness and Response was developed to facilitate sharing health information among participating states in response to a declared national disaster [16].

Reporting to Public Health Agencies

Because public health agencies depend on accurate and timely reporting, activities that facilitate information sharing are extremely important. HIEs can help improve the reporting rate and timeliness of these activities. The Meaningful Use criteria include several public health objectives that support reporting: immunization, syndromic surveillance, reportable laboratory results, cancer reporting, and specialized registries [17]. Because of their inclusion in the Meaningful Use regulations, EHRs are likely to support reporting functionality for these items.

HIEs can support public health reporting. It is a mandatory requirement to report some positive laboratory test results [13,18]. Other results are not mandatory but can be helpful for public health activities. HIEs can help improve the reporting rate and timeliness of these activities. With electronic reporting, data are more likely to be complete [19,20]. For nonmandatory reporting, having information available can help identify patterns [15].

Electronic laboratory reporting does not include reporting of physician diagnoses. Such reporting is a separate process with physician-based diagnoses that are mandatory to report and others that are not. Some pieces of clinical information can supplement a diagnosis that is identified through laboratory testing [13,15]. HIEs can facilitate this reporting on the basis of diagnoses, medications, or other identifying factors, which can provide valuable situating information to guide public health activities.

Implementation of HIEs can avoid significant administrative costs of this mandatory reporting to public health departments. Walker et al. [21] estimate that national implementation of interoperable HIEs could reduce reporting costs by $195 million (2003 dollars) annually.

HIEs can also support immunization registries, which can result in improved tracking and reporting of vaccination rates and preventable disease. With the proposed move to barcoding of vaccine data, exchanging those data will become more important for tracking and reporting [22].

Syndromic surveillance depends on exchange of health information. Programs such as BioSense [10] provide a platform to collect and share information. The Kansas Health Information Network is connected to the BioSense syndromic surveillance system at the Centers for Disease Control and Prevention (CDC) in November 2012 [23]. Previously, the Kansas Department of Health and Environment had been manually collecting and reporting information, such as influenza data, using a system built for another purpose. Through this connection, Kansas can now use the BioSense Platform to track this type of information, rather than collecting it manually.

All of these uses of HIEs can help to better coordinate public health activities. By having more information available electronically and a mechanism to share it, public health agencies can have more accurate and timely information.

Public Health Alerting

Because of the importance of timeliness and accuracy in public health reporting, HIEs can be extremely useful. At the patient level, sharing information can help identify other affected individuals in the case of a reportable diagnosis. At the population level, HIEs can help ensure that public health alerts are accurate and sent in a timely fashion [24].

Traditional paper-based methods of alerting are time-consuming, rely on information that might be out of date, and are not immediate [24,25]. Thus, clinicians may not receive alerts at all or receive them too late to affect their clinical practices. In Indiana, HIE was used to facilitate a clinical messaging service to deliver public health alerts with improved efficiency and effectiveness of messaging [25].

Clinical Care

Clinical care is managed through public health agencies for some diseases, but it varies by jurisdiction. These diseases are typically communicable, such as TB and STIs, or characterized by settings with many people such as schools, jails, or shelters [15]. HIEs can ensure that referrals are made accurately and promptly. In addition, HIEs can support information sharing so that full identifiers and history are available. This exchange of information can facilitate coordination and improve outcomes [26].

Public Health Services

HIEs also support public health services such as investigations and quality measurement. Investigations rely heavily on information gathering and synthesizing. By having information about the patient and any other individuals available, public health agencies can conduct better epidemiological investigations. HIE can support public health investigations through improved information availability [13]. Disease clusters can more easily and quickly be identified.

Similarly, quality improvement activities such as chart audits are facilitated through HIEs. Electronic chart audits have been shown to provide reliable data [27]. However, these chart audits could not be completed offsite without a system logon or access through an HIE. Paper chart audits are manual and time intensive. With electronic information, chart reviews do not require travel to a site for review of copied paper charts, thus improving efficiency and effectiveness of review.

Increased EHR uptake and electronic exchange of that information can support public health activities in many ways, including catastrophic event response, reporting, alerts, and clinical care and public health services. As more providers implement EHRs, the benefits will continue to accrue for public health activities.

CASE STUDY MAIN CONTENT

Intervention, Planning, and Assessment

Although representatives from state and local public health departments were on the board of HEALTHeLINK, the HIE was not developed with public health in mind. Rather, public health officials used existing infrastructure to support public health activities. The improvements in communicable disease epidemiologic investigations were not the result of a planned intervention but were used by public health officials to leverage the capabilities of a well-conceived robust HIE.

In 1999, a core group of stakeholders defined the vision for HEALTHeNET as a for-profit network for the exchange of administrative data, which went live in 2002. HEALTHeNET is a collaboration that includes as stakeholders the three major payers (BlueCross BlueShield of Western New York, the Independent Health Association, and Univera Healthcare) and four major hospital systems (Kaleida Health, the Erie County Medical Center, the Catholic Health System, and the Roswell Park Cancer Institute) [28].

HEALTHeNet allows all providers (hospitals, clinics, and provider practices) in western New York to access administrative information such as eligibility and claim status. Providers could find the insurance information they needed quickly, easily, and in one place, which allowed them to improve efficiency. Insurance companies benefited from the decrease in telephone calls from providers requesting information. The effort demonstrated to key stakeholders in the region that collaboration could work. The number of participants, data sources, and functionalities continued to grow, when, in 2004 and 2005, these same key stakeholders defined the vision for HEALTHeLINK.

In 2004, a collaborative group conducted the Upstate New York Professional Healthcare Information & Education Demonstration Project and developed a white paper outlining a plan for regional interoperability. Participants included the Buffalo Academy of Medicine, members of the physician community, the State University of New York at Buffalo, the county and state public health departments, and HEALTHeNET. With additional support from the Agency for Healthcare Research and Quality and the Health Foundation for Western & Central New York, the group conducted a 1-year effort to collaborate as the Health Care Information Coordinating Council and developed a 5-year plan. They hired IBM to conduct an independent feasibility study and develop the business case to improve quality through a financially sustainable model. The support of these organizations individually and collectively culminated in western New York receiving funding from HEAL NY to create HEALTHeLINK.

HEALTHeLINK stakeholders include a broad representation of health care professionals and organizations throughout the eight-county western New York region, such as the Buffalo Academy of Medicine, ECDOH, the State University of New York at Buffalo, and the Western New York Rural Area Health Education Center.

HEALTHeLINK's success in sharing administrative data led to buy-in for sharing clinical data. Today, its mission is to create and maintain a secure and reliable infrastructure for the timely and accurate electronic exchange of clinical information among health care providers, insurers, and other medical professionals. HEALTHeLINK's vision is for western New York to have an electronic system for real-time sharing of clinical information among health care professionals to promote collaboration, limit duplication, control health care costs, and improve the delivery of services, clinical outcomes, and patient safety [29]. The support of the Beacon Community initiative, along with the P^2 Collaborative of Western New York, has enabled HEALTHeLINK to continue to build trust among the community and increase the number of participating data sources connected to the HIE.

One factor in building trust was disseminating the security protocols. Access to the system requires two-factor authentication. This includes a passcode plus either a token or a code received by text or voice message. Authorized access is strictly governed and enforced through audit reports. As a result, providers and patients felt confident that patients' health information was appropriately protected from unauthorized access or use and were willing to participate.

New York is an opt-in state regarding patient consent to share protected health information. HEALTHeLINK leveraged partnerships so that patients could opt-in at the community level. This means that if patients consent at a physician's office, they are also consenting for other participants in western New York and do not have to sign a consent form at every clinical location at which they receive care. Patients can also designate practices that do not have access to their information. This degree of specificity in opting in has enabled the HIE to gain traction and acceptance among providers and patients. As an indication of public acceptance, the number of patients consenting to share data via HEALTHeLINK rose from just less than 300,000 to more than 500,000 between 2010 and 2013, while the number of patient record queries rose from 100,000 to 600,000 during that time.

Health departments have access to all HEALTHeLINK data without consent, which is consistent with the Health Insurance Portability and Accountability Act of 1996 (HIPAA) Privacy Rule. Therefore, the high rate of patient consent ensures the robustness and utility of the data but is not required for public health access and use. High rates of provider participation ensure the completeness and utility of the data for public health investigations [1].

Implementation

HEALTHeLINK has been used in a variety of ways to improve public and population health, including communicable disease epidemiologic investigations conducted by the county and state departments of health, which routinely work closely together.

Laboratory results of reportable communicable diseases are reviewed by NYSDOH via ECLRS. NYSDOH staff receive automated reports, then manually sort them and send them to the appropriate counties for follow-up investigation. In Erie County, these reports go to the Epidemiology/Disease Control Program.

Erie County public health staff evaluate reports from NYSDOH for completeness of demographic information, such as address. If information is missing, they use HEALTHeLINK to identify or confirm the patient's city of residence, so that the appropriate county can be notified and follow-up can be routed accordingly. This process decreases the amount of time needed to identify the correct county, eliminating the time that would otherwise be needed to contact the ordering laboratory or associated physician to obtain basic demographic information. Staff indicated that time to obtain and correct information decreased from hours to minutes.

Uses of HEALTHeLINK to Provide Public Health Services

Although HEALTHeLINK does not generate reports of laboratory diagnoses, physician-based diagnoses, or immunization or surveillance data, it is used to follow up on reports and facilitate investigation. Public health staff receive automated reports of diagnoses through other surveillance systems and use HEALTHeLINK to follow up. Staff use HEALTHeLINK to access treatment information, patient contact information, and clinical encounter and laboratory test results that are relevant but not reportable. Examples of these uses follow.

CHLAMYDIA

HEALTHeLINK allows ECDOH to identify and follow up on priority chlamydia cases. Cases are manually identified using criteria including all untreated cases, pregnant females, repeaters (more than once in 90 days), and youth 16 years of age or younger. In 2012, Erie County had 5088 cases of chlamydia, of which 634 were assigned to epidemiologists for further investigation. Erie County uses HEALTHeLINK to look at pharmacy records to identify filled prescriptions. Thus, ECDOH can rapidly access information on treatment, treatment compliance (filled prescriptions), and the appropriateness of prescribed therapy. ECDOH can review the prescribed and filled prescription data to determine whether the clinician has prescribed a correct medication effective against chlamydia. Additionally, if the patient is of childbearing age, the HIE can be queried for information on pregnancy status.

GONORRHEA

HEALTHeLINK allows ECDOH to identify and follow up on gonorrhea cases. In 2012, Erie County had 1781 cases of gonorrhea, of which 1313 were assigned to disease investigators for investigation. ECDOH staff use HEALTHeLINK to retrieve pharmacy data on filled prescriptions, confirm appropriateness of treatment regimen, verify the name of the ordering physician if it is not on the laboratory report, and verify patient demographic information. ECDOH staff can intervene quickly to treat close contacts in a timely way.

SYPHILIS

ECDOH staff use HEALTHeLINK to retrieve pharmacy data on filled prescriptions, confirm treatment compliance and appropriateness of the treatment regimen, verify the name of the ordering physician if it is not on the laboratory report, and verify patient demographic information. Negative test results available through HEALTHeLINK are valuable to health department staff. The date of the last negative test can often allow investigators to stage the disease, which determines treatment. In the case of syphilis, if they can determine that the disease is in stage 1, only one treatment injection is required. If disease stage is unknown, three injections will be required, tripling the cost of treatment. ECDOH staff can intervene quickly to treat close contacts in a timely way.

HEPATITIS SURVEILLANCE

HEALTHeLINK allows health department staff to review all viral hepatitis laboratory tests, including negative results, which are not reportable but do encompass case definitions of reportable hepatitis. They can also review liver function tests to identify acute cases and prioritize cases. These data are also not reportable but are needed for case classification and follow-up. Staff use HEALTHeLINK to view the date of diagnosis and determine whether the case is new, which again enables them to prioritize their work. Being able to prioritize cases is critical: health department staff can intervene quickly and treat family members and close contacts in a timely way. In addition, they use HEALTHeLINK to view pregnancy test results and to determine hepatitis B status in pregnant and recently delivered women, which is required for the perinatal hepatitis B surveillance program. These cases require high-intensity follow-up. Health department staff need to ensure that the child is vaccinated for hepatitis B and subsequently tested to confirm antibody response to vaccination. Using HEALTHeLINK allows health department staff to manage these cases more effectively.

RABIES INVESTIGATIONS

ECDOH staff use HEALTHeLINK to access the most up-to-date information regarding addresses and phone numbers of the exposed victim, potential other victims, and the animal's owner (when applicable). HEALTHeLINK is a rich source of contact information because of the number of connected data sources. This information allows health department staff to begin public health work sooner by telephone and significantly reduces the number of field visits requested by epidemiologists.

FOODBORNE ILLNESS OUTBREAKS

Similar to their other uses of HEALTHeLINK, ECDOH staff access the HIE to retrieve contact information for persons to investigate outbreaks and conduct food history interviews. They also use it to retrieve laboratory testing on people involved. Improving the timeliness and completeness of these investigations allows ECDOH staff to complete mandatory reporting, follow-up with providers, and prevent infected people from handling food and infecting others.

TUBERCULOSIS

ECDOH epidemiologists send TB reports to a separate group of nurses at a TB clinic dedicated to these investigations. Nurses there access HEALTHeLINK to (1) view information on chest x-rays; (2) see other laboratory tests and results, track admission, and discharge dates; and (3) see medications prescribed and review discharge notes. They follow these techniques to rule out cases, follow the clinical path, and ensure proper treatment. Before HEALTHeLINK, the Department of Health would either send a nurse to the hospital to look through charts for this information or call the hospital to request visit information by fax. Both approaches were labor intensive and inefficient, requiring nurses to search through entire medical records.

QUALITY AUDITS TO TRACK INFECTION CONTROL IN HOSPITALS

One state public health function is quality auditing and reporting, which includes auditing and validating reports from hospitals, reviewing infection prevention practices, and ensuring consistent data across reporting hospitals. HEALTHeLINK allows NYSDOH to conduct audits remotely, significantly reducing time and expense. Before HEALTHeLINK, auditing required ECDOH staff to travel to 40 hospitals and review 60–70 charts per hospital. Onsite auditing required travel, lodging for 1–4 days, and per-diem expenses. Chart review occasionally identified the need for hospital staff to pull additional charts, requiring additional time. In addition to reducing costs associated with travel, HEALTHeLINK allows staff to monitor the details of admissions and readmissions, ensuring accurate reporting. Remote auditing has enabled staff to spend more time in the office and less time traveling, allowing them to keep pace with an increase in the types of surgical procedures that require reporting despite staffing reductions.

TRACKING NURSING HOME AND LONG-TERM CARE INFECTIONS

NYSDOH staff use HEALTHeLINK to support tracking and follow-up on health care–associated infections in nursing homes and long-term care facilities. Staff use

HEALTHeLINK to check address information to determine whether a patient is a resident of such a facility (which can be challenging because this population may not have a consistent address). Staff use HEALTHeLINK to conduct investigations in response to trends such as an increase in multidrug-resistant organisms. One such investigation of vancomycin-intermediate *Staphylococcus aureus* involved reviewing health information for 25 patients, including admission and discharge, underlying medical condition, demographics, laboratory results, and primary care physicians. HEALTHeLINK was particularly useful in these cases because these patients often travel from rural areas to cities for health care.

HIV INVESTIGATION AND CONTACT TRACING

Upon notification of HIV-positive status, NYSDOH staff use HEALTHeLINK to research cases. This includes identifying those with potential exposure to HIV. HEALTHeLINK can be used to identify those who might be exposed through demographic information such as spousal documentation. Once an HIV-positive individual has identified contacts that could result in transmitting HIV, health department staff can use HEALTHeLINK to contact those individuals and ensure that they get the testing and treatment they need.

In addition, ECDOH staff follow up with HIV-positive individuals who have not received treatment for the disease in the last 13 months. HEALTHeLINK provides an additional source of contact information for these individuals, allowing public health professionals to reach patients more quickly and avoid time-consuming field visits. In addition to time savings, additional information in HEALTHeLINK such as toxicology screens and provider comments on other medical conditions provide greater situational awareness to public health staff and allow them to target their approach to patient follow-up.

Implementation Analysis

Sustainability

HEALTHeLINK, established by the region's major hospital systems and health plans with the support of NYSDOH, serves as the foundation of the WNY Beacon initiative. Among other things, the functionality and data access provided by HEALTHeLINK enabled innovations in communicable disease epidemiologic investigation that are the focus of this case study.

HEALTHeLINK was founded on the shared recognition by key stakeholders that building the infrastructure and enabling the exchange of data would offer tremendous return on investment. Since 2005, HEALTHeLINK has enjoyed the financial support of three major payers and four major hospital systems. Thanks in large part to Beacon Community funding, payer and provider engagement has continued to grow. New opportunities for improving epidemiologic investigations continue to be explored as sources of data are added. WNY Beacon has passed the sustainability tipping point as penetration among major regional health care entities and integration with regional health care practices approach 100%.

The financial viability of HEALTHeLINK is overseen by the audit finance committee, which is composed of senior financial representatives from each of the seven participating entities, with the chair of the committee representing the largest payer. Their shared vision is that adoption of HIE services is the key to building value. The grant funding received to date has enabled HEALTHeLINK to create and expand their HIE infrastructure. Funding is needed to sustain operations. While local payers intend to continue their support for HEALTHeLINK, sustainability requires multiple funding streams and continuous demonstration of value to stakeholders (see chapter: "Managing the Business of Health Information Exchange: Toward Sustainability").

Challenges

Several challenges were associated with using HEALTHeLINK to support public health services, including access to information by public health workers, integration with other state regulatory requirements, and education for both providers and patients.

One reason for the high uptake is that users (eg, providers, provider staff, and payer staff) have role-based access control. This means that there is a mechanism to restrict HIE access to authorized users and to further restrict it so that people can see only the information they need for their jobs. Because the HIE was designed primarily for payers and providers, access for public health workers was not initially considered, and they did not have a profile for role-based access. This means that there was no set protocol for giving public health workers access. This issue, coupled with an initial misunderstanding of the HIPAA Privacy Rule, made access to data challenging for public health workers.

To combat concerns, NYSDOH established a workgroup consisting of its legal, public health, and IT staff, and included county public health representatives to help develop policies that would allow public health access to all RHIOs in New York State. The legal staff additionally developed one uniform public health contract statement based on input from the workgroup, which was designed to be incorporated by every RHIO when granting public health access to their systems. The policies were then submitted for review to the commissioner's advisory council on HIE, and after their input, the commissioner.

In the interim, the western region's associate commissioner used a workaround to grant access and spent a great deal of time on education and awareness. Public health staff were then given specific role-based access to do public health work. This workaround was eventually addressed, and the staff were given access. This issue is not unique to western New York, and other communities may need to consider similar issues for public health access.

Although the users of public health data made accessible via the HIE were pleased with the benefits realized to date, they identified opportunities to improve the usefulness of the data: more complete data, real-time availability, and improved access. Several changes could be made to improve effectiveness:

- Include vaccine information for children and adults.
- Connect additional area practices and hospitals to the network.
- Automate nightly updates of reportable disease diagnoses to ensure timely reporting.
- Automate alerts to public health staff based on prescribing certain drugs such as TB drugs so that public health staff can follow up.

Improvements in these areas would increase the timeliness and effectiveness of public health investigations and would simultaneously decrease the number of telephone calls to providers, which are often disruptive. Negative test results would allow regional public health agencies to calculate denominators needed for aggregate reporting. Otherwise, they are not easily able to determine, for example, if a doubling in positive test results represents an increase in disease or an increase in testing. In addition, access to total numbers tested for recommended preventive health screenings, such as mammograms, Pap tests, and colorectal cancer screenings, can provide community measures for compliance with recommended preventive health screenings among those who are eligible.

As mentioned previously, there is a continuing need to educate providers and consumers to explain public health workers' right to access the data and the privacy and security regulations they follow. Such clarification would help address vague uneasiness based on inaccurate perceptions of unlimited access to data.

Contributors to Success

Building on the vision of the core group of payers and hospitals that founded HEALTHeNET and demonstrated value from the outset, HEALTHeLINK now enjoys the participation of pharmacies, radiologists, laboratories, and physicians, and HEALTHeLINK itself participates in the Statewide Health Information Network of New York.

Developing and following a 5-year plan allowed the participants to apply successfully for funding and use it strategically to establish governance and policies as a foundation for trust. Representation of stakeholders in governance and oversight has enabled HEALTHeLINK to establish community-wide trust that data will be protected and used appropriately. Trust among providers has led to high rates of participation, which has yielded a critical mass of clinical information. Trust among patients has ensured low rates of opting out. Successful planning also allowed strategic engagement of data holders and addition of new data sources.

The result is an easy-to-use network that provides secure access to timely and accurate data. HIE users can define workflows that improve operational efficiency. Relationships between public health officials and physicians have been strengthened because physicians are not burdened with retrieving information, and calls placed by health departments can focus on more urgent issues.

Lessons Learned

Although HEALTHeLINK was in place before Beacon Community funding, the public health use cases were not considered from the start. One reason for this is that to maximize an HIE's public health benefit, there needs to be high participant uptake. Consequently, HEALTHeLINK initially focused on getting high participation, then focused on uses of information. However, including public health from the start could have helped in designing the HIE to support public health challenges. This would include developing a role profile for public health access, developing automated alerts, and sharing information. The board of directors had some representatives from the public health sector to facilitate public health access once the HIE had matured.

Other considerations include educating providers and patients about HEALTHeLINK. When HEALTHeLINK was first implemented, stakeholders were concerned about creating and controlling access to a huge repository of data. Although HEALTHeLINK is not a repository, a great deal of education was needed to explain how it works, who is authorized to access it, and how access is controlled. Stakeholders such as patients and clinicians had some concerns about public health staff having access to data, which further supports the importance of public health involvement. HEALTHeLINK had a champion in the NYSDOH associate commissioner, who conducted educational sessions and other activities to secure access for public health staff.

SUMMARY AND FUTURE DIRECTIONS

HEALTHeLINK is a case study of an existing, robust HIE for clinical care that was able to build on a solid foundation to support public health activity. This was possible because of several factors beyond a one-time public grant, including interdisciplinary stakeholder involvement and education. Because the Beacon Community funding supported increased participation in HEALTHeLINK, more records were available through the HIE which facilitated its use for public health.

To support the provision of core public health services, HIEs must have high levels of participation from a wide variety of providers. Beacon Community funding allowed western New York to add more providers, which was added to data availability. In addition to technical aspects, patient and provider education was required. Western New York worked with providers to help them understand how the HIE worked and to incorporate signing up into its workflow. This work was then augmented by a general awareness program.

Although HEALTHeLINK streamlined many public health functions, additional potential to improve public health remains untapped for the future. An automated reporting function does not exist, so HEALTHeLINK is used to augment data sources from existing systems. Going forward, electronic public health case reporting and HEALTHeLINK could be integrated more seamlessly. Using HEALTHeLINK for automated mandatory and nonmandatory public health reporting could streamline follow-up and research efforts. In addition, HEALTHeLINK could be used more broadly to facilitate chronic disease management throughout the region, not just for diseases for which the public health department provides care. The role of HEALTHeLINK can be identified and specified for disaster recovery planning. Integration of systems and automated reporting would add more value. Other public health departments should consider how HEALTHeLINK can help to provide public health services.

Acknowledgments

This project was funded under Contract 200-2011-F-40207 from the Centers for Disease Control and Prevention to RTI International.

DISCUSSION QUESTIONS

1. What are some other ways in which HEALTHeLINK could be used to support public health activities?
2. What would be necessary in other communities to use their health information exchange or regional health information organizations to support public health?
3. What are ways in which the use of HEALTHeLINK could be improved to maximize public health benefit?
4. Describe the efficiencies achieved by using HEALTHeLINK.
5. Is the use of HEALTHeLINK synchronous or asynchronous? Why?
6. How would involving public health stakeholders from the outset have changed uses of HEALTHeLINK for public health?
7. What are other ways in which HIE can be used for public health beyond what HEALTHeLINK is doing?
8. If you were a public health official involved in HEALTHeLINK, what would your next steps be?

References

[1] HEALTHeLINK. Participants. 2012 [cited January 27, 2014]. Available from: <http://www.wnyhealthelink.com/Physicians/Participants>.

[2] New York State's Empire State Development. Western New York Regional Office: Inside Western New York. 2010. Available from: <http://esd.ny.gov/RegionalOverviews/WesternNY/InsideRegion.html>.

[3] HEALTHeLINK. Who we are. Frequently asked questions. 2015. Available from: <http://www.wnyhealthelink.com/WhoWeAre/FAQs>.

[4] New York State Department of Health. Western New York Community Health Needs Assessment: Delivery System Reform Incentive Payment (DSRIP) Program: Volume 1: CNA Summary. 2014 [cited 2015]. Available from: <http://www.health.ny.gov/health_care/medicaid/redesign/dsrip/pps_applications/docs/erie_county/3.8_millenium_collaborative_care_pps_cna.pdf>.

[5] HealthIT.gov. Beacon Community Program. 2015. Available from: <http://www.healthit.gov/policy-researchers-implementers/beacon-community-program>.

[6] Western New York Beacon. The Western New York Beacon Community Report. 2014 [cited January 27, 2014]. Available from: <http://www.wnybeacon.com/>.

[7] Calderwood MS, Platt R, Hou X, Malenfant J, Haney G, Kruskal B, et al. Real-time surveillance for tuberculosis using electronic health record data from an ambulatory practice in eastern Massachusetts. Public Health Rep [Internet] 2010;125(6):843–50. Available from: http://www.ncbi.nlm.nih.gov/pubmed/21121229.

[8] Overhage JM, Grannis S, McDonald CJ. A comparison of the completeness and timeliness of automated electronic laboratory reporting and spontaneous reporting of notifiable conditions. Am J Public Health 2008;98(2):344–50.

[9] Centers for Disease Control and Prevention. BioSense Program. 2010 [cited November 26, 2013]. Available from: <http://www.cdc.gov/biosense>.

[10] Centers for Disease Control and Prevention. Public health information network: guides. 2013 [cited January 27, 2014]. Available from: <http://www.cdc.gov/phin/resources/PHINguides.html>.

[11] Centers for Medicare & Medicaid Services. Health Care Innovation Awards round two. 2014 [cited January 27, 2014]. Available from: <http://innovation.cms.gov/initiatives/Health-Care-Innovation-Awards/Round-2.html>.

[12] Kern LM, Kaushal R. Health information technology and health information exchange in New York State: new initiatives in implementation and evaluation. J Biomed Inform 2007;40(Suppl. 6):S17–20. PubMed PMID: 17945542. Epub September 7, 2007.

[13] Shapiro JS. Evaluating public health uses of health information exchange. J Biomed Inform [Internet] 2007;40(Suppl. 6):S46–9. Available from: http://www.ncbi.nlm.nih.gov/pmc/articles/PMC2137930/.

[14] Kass-Hout TA, Gray SK, Massoudi BL, Immanuel GY, Dollacker M, Cothren R. NHIN, RHIOs, and public health. J Public Health Manag Pract 2007;13(1):31–4. PubMed PMID: 17149097.

[15] Shapiro JS, Mostashari F, Hripcsak G, Soulakis N, Kuperman G. Using health information exchange to improve public health. Am J Public Health 2011;101(4):616–23.

[16] RTI International. ONC State Health Policy Consortium Project: health information exchange in disaster preparedness and response. Washington, DC: Office of the National Coordinator for Health Information Technology, U.S. Department of Health and Human Services; 2012 [cited January 27, 2014]. Available from: <http://www.healthit.gov/sites/default/files/pdf/SERCH-White-Paper.pdf>.

[17] Tandon S., Adhi S. Summary of public health objectives in stage 2 meaningful use ONC and CMS final rules. n.d. [cited January 27, 2014]. Available from: <http://www.cdc.gov/ehrmeaningfuluse/Docs/Summary%20of%20PH%20Objectives%20in%20Stage%202%20MU%20ONC%20and%20CMS%20Final%20Rules.pdf>.

[18] Centers for Disease Control and Prevention. 2013 National notifiable infectious conditions. 2014 [updated January 27, 2014]. Available from: <http://wwwn.cdc.gov/nndss/script/conditionlist.aspx?type=0&yr=2013>.

[19] Overhage JM, Suico J, McDonald CJ. Electronic laboratory reporting: barriers, solutions and findings. J Public Health Manag Pract 2001;7(6):60–6. PubMed PMID: 11713754.

[20] Silk BJ, Berkelman RL. A review of strategies for enhancing the completeness of notifiable disease reporting. J Public Health Manag Pract 2005;11(3):191–200. PubMed PMID: 15829831.

[21] Walker J, Pan E, Johnston D, Adler-Milstein J, Bates DW, Middleton B. The value of health care information exchange and interoperability. January 19, 2005; January–June 2005 (Suppl Web Exclusives):W5-10-W5-8.

[22] O'Connor AC, Haque SN, Layton CM, Loomis RJ, Braun FM, Amoozegar JB, et al. Impact of a two-dimensional barcode for vaccine production, clinical documentation, and public health reporting and tracking. Atlanta, GA: Centers for Disease Control and Prevention; 2012. Available from: <http://www.cdc.gov/vaccines/programs/iis/activities/downloads/2d-barcode-trkg-rpt.pdf>.

[23] Kansas Health Institute. Kansas HIE first to connect to CDC surveillance system. 2012 [cited November 21, 2012]. Available from: <http://www.khi.org/news/2012/nov/21/kansas-hie-first-nation-connect-cdc-outbreak-surve/>.

[24] Dixon BE, Gamache RE, Grannis SJ. Towards public health decision support: a systematic review of bidirectional communication approaches. J Am Med Inform Assoc 2013;20(3):577–83.

[25] Gamache R, Stevens KC, Merriwether R, Dixon BE, Grannis S. Development and assessment of a public health alert delivered through a community health information exchange. Online J Public Health Inform 2010;2(2) PubMed PMID: 23569583. Epub October 29, 2010.

[26] Mäenpää T, Asikainen P, Gissler M, Siponen K, Maass M, Saranto K, et al. Outcomes assessment of the regional health information exchange: a five-year follow-up study. Methods Inf Med 2011;50(4):308–18.

[27] Muehlenbein CE, Hoverman JR, Gruschkus SK, Forsyth M, Chen C, Lopez W, et al. Evaluation of the reliability of electronic medical record data in identifying comorbid conditions among patients with advanced non-small cell lung cancer. J Cancer Epidemiol 2011;2011:983271. PubMed PMID: 21765829. PMCID: 3134088.

[28] Western New York HEALTHeNET. Welcome to WNY HEALTHeNET. 2001 [cited January 27, 2014]. Available from: <http://www.wnyhealthenet.org/>.

[29] HEALTHeLINK. Mission. 2012 [cited January 27, 2014]. Available from: <http://wnyhealthelink.com/>.

CASESTUDY

3

Creating a 21st Century Health Information Technology Infrastructure: New York's Health Care Efficiency and Affordability Law for New Yorkers Capital Grant Program

Joshua R. Vest[1] *and Erika G. Martin*[2]

[1]Indiana University Richard M. Fairbanks School of Public Health; and the Regenstrief Institute, Inc., Indianapolis, IN [2]Nelson A. Rockefeller Institute of Government and Rockefeller College of Public Affairs and Policy, University at Albany, Albany, NY

OUTLINE

MAJOR THEMES

- Organization design of health information exchange
- Public funding
- Program evaluation
- Policy development and implementation
- Governance of health information exchange

INTRODUCTION

Health information exchange (HIE), the electronic sharing of patient information among providers, began in the United States as local activity. Starting in the 1990s, numerous collaborations of health care organizations, community organizations, and government agencies started the technical infrastructure and organizational relationships necessary to share patient information within their communities. These initiatives differed in their technology architectures, types of leading organizations and community sizes, but all focused on supporting HIE for a local community or geographically defined population [1]. These efforts had high failure rates, but throughout the decade, organizing HIE activity at the community level was the consistent approach [2]. HIE organizations serving local communities even demonstrated some ability to impact the cost of care [3,4].

In the early to mid-2000s, a small but growing number of operational local HIE organizations were serving as effective success stories [5] and the United States began formulating a national HIE strategy. The Office for the National Coordinator (ONC) for Health Information Technology's Framework for Strategic Action envisioned a "consumer centric and information-rich" health care industry, where health data follow patients and are used for medical decision making. Strategic goals included: improving the adoption and use of electronic health records in clinical practice, developing an interoperable health information technology infrastructure to connect clinicians, promoting the use of information to personalize health care, and improving public health surveillance and monitoring. The second goal, to interconnect clinicians, focused on fostering regional collaborations as the organizational mechanism for this activity [6]. The label applied to these local HIE organizations was "regional health information organizations" (RHIOs).

Organizing exchange activities around RHIOs offered several operational and political advantages over the approaches that had failed in the previous decade [1,7]. First, RHIOs were collaborative organizations with multistakeholder governance, allowing them to act as neutral third parties between competing health care organizations [8]. RHIOs were focused on quality and "improving health and care in that community" [9]. Finally, RHIOs served defined geographic areas, usually a collection of adjacent counties, a metropolitan area, or a state [1], consistent with the idea that HIE should be a locally organized and controlled activity.

The national strategy envisioned at this time was a "network of networks" [10,11]. Numerous autonomous local organizations, primarily RHIOs, would be responsible for HIE activity within their communities and subsequently connected together at a national level [12]. RHIOs were identified as the "building blocks" [13] of this network, with the federal government providing standards and guidance on technology, interoperability, and policy to facilitate HIE across RHIOs [11]. By focusing on organizations providing service locally, the United States adopted a "bottom up" approach to HIE [14].

At the same time, researchers, practitioners, and policy makers were increasingly aware of the barriers inhibiting widespread HIE. Adopting health information technology is costly (including financial costs, retraining staff, and changing clinical workflow), the quality of vendor products can be difficult to assess, and adopters face negative externalities (ie, although providers purchase technologies, the benefits mostly accrue to patients and payers) [15]. The potential benefits to patient and public health, combined with limited financial incentives, made public funding to establish and maintain a data sharing infrastructure a logical option [1,16,17]. Consequently, funding and national coordination could further support a vision of broader information exchange [6]. It is within this context that New York State launched the nation's largest (at the time) single public investment in developing a health information technology infrastructure to support HIE.

BACKGROUND: THE HEALTH CARE EFFICIENCY AND AFFORDABILITY LAW FOR NEW YORKERS CAPITAL GRANT PROGRAM

In 2004, New York State passed the Health Care Efficiency and Affordability Law for New Yorkers Capital Grant Program (HEAL NY) [18]. HEAL NY was designed to "encourage improvements in the operation and efficiency of the health care delivery system within the state" [19] and part of a broader interest by the governor's office and legislature in improving New York State's health care system [20]. Although most capital grants funded activities such as hospital conversions and debt retirement [21], 5 of the 22 phases aimed to expand the adoption and implementation of interoperable health information technology and HIE [22]. HEAL NY was jointly administered by the New York State Department of Health and the Dormitory Authority of the State of New York.

HEAL NY funds were disbursed through a series of competitive grant opportunities released in so-called "Phases"[1] (Fig. 1). In addition to funding health information technology, Phases were responsive to the hospital and nursing home reconfiguration recommendations in the Berger Commission report [21] and goals of the Federal-State Health Reform Partnership (F-SHRP) Medicaid Section 1115 waiver, which aimed to right-size the acute care system, shift long-term care to community-based settings, promote health information technology, improve the provision of ambulatory and primary care, and expand Medicaid managed care [23]. HEAL NY and F-SHRP, representing a mix of state and federal funds, were used to implement the Berger Commission's recommendations on health care restructuring across six regions and to expand health information technology. In 2006, HEAL NY Phase 1 provided $52.9 million to 26 projects. In 2008, 21 projects received $104.9 million under HEAL NY Phase 5. HEAL NY Phase 10's $99.9 million went to 11 projects in 2009. HEAL NY Phase 17 made $116.8 million in funding available to 14 projects in 2010. Finally, HEAL NY Phase 22 made $38.2 million available to 2 projects (Table 1) [24].[2] The focus and intent of each Phase differed.

Phases 1 and 5 were most directly related to establishing the state's initial HIE structure and promoting the adoption of electronic health records. These Phases funded RHIOs and supported community-wide adoption of electronic health records and other interoperable health information technologies. Phases 10 and 17 focused on health information technology for Patient Centered Medical Homes and care coordination. The last Phase (22) supported electronic health records for behavioral health (Table 2) [18].

[1] Only those Phases of HEAL NY related to health information technology are described here.

[2] In Phases 5, 10, and 17, two awards each were made to the New York eHealth Collaborative and Health Information Technology Evaluation Collaborative for evaluation and implementation; these awards are included in these counts.

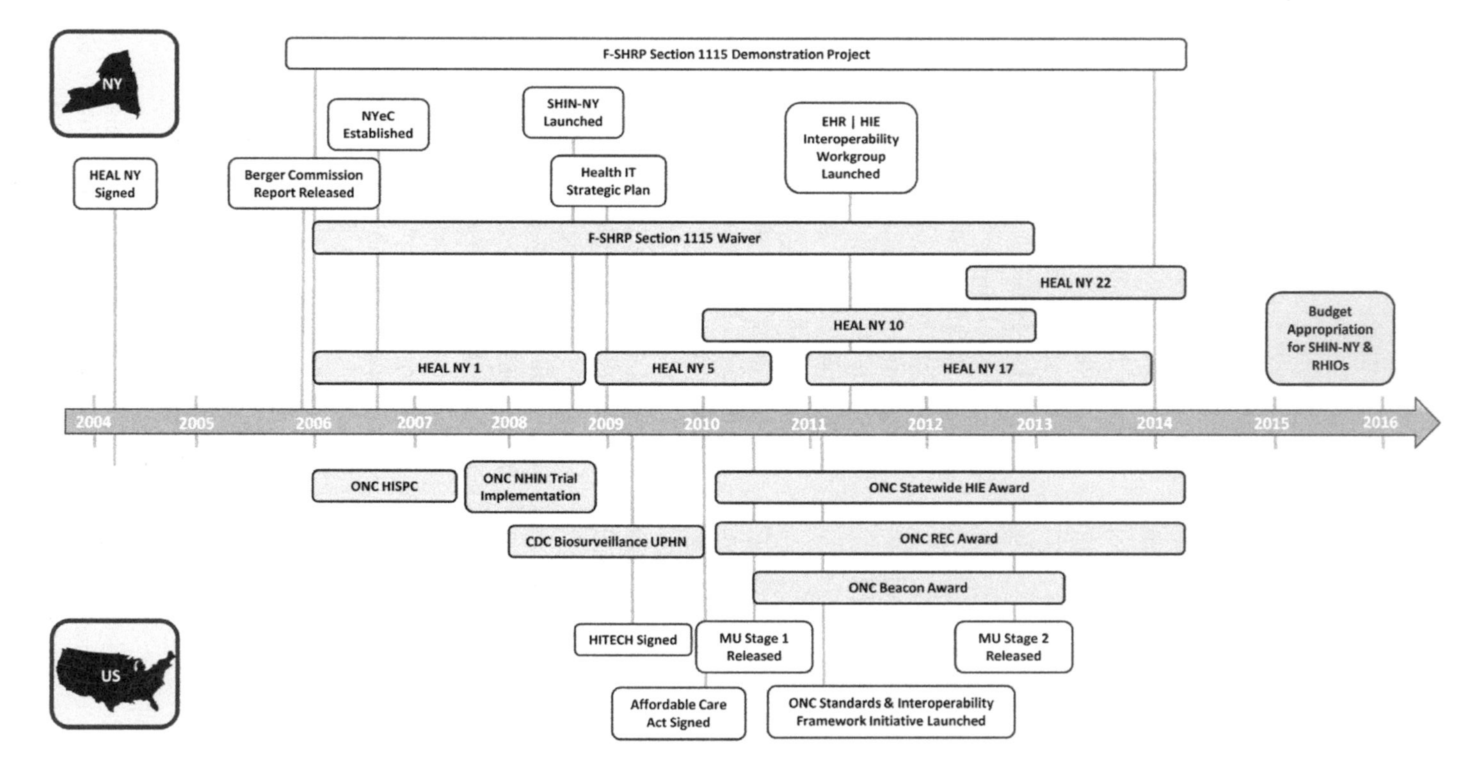

FIGURE 1 Chronology of HEAL NY Health Information Technology Grants. *Notes*: Green boxes represent funding sources, and white boxes represent policies and activities. *Abbreviations*: Electronic health records (*EHR*), Federal-State Health Reform Partnership (*F-SHRP*), Health Care Efficiency and Affordability Law for New Yorkers (*HEAL NY*), health information exchange (*HIE*), Health Information Security and Privacy Collaboration (*HISPC*), meaningful use (*MU*), Nationwide Health Information Network Exchange (*NHIN*), New York eHealth Collaborative (*NYeC*), Office of the National Coordinator for Health Information Technology (*ONC*), Regional Extension Center (*REC*), State Health Information Network of New York (*SHIN-NY*), Universal Public Health Node (*UPHN*). (For interpretation of the references to colour in this figure legend, the reader is referred to the web version of this book.) *Source: Adapted with permission from the New York State Department of Health [25].*

TABLE 1 HEAL NY Funding for Health Information Technology by Phase and Berger Commission Region

Characteristic	Awards, *N* (%)	Funding, $
Phase		
1	26 (35.1)	52,875,000
5	21 (28.4)	104,944,003
10	11 (14.9)	99,914,713
17	14 (18.9)	116,775,701
22	2 (2.7)	38,200,000
Berger Commission Region		
Central	9 (12.2)	35,311,990
Hudson Valley	7 (9.5)	31,985,788
Long Island	9 (12.2)	49,798,625
New York City	25 (33.8)	174,100,093
Northern	8 (10.8)	17,713,669
Western	11 (14.9)	61,494,205
Statewide	5 (6.8)	42,305,047
Types of health information technology		
Adoption or promotion of e-prescribing	12 (16.2)	73,070,183
Adoption or promotion of EHRs	56 (75.7)	312,453,255
Adoption of new EHRs	43 (58.1)	250,824,226
Expanded capacity of existing EHRs	33 (44.6)	184,204,077
Adoption or promotion of health information exchange	65 (87.8)	341,818,279
Adoption or promotion of consumer-mediated health information exchange	25 (33.8)	170,475,694
Evaluation	3 (4.1)	11,820,505
Implementation	3 (4.1)	51,684,542
Total, all awards	74 (100)	412,709,417

Rockefeller Institute of Government's analysis of HEAL NY grant materials [24].

TABLE 2 Categories of HEAL NY Grants for Health Information Technology, by Phase

Phase	Start Year	Application Categories
1	2006	– Creating e-prescribing capabilities – Furthering the use of EHRs – Developing community-wide clinical data sharing
5	2008	– Reference architecture and pilot implementations of the Statewide Health Information Network for New York (SHIN-NY) – Pilot implementations of Clinical Informatics Services, automated tools that aggregate, analyze, measure, and report clinical data for uses such as quality and population health reporting – Pilot implementations of community-wide interoperable EHRs
10	2010	– Implementing EHRs and facilitating HIE for patient-centered medical homes for patient populations with chronic and complex health conditions
17	2011	– Implementing EHRs and facilitating HIE for patient-centered medical homes for patient populations with chronic mental health conditions
22	2012	– Facilitating EHRs for behavioral health

Rockefeller Institute of Government's analysis of HEAL NY grant materials [24].

Although certain elements remained constant, HEAL NY was dynamic. For example, a goal of sharable patient information through interoperable health information technology was explicitly articulated in every HEAL NY Phase [15,26–28]. Additionally, under a requirement of "statewide geographic distribution of funds" [19], each HEAL NY Phase funded communities across the state, with each Berger Commission region receiving at least one award (Table 1). Importantly, RHIOs were the model of HIE organization. Even later Phases that did not provide direct funding to support RHIOs required grantees to be participants in one of the HEAL NY-funded RHIOs [15,28].

However, HEAL NY did evolve over time, with later Phases building on prior work (Table 2). Although Phase 1 had a large focus on e-prescribing and electronic health records [29], Phase 5 introduced the idea of and funding for the Statewide Health Information Network of New York (SHIN-NY), a statewide "network of networks" to connect RHIOs [30]. As Patient Centered Medical Homes were promoted through the Affordable Care Act, subsequent Phases focused on implementing electronic health records and facilitating HIE in these organizations especially among behavioral health and long-term care providers. This shift from building technology infrastructure to encouraging HIE across specific health care organizations was intended to "integrate this infrastructure with reimbursement reforms and innovative delivery reforms" [15].

CASE STUDY: THE EVOLUTION OF HEALTH INFORMATION EXCHANGE ORGANIZATIONS IN NEW YORK STATE

The landscape of HIE organizations in New York State changed dramatically over a relatively short period of time. In the summer of 2006, HEAL NY Phase 1 provided $52.9 million to 26 projects. By 2015, New York State was home to nine HIE organizations, a public–private state-wide exchange entity and a total public–private investment nearing $1 billion. New York's current state of HIE is the result of the interaction of HEAL NY with changes in state administration, changes in state and federal policy, new technology developments, sustainability needs, and organizational growth and development.

HEAL NY Phase 1 (2005–2008)

Phase 1 funded three categories of health information technology projects: HIE, e-prescribing technologies, and EHR adoption and implementation. HIE funding provided capital costs and targeted projects committed to interoperability. In contrast to the later Phases (which were more focused on HIE and promoting health information technology adoption more generally), e-prescribing received a heavy emphasis because at the time this activity had more advanced standards and clearer quality and efficiency returns [29].

There were a few additional requirements, also included in subsequent Phases. Each project required 50% matching funding (with reductions for financially distressed organizations) and applications described the financial viability and sustainability of their business models. This matching requirement was designed to ensure that applicants would be committed to the continued use of health information technology after HEAL NY grants ended [24]. Additionally, projects had to be collaborative. Grantees had to involve multiple stakeholders, at least one independent organization (ie, all organizations on the project could not be controlled by the same entity), and organizations of different types (eg, hospitals, physician groups, etc.) [26]. Lastly, all phases sought a "broad" geographic distribution of funds [31], which was accomplished by allocating funds to all six Berger Commission regions (Table 1).

The result was a very diverse set of initiatives by 26 grantees across the state (Fig. 2). New York City alone was home to nine projects. The average award was $2 million and ranged from about $175,000 up to $5 million [32]. Nearly all grantees reported supporting some type of HIE and described their activities as "regional connectivity," "community exchange," "regional information network," "clinical data exchange," or "information sharing" [32,33].

HEAL NY Phase 1 projects were led by two types of grantees: existing health care

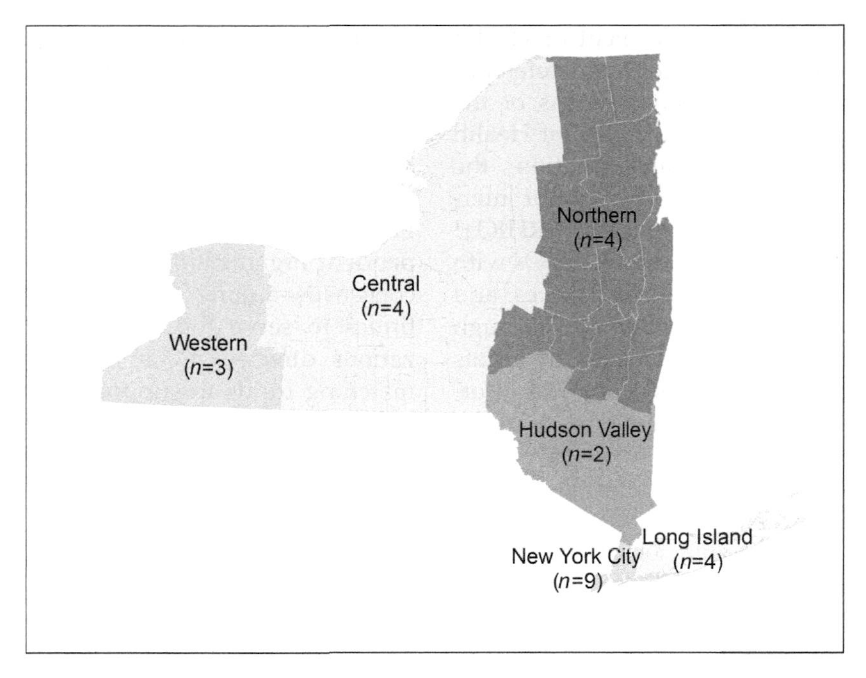

FIGURE 2 Number of HEAL NY Phase 1 Grantees per Region.

organizations and health information organizations created to facilitate HIE [33]. The health care organizations leading Phase 1 projects were hospitals, academic medical centers, health systems, and large physician practices. However, projects also included many other organizations such as physician offices, imaging centers, long-term care providers, and health plans. Eleven of the grantees had the governance structure and activities to be classified as RHIOs [22]. After 2 years all 26 grantee organizations were still in existence, but only 11 would subsequently receive funding under HEAL NY Phase 5 [33].

HEAL NY Phase 5 (2007–2010)

With HEAL NY Phase 5, New York State adopted a much more coordinated approach to health information technology policy and funding [22]. The new governor established the Office of Health Information Technology Transformation within the Department of Health to coordinate health information technology policies and programs [27]. Additionally, in line with the new administration's policy, New York State would establish a public–private partnership to develop and govern state-wide HIE rather than having the health department assume policy guidance [34,35]. Overall, the long-term goal was an health information technical infrastructure to enable state-wide information sharing and widespread EHR adoption, and support public and population health [36]. Phase 5 funding reflected this new policy direction.

HEAL NY Phase 5 articulated New York's network-of-networks approach to HIE across the entire state [27]. This Phase funded RHIOs as the foundational components for developing cross-sectional interoperability. Grants fell into three categories with corresponding use cases developed by the Department of Health (Table 1).The first grant category was reference architecture and pilot implementations of the SHIN-NY. As described by the Office of Health Information Technology Transformation, the SHIN-NY was envisioned as "the sum of interoperable regional HIEs governed by RHIOs" [37]. These grants supported the 10 RHIOs with common software protocols, core services, and standards that could later support HIE through the SHIN-NY. The second category of grants funded pilot implementations of clinical informatics services, tools to aggregate, analyze, measure, and report clinical data for quality and population health reporting. Remaining grants funded pilot implementations of community-wide interoperable electronic health records. Overall, this phase moved away from the initial focus on e-prescribing and towards the creation of RHIOs and improved penetration of electronic health records (Table 1).

At the onset New York State envisioned HIE as a local activity. "Design globally, implement locally" was a common refrain among those leading HEAL NY [15,38]. New York's conceptualization of the SHIN-NY as a network of networks reflects this all-health-care-is-local perspective and the political necessity of ensuring a statewide distribution of public funding.

RHIOs were the cornerstone of developing a state-wide HIE. To receive state funding, RHIOs had to be nonprofit (and nongovernmental), have multistakeholder governance and participation, serve a defined geographical area, have a sustainability plan, provide matching funds, agree to be interoperable, and participate in a statewide collaboration process to develop common exchange protocols, services, and standards [27]. New York allocated $60.4 million to 8 RHIOs (minimum $4.7 million and maximum $10 million) under Phase 5 as part of the SHIN-NY development [39]. All funded RHIOs had also received Phase 1 funding [22] (Fig. 3.)

To support the SHIN-NY development, Phase 5 funded the New York eHealth Collaborative (NYeC) to facilitate the statewide collaboration process [27]. NYeC was founded in 2006 as a nonprofit organization with funding and oversight from New York State (eg, a public–private partnership) focusing on policy and standards development [40]. Under Phase 5, NYeC became the designated independent organization to coordinate and obtain consensus among the RHIOs [41], and continues to serve this function. Funded organizations directed 5% of their reimbursable or matching funds to support NYeC [27]. NYeC's early activities including convening stakeholders (vendors, healthcare organizations, patients, public health departments, etc.) to formulate statewide HIE policies, including the consent policy that specified an opt-in model with exceptions for emergency access [42].

Phase 5 funded two additional entities that supported the adoption and implementation of health information technology. First, the program introduced a new type of entity called a Community Health Information Technology Adoption Collaboration (CHITA). CHITAs were less formally organized than RHIOs, typically alliances of local providers working to adopt health information technology tools. The HEAL NY Phase 5 request for grant applications describes CHITAs as "primarily responsible for achieving adoption and effective use of health IT tools, especially EHRs, by clinicians at the point of care" [27]. CHITAs purchased software licenses for quality reporting, point-to-point exchange connections, and EHR adoption [35]. With their focus on technology adoption, the eight CHITAs were in some ways a precursor to the ONC's Regional Extension Centers.

Phase 5 also developed new processes to improve effectiveness and accountability. First, the Health Information Technology Collaborative (HITEC) was formed to provide consistent statewide evaluation, which differed from the more informal final reports from Phase 1 grantees. HITEC, an academic collaborative of Cornell University, Columbia

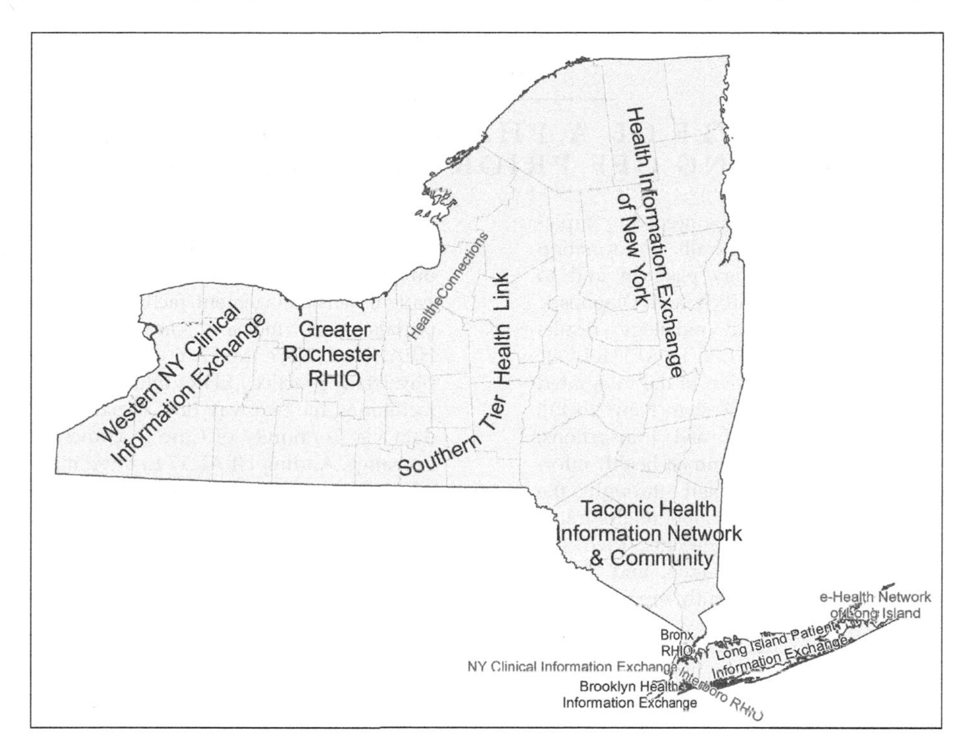

FIGURE 3 New York's Regional Health Information Organizations ca 2008–2009. *Note*: RHIOs funded under HEAL Phase 5 as part of the Statewide Health Information Network for New York are in blue. (For interpretation of the references to colour in this figure legend, the reader is referred to the web version of this book.)

University, the University of Rochester, the State University of New York at Buffalo, and the State University of New York at Albany, was tasked with establishing common measurement approaches and conducting evaluations of policy, implementation, and impact [43]. HITEC evaluated cross-cutting issues across projects such as adoption, implementation, costs, utilization, safety, and quality. All HEAL NY grantees had to cooperate with these evaluation activities [27]. Second, the HEAL NY program office developed a new pay-for-performance approach to manage grants. Staff created "GAP Tool" spreadsheets that listed all activities that grantees committed to completing in their applications, which were used to track milestones. Grantees submitted documentation or else demonstrated a technical capability in a webinar as evidence of each activity's completion. Ten percent of committed grant funds were withheld until the completion of all deliverables.

HEAL NY Phases 10, 17, and 22 (2009–2014)

Starting in Phase 10, HEAL NY grants were more targeted and followed national interest in medical homes, which received funding through the Patient Protection and Affordable Care Act. This new health care delivery system and reimbursement model promoted coordinated care for people living with chronic diseases or high-cost diagnoses. Interoperable electronic health records were requisite for providers to exchange clinical information about these patients, who often saw multiple clinicians at different health care facilities.

BOX 1

EXAMPLE OF A PHASE 17 APPLICANT BUILDING OFF PRIOR HEAL NY PHASES

HEAL 1 provided funding needed to implement HEALHeLINK's Health Information Exchange (HIE) technology platform and to execute ePrescription ("eRx") and Diagnostic Data Exchange (lab and radiology results reporting). Through HEAL 5, HEALTHeLINK is accelerating the expansion of the integrated HIE platform in WNY [(Western New York)], standardizing connections and transactions, and leveraging CHIxP [(common health information exchange protocols)] through the SHIN-NY architecture. This supports the transfer of NYS Immunization Records, Medicaid Medication History Information, and Public Health data. HEAL 10 currently supports EHR adoption to: improve chronic care management as demonstrated by improved clinical outcomes performance measures; proactive patient self-management facilitated by patient portals; and increase care coordination… HEALTHeLINK's MSSNY grant is enabling physician practice EHR interoperability by facilitating the two-way flow of patient referral data via Continuity of Care Document (CCD) exchange. Adding HEAL 17 to these initiatives, which by design build on and enhance each other, will have a significant impact on the provision of mental health care in Erie County that can be replicated throughout WNY. -- *Applicant C026926*

Whereas HEAL NY Phase 10 supported projects to develop interoperable electronic health records and promote HIE in primary care medical homes, Phase 17 specifically focused on populations with mental health conditions [28]. Phase 17 aimed to integrate mental health, long-term care, and home health providers into medical homes. There were two categories: "limited" projects that expanded patient-centered medical homes to include at least one mental health diagnosis and "expanded" projects that included at least one chronic disease associated with mental health disorders in addition to a combination of mental health, long-term care, and home health care providers [28]. Phase 22, the last HEAL NY grant, provided funding to the state's two regional extension centers to facilitate electronic health records for behavioral health, a disease area with limited use of electronic health records [44]. Because behavioral health and long-term care providers were ineligible for Meaningful Use incentives, these Phases helped address a gap in HIT adoption in New York State [45].

Overall, grants in Phases 10, 17, and 22 built off the infrastructure developed in earlier phases, "moving [emerging health IT systems] from infancy to childhood" (p. 6) [15]. Applications became more sophisticated, following the incremental adoption of health information technology across the state. As an example, one Phase 17 applicant described how the award would build on Phases 1, 5, and 10, a past federal Beacon Community Program award, and initiatives from the Medical Society for the State of New York (Box 1). Other applicants from these later phases proposed advanced capabilities for their existing electronic health records, such as quality metrics and immunization reports that could be automatically generated and transmitted to the Department of Health, incorporating Medicaid administrative data into clinical charts, and clinical decision tools ranging from pop-up reminders to sophisticated

BOX 2

EXAMPLES OF PHASE 10 APPLICANTS COORDINATING HEALTH CARE SERVICES THROUGH INTEROPERABLE ELECTRONIC HEALTH RECORDS AND HEALTH INFORMATION EXCHANGE

HeR EMR: a PCMH Model for High Risk Obstetrics Using Electronic Medical Records will improve the coordination and management of [high risk pregnancy] patients through the use of interoperable health information. Participating providers in the [care coordination zone] will implement practice-based EMRs in their offices that will connect to specialists to whom they refer their high risk patients (for example cardiologists for hypertensive pregnant women, endocrinologists for patients with pre and post gestational diabetes), pediatricians, laboratories, home care. Additionally, individual practices will be able to connect electronically to the labor and delivery units and the well-baby nurseries and neonatal intensive care units of North Shore University Hospital, Long Island Jewish Medical Center, and Schneider Children's Hospital where an EMR is currently being deployed. -- ***Applicant C025952***

Under the [Southwest Brooklyn Patient Centered Medical and Mental Health Home Project], select outpatient primary and mental health clinics...will utilize electronic health records ('EHRs') and portal access to connect to the Brooklyn Health Information Exchange ('BHIX') and the State Health Information Network of New York ('SHIN-NY') to access information about their patients from disparate sources and to communicate/coordinate with necessary caregivers along the care continuum, thereby enabling them to provide patient centered medical and mental health home services to their schizophrenic patients...Inpatient, specialty, home health, case managers, and other providers and caregivers involved in the care of the target population will also be connected to BHIX and the SHIN-NY and will be provided a secure care coordination plan template ('CCPT'), brokered through BHIX, that offers a presentation layer that aggregates relevant patient diagnostic information and recommended next steps in care, and that enables providers to add relevant documentation and orders to the plan throughout the patient's course of care...Finally, the project proposes to enable certain stakeholders to provide their patients with access to a Personal Health Record ('PHR') and to supplement the connectivity above with video-conferencing abilities to further enable the provision of truly coordinated care. -- ***Applicant C025950***

algorithms and visualizations about patients' risks for future complications. These capabilities built off the emerging HIE networks (Box 2).

New York State's Evolution during the Period of Federal Action: HITECH Act and Meaningful Use Stages 1 & 2 (2008–2014)

From the beginning, New York sought consistency with national approaches [26]. For example, HEAL NY Phase 5 envisioned the SHIN-NY as part of the federal Nationwide Health Information Network (NHIN) [27] and both state policy makers and RHIO leaders looked to follow technology standards being adopted by the federal government, when available [46]. Also, Phase 5 use cases aligned with both the ONC's and the Centers for Disease Control and Prevention's HIE use cases. However, midway through Phase 5, federal health information technology policy changed dramatically with the introduction of the Meaningful Use Program under the Health

Information Technology for Economic and Clinical Health (HITECH) Act of 2009.

The introduction of this large program had consequences for HIE activities within New York State. Immediately, the state moved to become more aligned with the Meaningful Use Program. This is most evident in the language and expectations for the HEAL NY Phases released during this period. Phases 10 and 17 required that grantees adopt certified EHRs and to ensure that health IT usage complied with the Meaningful Use Program so that the healthcare providers benefiting from the state grant program would also be eligible for incentive payments [15,28]. Also, RHIOs saw certification, the requirements for interoperability, and a stronger federal role in standard setting necessary and beneficial [46]. The Meaningful Use Program also increased the adoption of EHRs within communities, thereby creating more potential participants for the RHIOs.

Yet not all effects of the Meaningful Use Program were welcome or beneficial. For one, Meaningful Use became the top health information technology priority. For individual physicians and hospitals, resources and time were often allocated towards adopting EHRs or attestations for incentive funding, not for connections with RHIOs [47]. This did not necessarily reflect devaluation of the RHIOs, but with limited resources, achieving Meaningful Use was perceived as more important. Likewise, health information technology vendors had more financial opportunities from the federal Meaningful Use Program, making them less responsive to HEAL NY [46]. This had predictable effects on operations as RHIOs reported challenges with vendor responsiveness. More importantly, the shift in attention limited the RHIOs' ability to grow and innovate. As single entities with less funding, RHIOs reported difficulty in finding vendors willing, or able, to develop new interfaces or tools [47].

The challenges from Meaningful Use were even more pronounced with respect to the federal Direct Project and the Stage 2 criteria.[3] The Direct Project's point-to-point, single-patient approach to HIE was different than the centralized data approach taken by most New York RHIOs and the states' focus on the application of information for public health purposes [48]. In New York, RHIOs had adopted query-based exchange [35]. Direct was a challenge because, while all RHIOs eventually offered Direct services, this additional approach did not necessarily further their use of query-based exchange nor address their existing operational challenges. Importantly, the Direct Program meant that providers could meet Meaningful Use Program's expectations for interoperable patient information and HIE without participating in a RHIO [48].

In part because of Meaningful Use, this period also saw significant changes in the national thinking on the organization of HIE activities. For most of the decade, and throughout Phases 1 and 5, the US Department of Health and Human Services promoted a "network of networks" approach for HIE [49]. In 2009, that approach was abandoned [11]. RHIOs were no longer identified as the primary building blocks for national exchange activities and fewer federal resources were dedicated to RHIOs [12].

The HITECH Act also promoted increased centralization of HIE activities within New York State by funding states or their "State-designated entities" (SDEs) to "facilitate and expand the electronic movement and use of health information among organizations" [50]. To be eligible to receive federal funding, an SDE had to be named by the state, a nonprofit with collaborative governance, and focused on health information

[3] For more on the Direct Project see chapter "Standardizing and Exchanging Messages."

technology and exchange to improve care [50]. In 2009, NYeC was named as the SDE, due to its nonprofit status and existing work in facilitating collaboration among RHIOs [38].

In part to comply with the federal requirements, NYeC revised the state's Policy and Governance Structure to establish a certification process for organizations that could participate in the SHIN-NY. Organizations that met these criteria were known as "Qualified Health IT Entities" or QEs. QE requirements were very similar to the organizational and governance structure of the state's existing RHIOs, although QE membership was not restricted to RHIOs [51].

The New York HIE experience became marked by consolidation and moved towards centralization. Mergers between RHIOs were not new; two HEAL NY Phase 1 grantees merged to become a Phase 5 RHIO [9]. However, consolidation was more pronounced and focused in the downstate region. In 2011, the Manhattan-based New York Clinical Information Exchange (NYCLIX) and the Long Island Patient Information eXchange (LIPIX) merged to form Healthix. Within 2 years, the Brooklyn Health Information Exchange (BHIX) became part of Healthix, resulting in an RHIO with more than 9 million patients [52]. In 2014, Southern Tier Healthlink (STHL) and the Taconic Health Information Network and Community (THINC), Phase 5 RHIOs, formed HealthlinkNY to serve southern New York [53].

In another move toward centralization that coincided with many of the mergers, NYeC assumed responsibility for consolidating and operating core technology services for the QEs/RHIOs. To participate in the SHIN-NY network, QEs/RHIOs could either maintain their own existing technology infrastructure or else contract to use the infrastructure supplied by NYeC [51]. A total of six QEs/RHIOs signed service agreements to use NYeC's shared service platform; all of these "service QEs" were downstate. However, 2 years later in 2014, NYeC, in conjunction with the New York State Department of Health and the leaders of the "service QEs," decided to discontinue offering technology services for QEs. After this change, each QE was again responsible for contracting its own technology services, which was a slight shift from centralization.

The Current State of Health Information Exchange in New York State

By 2015, New York State was home to nine Qualified Entities (QEs), a public–private statewide exchange entity and a total public–private investment nearing $1 billion. Additionally solidifying the HIE infrastructure, the 2015–2016 state budget included $45 million for NYeC and the 9 RHIOs [54], and the New York State Department of Health proposed regulations requiring all providers using ONC-certified EHRs to connect to the SHIN-NY. Continuing support for the RHIO's role in state health objectives was further evidenced by the Delivery System Reform Incentive Payment Program Medicaid Section 1115 waiver requirements that recipient health care organizations connect to an RHIO [55]. The QEs currently offer HIE services to healthcare organizations and are largely supported by membership dues. To create sustainable business plans, QEs have also been developing "value-added" services for participating health care organizations, such as electronic master-patient index (eMPI) technologies. Together, these activities have allowed New York to have continuing HIE activity even after HEAL NY funding ended (Fig. 4). There is no RHIO-to-RHIO data exchange to date, but the SHIN-NY standards, policies, and relationships are in place to support a genuine statewide network.

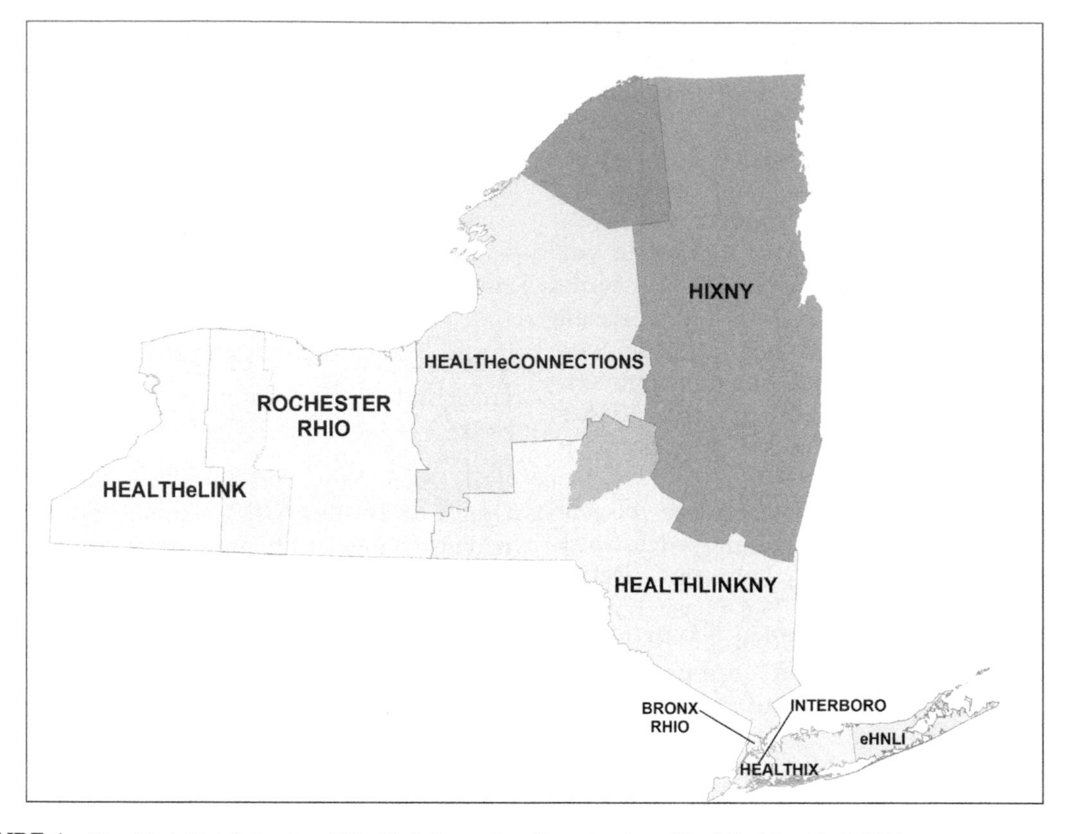

FIGURE 4 New York State's Regional Health Information Organizations (Qualified Entities), 2015.

SUMMARY

While HEAL NY's full impact will probably not be evident for several years, the program has been a successful policy intervention on numerous fronts. At a minimum, it expanded the adoption and implementation of interoperable health information technology and HIE across the state. More than 10 years later, the state is home to not only operational HIE organizations, but some of the leading HIE activities in the nation and is a Centers for Medicare & Medicaid Services innovation grantee. When the ONC began measuring national HIE activity in 2012, New York State led the adoption of query-based HIE [56] and was also a leader in directed exchange [57]. Providers who benefited from HEAL NY funding were more likely to become Meaningful Users of EHRs, compared to other New York State providers [58]. Along the way, the evaluations of grantees' adoption and implementation efforts provided important insights into the usage of health information technology [35,59,60], the integration of technology into workflows [61,62], patient perspectives on privacy and technology [63], success factors in health IT implementation [64], policy and implementation barriers to new HIE initiatives [65], the functioning of organizations in response to health information technology policy [33,46,48], and the practice of community-based research [66,67].

Substantial evidence exists to conclude that the program made significant progress towards the goal of encouraging "improvements in the operation and efficiency of the health care delivery system within the state" [19]. For example, studies of the Rochester RHIO found that HIE usage was associated with reduced hospital admissions via the emergency department, readmissions, and repeat imaging [68–70]. The public health benefits of the state's investment in health information technology included improved reporting efficiency and use of an immunization registry from EHRs [71] and that Southern Tier HealthLink provided emergency access to medical records for individuals displaced during the 2001 flood [72]. Additionally, NYeC participated in the NHIN Trial Implementations project [73].

No health policy, nor technology project, is implemented in a vacuum, and over time HEAL NY was influenced by and changed in response to internal and external developments. During the course of the HEAL NY program, New York State experienced multiple changes in executive leadership and program staff. The role of the public–private partnership increased and became formalized at the SDE. Most importantly, the federal government changed the entire industry landscape with HITECH and the Meaningful Use Program.

While the many of the experiences of New York State are similar to those had by other states and organizations working to facilitate HIE, in total New York's experience with health information technology and exchange adoption is unique. It stands alone in its cumulative scope, scale, total financial investments, public sector leadership, evolution and interaction with federal policy.

DISCUSSION QUESTIONS

1. Is the assertion "all health care is local" valid?
2. What are the strengths and weakness of a centralized versus a decentralized approach to health information exchange organization within a state?
3. What are the challenges or advantages for states on the cutting-edge of new policies?
4. Given the history of the HEAL NY program, what would you have changed, when, and why?
5. What factors contributed to the success of the HEAL NY program?
6. What should other states take away from the HEAL NY program? What lessons are applicable to the ongoing effort to develop nationwide HIE?

Acknowledgments

Thanks to Jessica Ancker, Thomas Campion Jr., and Alex Low for their comments and insights. Parts of this chapter have been adapted from *Evaluation of New York's Federal-State Health Reform Partnership (F-SHRP) Medicaid Section 1115 Demonstration* (Albany, NY: Rockefeller Institute of Government, 2015, Unpublished). Co-author E.G.M. was a coprincipal investigator on the Medicaid evaluation report.

References

[1] Vest J, Gamm LD. Health information exchange: persistant challenges & new strategies. J Am Med Inform Assoc 2010;17(3):288–94.

[2] Rubin RD. The community health information movement: where it's been, where it's going O'Carroll PW, Yasnoff WA, Ward ME, Ripp LH, Martin EL, editors. Public health informatics & information systems. New York: Springer; 2003.

[3] Overhage J, Deter P, Perkins S, Cordell W, McGoff J, McGrath R. A randomized, controlled trial of clinical information shared from another institution. Ann Emerg Med 2002;39(1):14–23.

[4] Lassila KS, Pemble KR, DuPont LA, Cheng RH. Assessing the impact of community health information networks: a multisite field study of the Wisconsin Health Information Network. Top Health Inf Manage 1997;18(2):64–76.

[5] eHealth Initiative Emerging trends and issues in Health Information Exchange: select findings from eHealth Initative Foundation's second annual survey of state, regional and community-based Health Information Exchange initatives and organizations. Washington, DC: Foundation for eHealth Initative; 2005.

[6] Brailer DJ. The decade of health information technology: delivering consumer-centric and information-rich health care. In: Services DoHaH, editor. Washington, DC; 2004.

[7] Adler-Milstein J, McAfee AP, Bates DW, Jha AK. The state of regional health information organizations: current activities and financing. Health Aff 2008;27(1):w60–9.

[8] Healthcare Information & Management Systems Society. RHIO/HIE: definitions & acronyms. Available from: <http://www.himss.org/content/files/RHIO_Definitions_Acronyms.pdf>; 2008 [cited July 3, 2008].

[9] The National Alliance for Health Information Technology. Report to the Office of the National Coordinator for Health Information Technology on Defining Key Health Information Technology Terms. Department of Health & Human Services. Available from: <http://healthit.hhs.gov/portal/server.pt?open=18&objID=848133&parentname=CommunityPage&parentid=5&mode=2&in_hi_userid=10741&cached=true>; 2008 [updated April 28, 2008; March 3, 2010].

[10] National Committee on Vital Health & Health Statistics. Functional requirements needed for the initial definition of a Nationwide Health Information Network (NHIN). Hyattsville, MD; 2006.

[11] Office of the National Coordinator for Health Information Technology (ONC), Department of Health and Human Services. Nationwide health information network: conditions for trusted exchange federal register. 2012;77(94):25843–8560.

[12] Lenert L, Sundwall D, Lenert ME. Shifts in the architecture of the Nationwide Health Information Network. J Am Med Inform Assoc 2012;19(4):498–502.

[13] Conn J, Robeznieks A. IT at center stage: HIMSS conference draws record attendees, vendors. Modern Healthcare. Available from: <http://www.modernhealthcare.com/article/20060220/MAGAZINE/602200301>; 2006 [cited February 13, 2015].

[14] Coiera E. Building a national health IT system from the middle out. J Am Med Inform Assoc 2009;16(3):271–3.

[15] New York State Department of Health and The Dormitory Authority of the State of New York. HEAL NY Phase 10—Improving Care Coordination and Management Through a Patient Centered Medical Home Model Supported by an Interoperable Health Information Infrastructure; 2009.

[16] New York eHealth Collaborative. SHIN-NY the Network of Networks: 'Better Healthcare through Technology'. Available from: <https://www.health.ny.gov/health_care/medicaid/program/medicaid_health_homes/docs/2014-10-01_hh_shiny_webinar.pdf>;2014 [November 24, 2014].

[17] Adler-Milstein J, Bates DW, Jha AK. U.S. regional health information organizations: progress and challenges. Health Aff 2009;28(2):483–92.

[18] New York State Department of Health. Health Care Efficiency and Affordability Law for New Yorkers Capital Grant Program. Available from: <https://www.health.ny.gov/technology/efficiency_and_affordability_law/>; 2010 [cited February 13, 2015].

[19] Health care efficiency and affordability law of New Yorkers (HEAL NY) capital grant program, Stat. 28 (2004).

[20] Governor George Pataki's Remarks: 2005 Budget Address. Gotham Gazette. Available from: <http://www.gothamgazette.com/index.php/economy/2678-governor-george-patakis-remarks-2005-budget-address>; 2005 [cited February 13, 2015].

[21] Commission on Health Care Facilities in the 21st Century. A plan to stabilize and strengthen New York's Health Care System: final report of the Commission on Health Care Facilities in the 21st Century. Available from: <http://www.nyhealthcarecommission.org/docs/final/commissionfinalreport.pdf>; December 2006 [June 24, 2015].

[22] Kern LM, Barron Y, Abramson EL, Patel V, Kaushal R. HEAL NY: promoting interoperable health information technology in New York State. Health Aff 2009;28(2):493–504. Epub March 12, 2009.

[23] New York State Department of Health. Federal-State Health Reform Partnership (F-SHRP). Available from: <http://www.health.ny.gov/health_care/managed_care/partner/operatio/docs/chapter_27.pdf>; [June 24, 2015].

[24] Rockefeller Institute of Government Evaluation of New York's Federal-State Health Reform Partnership (F-SHRP) Medicaid Section 1115 Demonstration. Albany, NY: Rockefeller Institute of Government; 2015.

[25] Smith S. Overview: State Health Information Network of New York (SHIN-NY). Available from: <https://www.health.ny.gov/technology/innovation_plan_initiative/docs/09-11-14_hit_wrkgrp_slides_final.pdf>; September 19, 2014 [June 24, 2015].

[26] New York State Department of Health and The Dormitory Authority of the State of New York. HEAL NY Phase 1: Health Information Technology (HIT) Grants; 2005.

[27] New York State Department of Health and The Dormitory Authority of the State of New York. HEAL NY-Phase 5 Health Information Technology Grants: Advancing Interoperability and Community-wide EHR Adoption; 2007.

[28] New York State Department of Health and The Dormitory Authority of the State of New York. HEAL NY Phase 17: Expanding Care Coordination Through the Use of Interoperable Health IT; 2010.

[29] New York State Department of Health. Request for Grant Applications. HEAL NY Phase 1: Health Information Technology (HIT) Grants. Available from: <https://www.health.ny.gov/funding/rfa/inactive/0508190240/>; 2005 [June 25, 2015].

[30] New York State Department of Health. HEAL NY—Phase 5: Health Information Technology Grants. Applicant Conference. Available from: <https://www.health.ny.gov/funding/rfa/inactive/0708160258/applicant_conference/docs/transcript.pdf>; 2007 [cited February 17, 2015].

[31] New York State Department of Health. HEAL NY hit RGA questions and answers—Set 1. Available from: <https://www.health.ny.gov/funding/rfa/inactive/0508190240/questions_and_answers.pdf>; 2005 [March 16, 2015].

[32] New York State Department of Health and The Dormitory Authority of the State of New York. Health Information Technology (Health IT) Grants—HEAL NY Phase 1. Available from: <https://www.health.ny.gov/technology/awards/>; 2006 [March 13, 2015].

[33] Kern LM, Wilcox AB, Shapiro J, Yoon-Flannery K, Abramson E, Barron Y, et al. Community-based health information technology alliances: potential predictors of early sustainability. Am J Manag Care 2011;17(4):290–5. Epub May 28, 2011.

[34] Conn J. EHR systems key to Spitzer's healthcare agenda. Modern Healthcare. Available from: <http://www.modernhealthcare.com/article/20080111/NEWS/717373599>; 2008 [cited March 23, 2015].

[35] Campion Jr. TR, Vest JR, Kern LM, Kaushal R, for the HITEC investigators. Adoption of clinical data exchange in community settings: a comparison of two approaches. AMIA Annu Symp Proc 2014;2014:359–65.

[36] New York State Department of Health. HEAL NY—Phase V Health IT Grant Program: Advancing Interoperability and Community-wide EHR Adoption. Available from: <https://www.health.ny.gov/technology/projects/docs/overview.pdf>;2008 [cited March 23, 2015].

[37] New York State Office of Health Information Technology Transformation. Technical Discussion Document: Architectural Framework for New York's Health Information Infrastructure; 2007.

[38] New York State Department of Health. State HIE Cooperative Agreement Program: Strategic Plan; 2009.

[39] New York State Department of Health. HEAL NY Phase 5—Advancing Interoperability and Community-wide EHR Adoption in New York State. Available from: <https://www.health.ny.gov/technology/projects/>; 2015 [cited March 23, 2015].

[40] New York eHealth Collaborative. About NYeC. New York eHealth Collaborative. Available from: <http://nyehealth.org/about-nyec/>; 2015 [cited March 23, 2015].

[41] Beaton BJ. Walking the Federalist Tightrope: a national policy of state experimentation for health information technology. Columbia Law Rev 2008;108(7):1670–717.

[42] Anonymous Privacy and security policies and procedures for RHIOs and their participants in New York State, v 2.2. Albany, NY: New York eHealth Collaborative and the New York State Department of Health; 2010. <http://nyehealth.org/images/files/File_Repository16/pdf/final%20pps%20v2.2%204.1.11.pdf> [accessed 02.09.12].

[43] New York State Department of Health. Health Information Technology Evaluation Collaborative (HITEC). Available from: <https://www.health.ny.gov/technology/goals_and_activities/evaluation.htm>; 2008 [cited March 23, 2015].

[44] New York State Department of Health and The Dormitory Authority of the State of New York. HEAL 22 Questions and Answers; 2012.

[45] Abramson EL, Edwards A, Silver M, Kaushai R, for the HITEC Investigators. Trending health information technology adoption among New York nursing homes. Am J Manag Care 2014;20(11 Spec No. 17):eSP53-9. Epub March 27, 2015.

[46] Vest JR, Campion TR, Kern LM, Kaushal R, for the HITEC Investigators. Public and private sector roles in health information technology policy: insights from the implementation and operation of exchange efforts in the United States. Health Policy Technol 2014;3(2):149–56.

[47] Vest J, Kash B. Differing strategies to meet information sharing needs: the publicly supported community health information exchange versus health systems' enterprise health information exchanges. The Milbank Quarterly. *In press*.

[48] Vest J, Campion Jr. TR, Kaushal R, for the HITEC Investigators. Challenges, alternatives, and paths to sustainability for health information exchange efforts. J Med Syst 2013;37(6):9987.

[49] US Department of Health & Human Services, Office of the National Coordinator. Summary of Nationwide Health Information Network (NHIN) Request for Information (RFI) Responses. Washington, DC; 2005.

[50] American Recovery and Reinvestment Act of 2009; 2009.

[51] New York eHealth Collaborative. Policy and Governance Structure; 2012.

[52] Healthix. Healthix, Inc. and the Brooklyn Health Information Exchange (BHIX)

announce their merger, effective December 1. Available from: <http://healthix.org/healthix-inc-and-the-brooklyn-health-information-exchange-bhix-announce-their-merger-effective-december-1/>; 2013 [cited March 27, 2015].

[53] healthlinkny. About us. Available from: <http://www.healthlinkny.com/about-us.asp>; 2015 [cited March 27, 2015].

[54] New York eHealth Collaborative. Final State Budget Funds Statewide Health Information Network of New York. Available from: <http://nyehealth.org/wp-content/uploads/2015/04/SHIN_NY_Budget-PR_2015_FINAL.pdf>; 2015 [cited April 3, 2015].

[55] New York State Department of Health. New York State Delivery System Reform Incentive Payment Program Project Toolkit. Available from: <http://www.health.ny.gov/health_care/medicaid/redesign/docs/dsrip_project_toolkit.pdf>; [June 25, 2015].

[56] Office of the National Coordinator for Health IT. Program Measures Dashboard: Query-Based Exchange Adoption. Available from: <http://www.healthit.gov/policy-researchers-implementers/query-based-exchange-adoption>; 2014 [cited March 27, 2015].

[57] Office of the National Coordinator for Health IT. Program Measures Dashboard: Directed Exchange Adoption. Available from: <http://www.healthit.gov/policy-researchers-implementers/directed-exchange-adoption>; 2014 [cited March 27, 2015].

[58] Jung H-Y, Unruh MA, Kaushal R, Vest JR. Growth of New York physician participation in meaningful use of electronic health records was variable, 2011–12. Health Aff 2015;34(6):1035–43.

[59] Campion Jr. TR, Vest JR, Ancker JS, Kaushal R, for the HITEC Investigators. Patient encounters and care transitions in one community supported by automated query-based health information exchange. AMIA Annu Symp Proc 2013;2013:175–84. Epub February 20, 2014.

[60] Vest J, Grinspan ZM, Kern LM, Campion Jr. TR, Kaushal R, for the HITEC Investigators. using a health information exchange system for imaging information: patterns and predictors. AMIA Annu Symp Proc 2013;2013:1402–11.

[61] Kierkegaard P, Kaushal R, Vest J. Patient information retrieval in multiple care settings: examining methods of exchange in emergency departments, primary care practices, and public health clinics? Am J Manag Care 2014;20(11 Spec No. 17):SP494–501.

[62] Kierkegaard P, Kaushal R, Vest JR. How could health information exchange better meet the needs of care practitioners? Appl Clin Inform 2014;5(4):861–77.

[63] Ancker JS, Edwards AM, Miller MC, Kaushal R. Consumer perceptions of electronic health information exchange. Am J Prev Med 2012;43(1):76–80. Epub June 19, 2012.

[64] Ancker JS, Singh MP, Thomas R, Edwards A, Snyder A, Kashyap A, et al. Predictors of success for electronic health record implementation in small physician practices. Appl Clin Inform 2013;4(1):12–24.

[65] Ancker JS, Miller M, Patel V, Kaushal R, for the HITEC Investigators. Sociotechnical challenges to developing technologies for patient access to health information exchange data. J Am Med Inform Assoc 2013.

[66] Ancker JS, Kern LM, Abramson E, Kaushal R. The Triangle Model for evaluating the effect of health information technology on healthcare quality and safety. J Am Med Inform Assoc 2012;19(1):61–5. Epub August 23, 2011.

[67] Kern LM, Ancker JS, Abramson E, Patel V, Dhopeshwarkar RV, Kaushal R. Evaluating health information technology in community-based settings: lessons learned. J Am Med Inform Assoc 2011;18(6):749–53. Epub August 3, 2011.

[68] Vest J, Kaushal R, Silver M, Hentel K, Kern L. Health information exchange and the frequency of repeat medical imaging. Am J Manag Care 2014;20(11 Spec. 17):eSP16–24.

[69] Vest J, Kern L, Campion Jr. TR, Silver M, Kaushal R, for the HITEC Investigators. Association between use of a health information exchange system and hospital admissions. Appl Clin Inform 2014;5(1):219–31.

[70] Vest JR, Kern LM, Silver MD, Kaushal R. The potential for community-based health information exchange systems to reduce hospital readmissions. J Am Med Inform Assoc 2014.

[71] Merrill J, Phillips A, Keeling J, Kaushal R, Senathirajah Y. Effects of automated immunization registry reporting via an electronic health record deployed in community practice settings. Appl Clin Inform 2013;4(2):267–75. Epub July 23, 2013.

[72] Southern Tier HealthLink. Southern Tier HealthLink Appreciation Day. Available from: <http://www.sthlny.com/news/viewarticle.asp?a=1829>; 2012 [cited April 3, 2015].

[73] Office of the National Coordinator for Health IT. NwHIN Trial Implementations. Available from: <http://www.healthit.gov/policy-researchers-implementers/nwhin-trial-implementations>; 2013 [cited July 3, 2015].

CASESTUDY

4

Use of HIEs for Value-Based Care Delivery: A Case Study of Maryland's HIE

Hadi Kharrazi[1,2], *David Horrocks*[3] *and Jonathan Weiner*[1]

[1]Johns Hopkins School of Public Health, Department of Health Policy and Management, Center for Population Health IT (CPHIT), Baltimore, MD [2]Johns Hopkins School of Medicine, Division of Health Sciences Informatics, Baltimore, MD [3]Chesapeake Regional Information System for our Patients (CRISP), Baltimore, MD

OUTLINE

INTRODUCTION

Continued growth in healthcare costs is unsustainable. Poor levels of efficiency and mixed attainment of quality indicators and patient outcomes have accelerated the adoption of value-based care among US healthcare delivery systems. The Affordable Healthcare Act (ACA) has propelled the adoption of value-based care by promoting and incentivizing new care delivery models such as so-called Accountable Care Organizations (ACOs) and

Patient-Centered Medical Homes (PCMHs). These value-based healthcare delivery models focus on the achievement of the "Triple Aim" of patient satisfaction, improved population health, and increased cost efficiency. The U.S. Centers for Medicare and Medicaid Services (CMS)-sponsored ACOs attempt to achieve this in large part through a "shared saving" model, where clinicians receive increased incentive payments when the services they provide to a target population are lower in cost and higher in quality.

ACOs, PCMHs, and other similar "integrated" delivery systems have experienced challenges in collecting and analyzing the information needed to better manage the populations they serve. This has been partly due to a lack of alignment of the Meaningful Use (MU) program with most ACO/PCMH goals. The MU program—funded by the HITECH Act and managed by CMS—has been the main driver to increase the adoption of electronic health record (EHR) systems among professionals and hospitals, but it has never been intended to provide a turnkey solution for value-based healthcare systems. Consequently, ACOs have often found themselves working closely with a diverse set of healthcare providers who do not necessarily have interoperable information with which to draw a comprehensive picture of their attributed patient populations.

Health Information Exchanges (HIEs) have the potential to fill in the population-wide informational gap for ACOs and play a pivotal role to enhance value-based care. An HIE can collect, analyze, and provide critical information from a range of information systems about patients associated with an ACO network. HIEs can also provide information about the events that ACO patients experience out of the ACO's network. Furthermore, HIEs can provide ACOs with broader population-wide health information that goes beyond the ACO providers' medical data (eg, information derived from the surrounding community). This will enable ACOs to strategically plan ahead for potential patient populations that might be attributed to them in the future.

Maryland underwent a major healthcare payment reform in 2014. The all-payer waiver program, where all public and private payers pay the same rate for inpatient and outpatient hospital services, is now extended to all Maryland hospitals, which now face a fixed cap for any annual increase in expenditures. This cap is set relative to state's gross domestic product (GDP) and, consequently, the vast majority of Maryland hospitals now operate under a value-based global budget. This global budget is adjusted based on various metrics including population health measures within the hospital's target communities, as well as inpatient quality indicators. One of the key tools being used to achieve such an ambitious value-based program in Maryland is a statewide HIE. The Maryland HIE offers a set of informational and health information technology (HIT) resources to assist the hospitals and other organizations to better manage their patient populations.

The Maryland designated HIE is known as the Chesapeake Regional Information System for our Patients, or CRISP for short. CRISP covers a diverse set of stakeholders such as hospitals, ambulatory settings, and ancillary providers. CRISP is one of the few HIEs with 100% real-time participation of all hospitals. CRISP provides a number of services that are deemed essential to the operations of the inpatient all-payer waiver program and are also quite valuable to ACOs/PCMHs and other organizations moving toward value-based models. Some of these initiatives include: real-time encounter notification of significant events; a centralized care coordination infrastructure; automated reporting of quality metrics; and population-based health risk stratification and predictive analytics.

The remainder of this chapter will discuss the role of information exchange and population health analytics support for value-based initiatives including ACOs. The role of Maryland's HIE—CRISP—will be featured within the context of Maryland's unique population-based value-based reform initiative.

VALUE-BASED CARE AND ACCOUNTABLE CARE ORGANIZATIONS

Background

US healthcare has historically been delivered based on a fee-for-service (FFS) basis [1,2]. In this model, healthcare providers are incentivized to focus on each distinct encounter, diagnosis, or procedure regardless of the broader population health implications. Most policy experts agree that the major ramification of this model has been an increasing number of clinical interventions with minimal improvement in population health. Indeed, by adopting the volume-driven FFS model, overall US healthcare expenditure has risen from $2 trillion to more than $3 trillion in less than a decade [3]. The FFS model has also spurred fragmentation in care as parties involved in the care process have few effective means to coordinate care [4]. The net effect of FFS has led the US healthcare system to become the most costly system in the world, accounting for more than 17% of the nation's current GDP with an estimated ~20% of GDP by 2020 [3].

The "Triple Aim" is a unifying framework developed by the Institute for Healthcare Improvement (IHI) that describes an approach to optimizing health system performance [5]. The three dimensions of the Triple Aim include: (1) improving the patient experience of care (including quality and satisfaction); (2) improving the health of populations (and not just patients under care); and (3) reducing the per capita cost of care [6]. Unfortunately, until recently, most of the US healthcare delivery systems and providers (other than a few Health Maintenance Organizations where payment and delivery of care are integrated) were not accountable for all three dimensions of the Triple Aim. For example, hospitals were not responsible for the overall health of their target population which would entail a focus on community determinants of health, empowering patients and their families, and an emphasis on community-based primary care. However, recent initiatives, in part promoted by the ACA, have propelled the establishment of healthcare delivery systems that are "accountable" for all dimensions of the Triple Aim. ACOs and PCMHs, as well as several dozen CMS-sponsored "innovations" such as the Maryland Waiver, are the most widely adopted emerging models of value-based delivery systems [7].

ACO Concept

ACOs are networks of providers with unified governance that assume risk for the quality and total cost of the care they deliver. ACOs may include a variety of healthcare providers from inpatient or outpatient settings. Participation in an ACO is voluntary, and the main goal is to achieve the Triple Aim. Some of the priorities of ACOs include operational tasks such as: effective care coordination of patients with chronic conditions, avoiding duplications of services, and preventing medical errors [8].

Though there are many non-Medicare ACOs as well, CMS has been the main gateway to support ACOs. CMS reimburses most ACOs through a type of pay for performance (P4P) program termed the "Medicare Shared Savings Program" (MSSP), although there are also similar ACOs termed as Advanced Payment ACO Models, and the Pioneer ACO. The MSSP model basically shares the "savings" with physicians for a target "attributed" Medicare patient population when actual cost FFS are lower than risk-adjusted predicted costs for the cohort, and when quality targets are also met [9].

There are predefined conditions that CMS uses to approve providers as an MSSP ACO [10–12]. These include:

(1) ACO providers must coordinate care for their attributed Medicare FFS beneficiaries and be accountable for quality and cost of these patients
(2) ACOs must meet or exceed a minimum cost saving rate established by CMS in order to receive shared savings payments
(3) ACO participants should include at least one provider/supplier from a specific type of delivery network
(4) ACOs must be a legal entity with an identifiable governing body, and at least 75% of the ACO's governing board must be held by ACO participants
(5) The ACO must include primary care professionals that are sufficient for the attributed Medicare population
(6) ACOs should promote evidence-based medicine, focus on patient-centeredness, have an established quality assurance program, evaluate their process regularly, coordinate care across participating providers, and promote patient engagement
(7) An ACO must have at least 5000 Medicare beneficiaries who receive the majority of their care from them
(8) ACO providers may not participate in other ACOs.

Unlike health maintenance organizations (HMOs), ACO patients are not locked into the ACO provider network and can seek care elsewhere while the ACO is still liable to achieve the overall quality metrics and financial savings. Note that other organizations, such as the National Committee for Quality Assurance (NCQA), may have different eligibility criteria to grant ACO status [13], and these criteria are often used for ACOs targeting non-Medicare patients.

The total number of registered ACOs under the CMS programs has grown from 64 in 2011 to 447 in 2013 and surpassed 744 by mid-2015. The population covered under ACOs (Medicare, Medicaid, and commercial) has also grown considerably from 2.6 million in 2011 to more than 23.5 million in mid-2015. As of 2015, ACOs exist and operate in all 50 US states, Washington, DC, and Puerto Rico. The number of ACOs correlates strongly with the underlying population of each state; hence California, Texas, and Florida have the highest number of ACOs. However, it is important to note that on a smaller geographical scale there are still regions where there is negligible ACO activity. Besides CMS, commercial payers also contract with ACOs and their numbers have also raised over time from 44 payers in 2011 to 132 payers in 2015 [14].

Value-Based Metrics

Tracking the quality of care provided by ACOs is critical to ensure that quality is not compromised while achieving reduced cost. CMS, NCQA, National Quality Forum (NQF), and other organizations that promote quality measures have published their set of metrics to track the performance and outcomes of ACOs in achieving value-based care. CMS measures for ACOs include a number of quality metrics that cover various domains such as patient and caregiver experience, care coordination, patient safety, preventative health, and at-risk populations of certain chronic conditions [15]. CMS envisions that in the near future the ACO metrics, which currently focus on performance and outcome attributes, will be further refined by comprehensive population health measures [16]. This is partly due to the fact that population health metrics are the most appropriate approach to evaluate the population health dimension of the Triple Aim [17].

Role of Population Health

Population health is a major but yet ambiguous target of value-based care [18]. As discussed earlier, value-based care intends to address each of the three Triple Aim dimensions including the one that emphasizes the improvement of population health. This aim, however, has not been well defined in the past mainly due to the ambiguity of what exactly population health is, what outcomes should be measured, and what interventions are available to improve it [19]. Despite efforts to identify various aspects of population health and to standardize related concepts and terminologies [20], the theoretical and operational complexities of population health have led to lack of clarity associated with its application within the value-based care context. Some challenges have included: unclear definition of the theoretical population "denominator"; complex population attribution algorithms; lack of standardization of population-focused metrics, outcomes, and timelines; and the overlapping population health goals of value-based medical providers, public health and social services government agencies [21]. Perhaps the main distinction between traditional public health and population health relies on two factors: (1) population health is less directly tied to governmental public health agencies and (2) population health requires the involvement of the healthcare delivery system, thus making it relevant to value-based operations of ACOs/PCMH [17,22].

Population-focused "care management" is a subset of broader population health activities and it is essential to the long-term operations of value-based delivery systems. Population healthcare management is an organized, data-supported approach that emphasizes the achievement of health outcomes of individuals in a group, while assessing the distribution of outcomes across the target cohort [23]. Population health management is also critical for ACOs to effectively manage the care of a defined patient population across the continuum of care [24]. Currently the main users of population health management programs are large integrated delivery systems or advanced health maintenance organizations, such as Kaiser Permanente and the Veterans Health Administration, which have robust, centralized HIT infrastructures. Most of the emerging ACOs, however, often do not have such advanced HIT infrastructure to support the case finding and monitoring essential for such an intervention. This lack of HIT infrastructure will likely be a major challenge that new ACOs will face. Specifically without adequate HIT support, there will be challenges for ACOs to achieve: adequate risk stratification and case identification, effective cross-provider care coordination, efficient care management across the population cohort (and not just focusing on presenting patients), impactful patient and caregiver empowerment (eg, by sharing information), and meaningful community engagement (eg, to identify community needs).

ACO's Information Technology Needs

As discussed earlier, the ACA has incentivized healthcare providers to achieve value-based care. However, existing HIT policies, such as the "Meaningful Use" (MU) incentive program from CMS, have not been fully aligned with value-based care. For example, MU criteria, the metrics that establish whether or not an eligible hospital or provider receives an incentive payment for using EHRs, have not for the most part emphasized population health—a cornerstone of an ACO concept. So even though MU has resulted in the wide adoption of EHR systems among eligible hospitals and professionals, more work is needed in support of ACOs who need to address essential HIT challenges.

To operationalize population health, value-based providers need to perform a wide range of information management activities including: capturing population-wide health and medical information; linking, analyzing, and sharing patient-level information among participating providers; integrating nonclinical and clinical information; aggregating population-level data; measuring population health performance from multiple data sources and analyzing the outcomes from different perspectives; delivering actionable information to the population health management team as well as to the clinicians at the point of care; interacting effectively with the population (patients, caregivers, and the larger community); and using the generated knowledge to effectively change practice patterns when needed. These data related activities are all essential for ACOs to become a population-oriented healthcare system [25].

To address these and other related information support challenges for ACOs, HIT action items can include: (1) interoperability of the diverse set of HIT systems across all key ACO units; (2) consensus on the definition of population denominators and its extraction from local datasets; (3) reliability and validity of population health metrics that go beyond medical performance and outcome quality measures; (4) certified analytical tools that can provide in-depth risk stratification and "predictive modeling" of the covered population; (5) adoption of HIT solutions within the operational workflows of other non-ACO providers; and ultimately, (6) the integration of population health findings as part of the broader learning health system seeking to gain evidence on what care is linked to increase effectiveness and efficiency.

Current US HIT standards and incentives at-large do not always align with ACO mandates to use information to improve population health. For example, measuring and improving the quality of care provided to the covered population of an ACO requires the interoperability of HIT systems across all ACO units, not just a single hospital or physician practice. The interoperability challenges include both the effective integration of data generated or needed by ACO services across the continuum of care (eg, care coordination across various ACO units) and the effective exchange of data between ACO and other healthcare stakeholders (eg, sharing ACO data with out-of-ACO entities). As depicted in Fig. 1, a variety of HIT systems are used to manage patients within an ACO including information from organizations external to the ACO that can affect the health of those patients (eg, payers, public health departments). These challenges have prevented many ACOs from managing their patients effectively due to their incomplete population health data and unreliable analytics [26].

Multiple drivers associated with value-based models of care are now offering incentives and facilitators in support of population HIT solutions, thereby focusing attention and resources on the types of population health enhancing systems outlines above. Some of these drivers include: the consolidation of data exchange standards (eg, S&I Framework [27]) and their increased adoption by the vendor community (eg, HL7 FHIR [28]); supporting new interoperability initiatives for HIEs to connect disparate health data sources (eg, ONC's funding for HIE interoperability [29,30]); and advancements in the utilization and integration of multiple data sources for population health analytics on a community-wide level [30,31].

Potential Role of HIEs for ACOs

HIE organizations can and should play a central role in supporting the population health IT operations of ACOs and other related value-based care systems [32]. HIEs can support the operations of ACOs by connecting entities that use disparate clinical IT systems by providing some level of interoperability to help enable patient-centered and population-based care. More specifically, HIEs can support key population health domains such as streamlining patient-centered care coordination efforts among noninteroperable providers; providing population-level clinical decision support; identifying and reporting at-risk populations; spotting patient safety issues and tracking quality

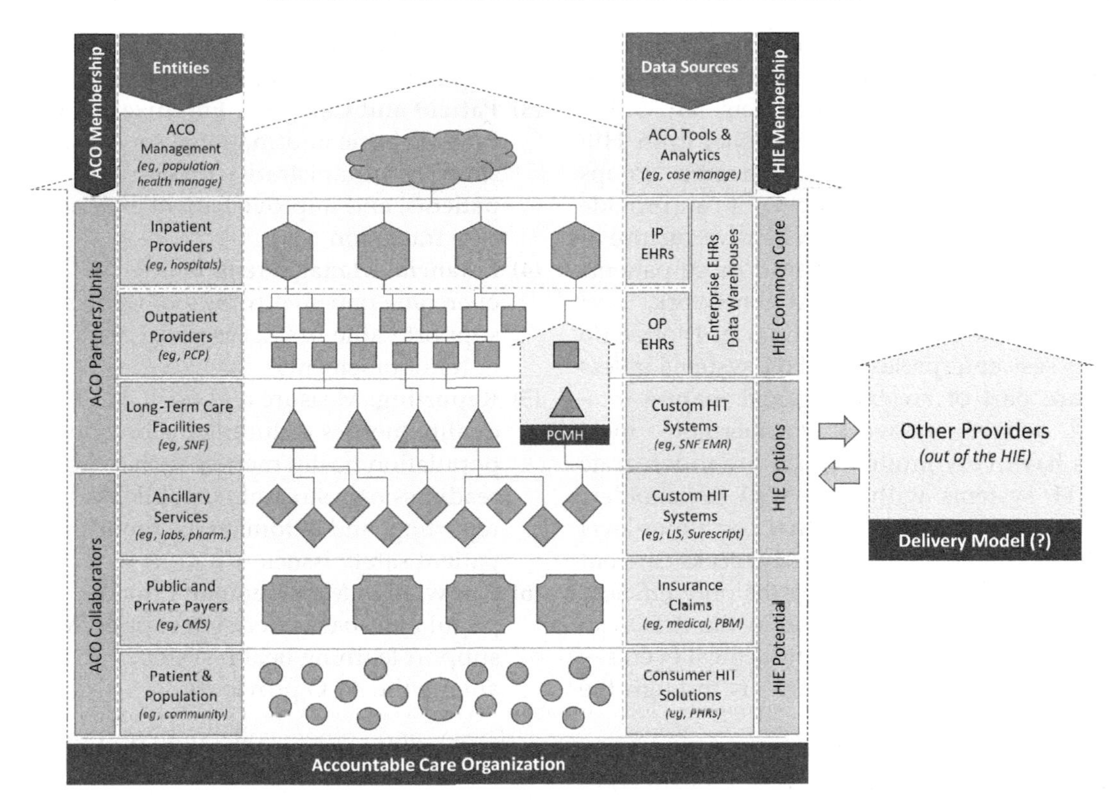

FIGURE 1 Diversity of health IT solutions among various healthcare providers operating under an ACO umbrella. Note that the HIE can be a viable solution for integrating the common core members; however, other stakeholders often lack the operational incentives and technical interoperability capabilities to integrate with the broader ACO. *ACO*, Accountable Care Organization; *CMS*, Centers for Medicare and Medicaid Services; *EHR*, Electronic Health Record; *EMR*, Electronic Medical Record; *HIE*, Health Information Exchange; *HIT*, Health Information Technology; *IP*, Inpatient; *LIS*, Laboratory Information System; *OP*, Outpatient; *PBM*, Prescription Benefit Management [System]; *PCMH*, Patient-Centered Medical Home; *PCP*, Primary Care Physician; *PHR*, Personal Health Record; *SNF*, Skilled Nursing Facility.

measures in real time; and informing and empowering patients/caregivers to be more involved with their own care [33]. Collectively, these HIE-derived IT capabilities can positively impact the measures that CMS and NCQA have adopted to evaluate ACO performance and outcomes.

HIE organizations have the potential to interconnect different entities that comprise an ACO. These entities will vary depending on the breadth and depth of the HIE and the ACO's existing stakeholders/members (Fig. 1) [34]. Hypothetically different groups of HIE stakeholders may include: (1) Common Core Members: include stakeholders from inpatient and outpatient settings such as hospitals, clinics, and primary care practices; (2) Optional Members: include long-term care facilities (eg, nursing homes and skilled nursing facilities) and ancillary providers (eg, diagnostic labs); and (3) Potential Members: include infrequent stakeholders such as payers, community-wide systems, public health departments, and patients/caregivers.

If an HIE includes a wide scope of member types and numbers, it will increase the likelihood that the HIE would be able to offer cross-provider services for an ACO entity if most of the component providers fall within the HIE's boundaries. For example, if an HIE integrates optional or potential member groups in addition to its core members, it can provide an ACO with a more comprehensive picture of its attributed population even if those patients have sought care out of the ACO network.

The core ACO entities/units (Fig. 1) often do not possess enterprise-level HIT systems unless they are part of an existing and mature integrated delivery network. Furthermore, most ACOs have very limited capability to integrate their IT systems with non-ACO stakeholders such as payers and individual consumer-level systems. For example, if a patient seeks care out of an ACO network, perhaps the only efficient approach that a provider within the ACO can access the patient's significant medical events—which has occurred elsewhere—is through the HIE services.

The HIE is central to ACOs in achieving the necessary degree of patient-centered care coordination; however, this requires the active participation of ACO members. Indeed, the ACO entities should not only provide the option of using the HIE infrastructure to obtain data to advance their population health management initiatives but they could also tightly integrate the HIE within their day-to-day population health management workflow (eg, case management, disease management, quality reporting).

Some of the key services that HIEs can provide to an ACO in this regard include [33]:

(1) **Care Coordination**: Share clinical data during transitions of care, identify social and community support, support the referral process, and improve clinical information reconciliation
(2) **Cohort Management**: Identify cohorts within the ACO patient population, monitor subpopulations for certain significant health events or quality metrics, and provide population-wide decision support
(3) **Patient and Caregiver Empowerment**: Provide basic informational services, simplify administrative processes for patients, and improve patient experience of care transition
(4) **Financial Management**: Enable ACOs to overcome patient attribution hurdles and support value-based case-mixed adjustment of reimbursements
(5) **Reporting**: Measure and track ACO quality metrics including the broader population health metrics such as hospital readmissions, streamline public health reporting, and automate the reporting of patient safety issues
(6) **Knowledge Management**: Provide population-based decision support and support learning health system initiatives among the ACO providers.

These and other collaborative opportunities of HIEs and ACOs are discussed in further technical detail within the context of Maryland's CRISP HIE.

ROLE OF MARYLAND'S HIE IN VALUE-BASED CARE

Background

The "Chesapeake Regional Information System for Our Patients," or CRISP, is a regional, community-based HIE serving Maryland and the District of Columbia. CRISP is a not-for-profit organization advised by a wide range of stakeholders who are responsible for healthcare throughout the region. CRISP has been formally designated as Maryland's statewide HIE by the Maryland Health Care Commission (MHCC) [35]. CRISP has also been named Maryland's Regional Extension Center for Health IT (REC) by the Office of the National Coordinator for HIT (ONC), with an objective of assisting 1000 primary care providers to deploy EHR systems and achieve meaningful use [36].

Mission and History

CRISP was chartered to improve health and wellness through HIT initiatives which are best pursued cooperatively. The mission of the organization is to enable and support the healthcare community of Maryland and the region to appropriately and securely share data in order to facilitate care, reduce costs, and improve health outcomes [37]. CRISP has achieved a great deal of its original mission since its inception. In 2009, shortly after being designated as the statewide HIE, CRISP implemented its cooperative governance model. In 2010, CRISP started the interconnectivity of hospitals, creating a statewide master patient index (MPI) and implementing a query portal for providers to retrieve past clinical events. By late 2011, CRISP was connected to every hospital in Maryland and focused on increasing its utilization among providers. In 2012, CRISP turned on the encounter notification system (ENS) which notifies providers about significant patient events for enrolled patient populations [38]. By 2013, CRISP achieved financial sustainability of HIE operations, no longer relying on the initial grant/seed funding, and turned its attention to connecting providers in the District of Columbia. In 2014, CRISP started offering population health IT services in addition to providing real-time reports (eg, hospital readmission reports) and hosting Maryland's statewide prescription drug monitoring program (PDMP) [39].

Types and Number of Stakeholders

As of 2015, CRISP serves all 47 Maryland acute care hospitals, 6 of the 8 DC hospitals, more than 40 long-term care facilities, 15 radiology centers, the national nonhospital labs, and 2 emergency medical facilities [40]. CRISP shares encounter information among all of its entities; however, inpatient lab, radiology, continuity of care document, and ENS (admission and disposition) data varies among hospitals. In June 2015, CRISP reached 6800+ active users, 111k+ queries per month by clinicians at the point of care, and almost 600k monthly notifications sent through the ENS system to more than 400 subscribed entities.

Governance

CRISP strives to build only services which are best pursued through cooperation and collaboration. This has led to operational sustainability of CRISP. In coordination with the MHCC, CRISP has developed a governance model that includes a Board of Advisors to provide guidance and input to the CRISP Board of Directors on certain key decisions during the development of services and operation of the HIE [41]. The Board of Advisors is intended to be broad based to ensure that a breadth of interested organizations have the opportunity to participate and represent their constituencies. There are currently over 30 organizations represented by 65 individual members in CRISP's several Advisory Board committees [42].

Patient Privacy policies are foundational to HIEs. CRISP operates under a combination of: Federal laws (eg, HIPAA and 42 CFR Part 2 [43]); State laws and regulations (eg, MHCC regulations); Stakeholder agreements (eg, Participation Agreement); and specific data use agreements with various State-based agencies. All participating organizations in CRISP HIE are required to (1) update their HIPAA Notice of Privacy Practices to include a paragraph on their participation with CRISP and (2) make CRISP informational brochures and opt-out forms available at intake areas. CRISP operates an opt-out model meaning that patients have the right to block electronic access to their information through CRISP. If a patient opts out, no information will be available through the portal (other than PDMP records, which by statute continue to be available to prescribers and dispensers). Notifications about hospitalizations for opt-out patients will also be blocked, even if a provider has requested them. To drop out, patients must contact CRISP by phone, by online, or by mail.

Information Flow and Architecture

CRISP uses a federated and harmonized information architecture. Mirth's open-source interface engine is used as the underlying data connector [44]. CRISP's MPI engine is built on top of IBM Initiate[1] and uses a variety of patient data for matching purposes [45]. As depicted in Fig. 2, CRISP delivers three major services to its stakeholders:

(1) Query Portal: The query portal allows credentialed users to search the HIE for clinical data. Users can search for patients using last name, date of birth or the medical record number of their practice or a hospital. The initial query returns information from the past 6 months but the user can query data as far back as 2012 or earlier. While a valuable tool, there are workflow challenges, primarily with the time required to manually check the portal. Over 100k queries are made per month, but this represent only a fraction of the total medical encounters in which a query might be helpful. The following types of data are available through the portal: patient demographics, lab results, radiology reports, PDMP and other prescription data, discharge summaries, history and physicals, operative notes, and consults.

(2) Encounter Notification System (ENS): CRISP receives information pertaining

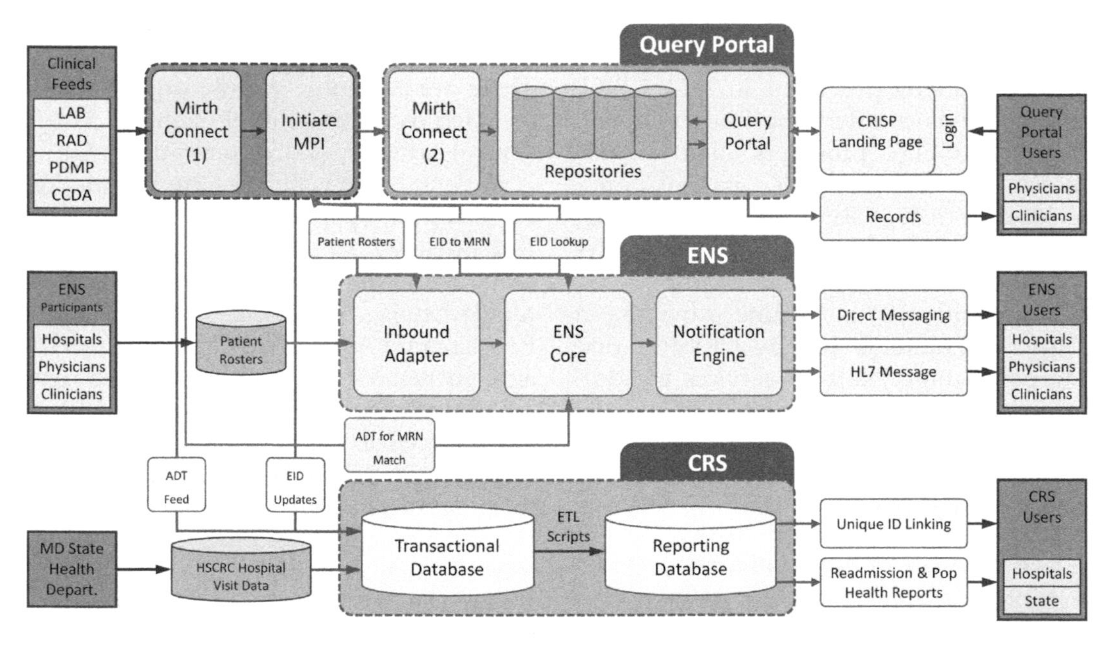

FIGURE 2 CRISP's technical and information architecture for its three major services. *ADT*, Admission Discharge and Transfer; *CCDA*, Consolidated Clinical Document Architecture; *CRS*, CRISP Reporting System; *EID*, Enterprise Identifier; *ENS*, Encounter Notification System; *ETL*, Extract Transform and Load; *HL7*, Health Level 7; *HSCRC*, [Maryland] Health Services Cost Review Commission; *MPI*, Master Patient Index; *MRN*, Medical Record Number; *PDMP*, Prescription Drug Monitoring Program; *Pop*, Population; *RAD*, Radiology.

to ER visits and inpatient admissions or discharges in real time from all Maryland and most DC hospitals. Through ENS, CRISP has the ability to communicate this information in the form of real-time hospitalization alerts to primary care physicians, care coordinators, and others responsible for patient care. As of 2015, CRISP routes roughly 20,000 notifications per day. Full continuity of care documents are also routed through ENS to support transitions of care (including supporting hospitals in meeting stage 2 MU measures). Hospitals can also "auto-subscribe" to receive various reports based on certain patient events. Once the sign up is complete, any time CRISP receives admission, discharge, transfer (ADT) messages for patients on a patient panel, physicians and care coordinators automatically receive an electronic notification. Recipients can receive notifications as read-only PDF attachments in electronic inboxes (like secure email), or merged directly into their EHR systems as HL7 messages. CRISP uses the Direct Project[1] protocol to securely transport the notifications [46,47].

(3) **CRISP Reporting System (CRS)**: The CRS enables linking of healthcare datasets in support of population health reporting and performs statewide health information analytics and reporting. A key element of the infrastructure is the region-wide MPI, used to combine information at a patient level. Furthermore, CRS has evolved in the last 2 years to support a variety of users ranging from hospitals to state policy makers who need more in-depth analysis of health data for the state of Maryland. The reporting system includes a temporary reporting database that updates routinely. This database is used for analysis and generating reports such as 30-day hospital readmission reports, inpatient and ER utilization reports, and other population health reports. In light of Maryland's new Medicare waiver, which targets controlling costs while improving quality, reducing readmissions, and decreasing the number of unnecessary hospitalization that can be better and more cost-effectively treated in an outpatient setting, regular reporting from CRS on hospital performance has become especially important. In 2014, CRS began providing monthly reports via a secure web portal. In late 2015, an enhanced portal that provides more interactive and sophisticated analysis was launched by CRISP. The scope of CRS has expanded substantially over time by incorporating data from more sources, such as detailed visit information submitted by hospitals for rate setting purposes. CRS is uniquely innovative given the depth and breadth of data available to the solution. Moreover, CRS combines data from different sources to allow the analysis of clinical and financial data by demographic groups and geographic regions and to provide more insight into overall healthcare utilization and population health management in Maryland [48].

Maryland All-Payer Waiver Program and CRISP

The state of Maryland has recently extended a longstanding CMS Medicare waiver for all of its hospitals, authorizing its Health Services Cost Review Commission (HSCRC) to manage hospital rates for all-payers, while maintaining an annual rate growth cap [49]. Through the efforts of HSCRC, currently all of Maryland's hospitals are operating under a global budget—fixed annual revenue based on the population served, rather than the volume of services. Therefore population health is considered a key, if not the only, approach for Maryland's hospitals to improve financial performance.

However, Maryland's hospitals will be challenged to achieve the mandated quality goals without the underlying HIT and analytical tools to provide them with a complete picture of their attributed populations [50]. This challenge is mainly due to the fact that these hospitals cannot track their patient population across multiple providers and payers. To overcome these challenges, the HSCRC recognized the important role of HIT and particularly population health IT solutions, and has decided to invest resources to expand the statewide HIT infrastructure by (1) developing new population health measures based on existing data captured across various HIT systems; (2) increasing the role of CRISP to capture the data necessary to measure the population health metrics; and (3) utilizing various statewide HIT systems, including CRISP, to provide hospitals with a high-level statewide care coordination platform [51].

CRISP's Population Health IT Services

CRISP offers a range of population HIT services, and it is planning to add more services due to the underlying need created by Maryland's unique waiver program. Fig. 3

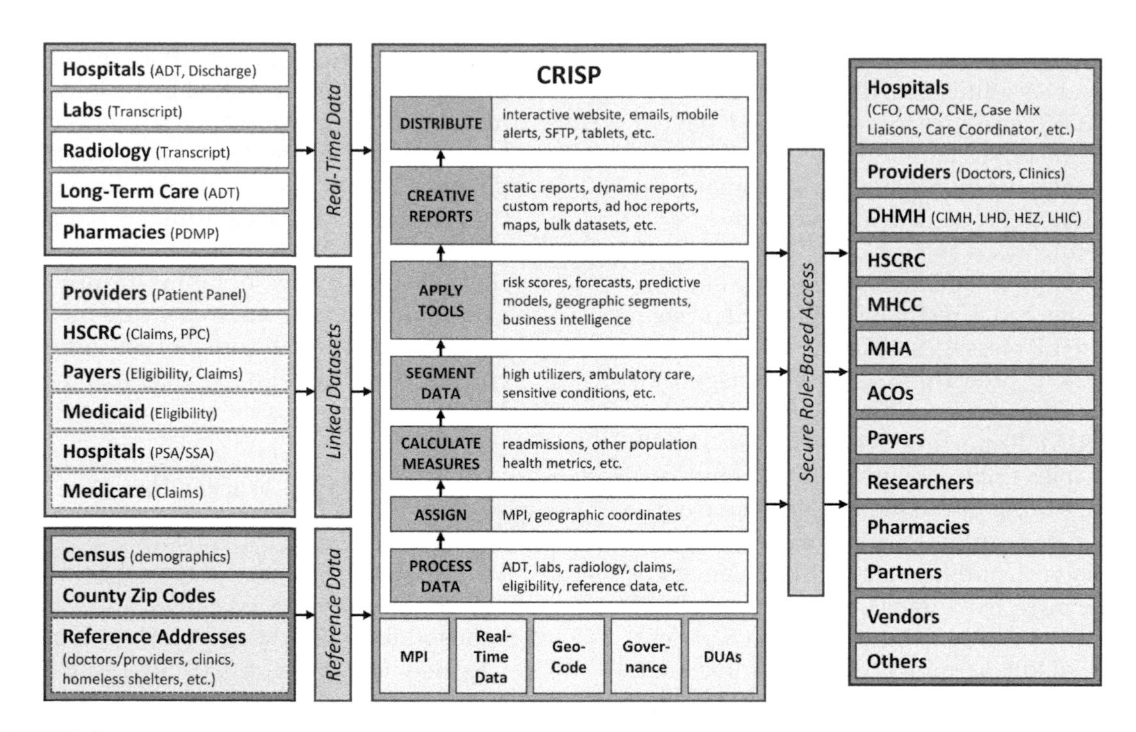

FIGURE 3 CRISP's population health IT services framework. *ACO*, Accountable Care Organization; *ADT*, Admission, Discharge, and Transfer; *CFO*, Chief Financial Officer; *CIMH*, [DHMH] Community Integrated Medical Home; *CMO*, Chief Medical Officer; *CNE*, Chief Nursing Executive; *DHMH*, [Maryland] Department of Health and Mental Hygiene; *DUA*, Data Use Agreement; *HEZ*, [DHMH] Health Enterprise Zones; *HSCRC*, [Maryland] Health Services Cost Review Commission; *LHD*, [DHMH] Local Health Department; *LHIC*, [DHMH] Local Health Improvement Coalition; *MHA*, Maryland Hospital Association; *MHCC*, Maryland Health Care Commission; *MPI*, Master Patient Index; *PDMP*, Prescription Drug Monitoring Program; *PPC*, Potentially Preventable Complications; *PSA*, Professional Services Agreements; *SFTP*, Secure File Transfer Protocol; *SSA*, Social Security Act (Medicare and Medicaid).

depicts a framework that lists the current and potential data sources (left), the population health analytic platform (middle), and a number of stakeholders that would use these population HIT services (right).

The main sources of data for CRISP's population health framework are:

(1) **Real-Time Data**: This group of data includes the common core of information that CRISP receives from hospitals, labs, radiology centers, long-term care facilities, and pharmacies. These data sources already exist in CRISP. Note that message types differ across the data sources (eg, hospitals send ADT data while labs send transcripts).
(2) **Linked Datasets**: These datasets include panels of patients that outpatient providers add voluntarily, HSCRC's hospital case-mix data (structured like claims data), MHCC's all-payer claims database, Medicaid and Medicare datasets, and other sources of data. These datasets include delayed (sometimes by a couple of months) information that will be linked to CRISP's population health core. Note that CRISP has already indexed some of these datasets (eg, MHCC and HSCRC datasets) with CRISP's MPI in order to operationalize the linkages.
(3) **Reference Data**: In order to expand population health data to include the determinants of health (eg, social and environmental factors), CRISP has linked census and zip-level geodata with the core population-level data collected from MHCC and HSCRC. The linkage of the reference datasets is mainly based on geotriangulation methods [52,53] but actual latitude and longitude distance matching is also planned.

CRISP's population HIT platform includes the following core processes: ingesting the data, assigning MPIs, calculate value-based measures, segmenting data into relevant categories, applying analytical tools, creating targeted reports, and distributing the reports to stakeholders within an ACO. Depending on the population health goals, CRISP's platform will generate relevant reports/alerts. For example, if the goal of the services fed by the platform is to risk stratify a subpopulation, all steps from processing the data to distributing the results should be targeted accordingly. In this case, relevant data for risk stratification (eg, ADT, claims, hospitals discharges) will be segmented into relevant fields for risk stratification (eg, diagnosis, medications, procedures, utilization, and cost). Then a risk adjustment tool (eg, Johns Hopkins ACG [54]) will be used to group the population into risk categories and assign them with risk scores. Finally, these scores can be used to generate reports, including geoadjusted maps, which can be shared with relevant parties such as providers operating under an ACO umbrella. The reports may vary in their timeliness from real-time hospital readmission reports/alerts to monthly inpatient utilization maps.

CRISP communicates the population health results with a number of healthcare stakeholders in Maryland. Hospitals, mainly due to Maryland's all-payer waiver program, are deeply engaged with CRISP and HSCRC to improve their population health outcomes. Other providers, especially if part of a larger ACO or PCMH system, also receive vital population health information from CRISP. Naturally, state agencies such as the Department of Health and Mental Hygiene (DHMH), HSCRC, and MHCC are also heavily invested to learn from the statewide population health results in order to adjust various statewide programs including the reimbursement of case-mixed plans under the waiver program. The following are a select number of population health services that CRISP is offering or is planning to offer in the near term to its stakeholders:

Hospital Readmission Reporting and Prediction

Maryland's readmission rates are high compared to the nation. Indeed, based on a 2013 CMS report, the majority of Maryland hospitals were ranked below the national average for Medicare's Hospital Readmission indicators, and many were in the lowest 25% [55]. The all-payer program establishes a readmission reduction target that requires Maryland Medicare rates to be equal or below national Medicare rates by 2018 [56].

Historically, CRISP's readmission reports have relied on basic interhospital readmission logic using ADT data. This allowed hospitals an early view of interhospital readmissions. Currently CRISP is aligning the readmission logic based on HSCRC's definitions and limitations set by Maryland's all-payer waiver program. Under this realignment, CRISP will offer several reports of Intra-Hospital and Inter-Hospital readmissions to help track performance on: monthly trends with Medicare FFS; statewide comparisons by clinical service line; and monthly patient-level drill down [57]. This is made possible as each month the CRISP MPI is linked to the inpatient and outpatient case-mix data enabling HSCRC to run the CMS readmission logic and to perform other interhospital analysis. CRISP and the Johns Hopkins Bloomberg School of Public Health are also funded by AHRQ to collaborate on the development of a real-time interhospital readmission prediction model that could be used to notify providers, specifically primary care physicians, of patients with high risk of readmission at the time of discharge [58].

CRISP's readmission analysis reports include: (1) monthly reports with patient drill downs; (2) year-to-year and monthly differentials; (3) comparison by hospital, zip, region, county, census block, and health enterprise zones [59]; and (4) grouping by diagnosis or disposition [60]. CRISP is also planning to provide a near real-time county readmission map for HSCRC and MHCC administrations.

Population Health Management Services

CRISP provides a series of case management and care coordination services. The general strategy of CRISP has been to: (1) identify high utilizer and high-risk Medicare patients (~40k beneficiaries) through a combination of case-mix and Medicare data; (2) use a methodology to associate these patients to hospitals (eg, hospital case-mix data) and to primary care practices (eg, Medicare data and CRISP's ENS panels); (3) engage hospitals to provide care management for their associated patients, either at a local level, through regional cooperatives, or through a statewide care management program; (4) engage ambulatory clinicians in the care management process; (5) ask clinicians who care for one of the 40k beneficiaries to create a sharable care profile or care plan; and (6) plan for future interventions to benefit a broader group of Medicare patients (~200k beneficiaries) [61].

To achieve care management services, CRISP covers the following service categories: (1) statewide reporting services; (2) point of care decision support; (3) case management interfaces; and (4) patient engagement initiatives. Currently CRISP offers a cadre of services for statewide reporting and point of care decision support, and is actively developing case management interfaces; however, CRISP's role in patient engagement such as patient portals has been limited to a few pilot studies [62].

A number of broader population health reports are also utilized by HSCRC, MHCC, and DHMH for statewide health planning. For example, CRISP generates monthly high utilization analysis reports that are categorized by the following: (1) number of visits, length of stay, and date; (2) census tract or neighborhood; and (3) diagnosis, disposition, or charges. See Fig. 4 for an interactive dashboard that is used by state administration to plan accordingly depending on various utilization plans such as ER services.

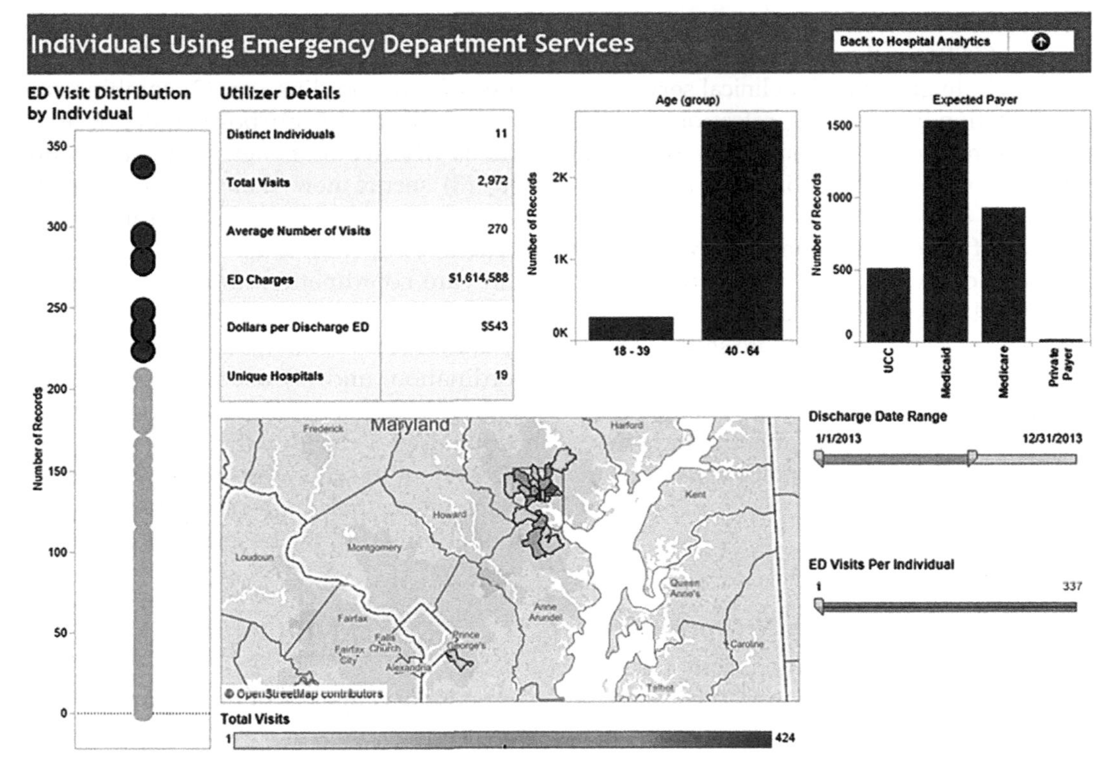

FIGURE 4 CRISP's utilization analysis dashboard.

Other Ongoing or Planned Population Health Services

CRISP has developed the capability to generate reports through a combination of CRISP and HSCRC data. A number of existing and planned reporting mechanisms include:

- **Public health feeds**: CRISP interfaces with providers to route certain types of information to DHMH, including syndromic surveillance data, immunizations, and reportable conditions.
- **Prescription Drug Monitoring Program (PDMP)**: CRISP operates the technical infrastructure of Maryland's PDMP and supports connectivity to every pharmacy licensed to dispense schedule II to IV drugs in Maryland. CRISP also serves as the access point for clinical providers, including prescribers, pharmacists, and other licensed healthcare practitioners [39].
- **Overdose analytics**: Based on certain overdose related questions, CRISP can produce reports relying on hospital data.
- **Newborn Early Hearing Detection and Intervention connectivity (EHDI)**: CRISP supports hospital integration with the system used by DHMH to submit newborn EHDI related information.
- **Patient attribution analysis**: CRISP is planning to provide reports with patient attribution levels categorized based on prior visits, percentage of visit allocation by patients, census tract or neighborhood, and by diagnosis or charges.

- **Market share analysis**: CRISP is going to provide HSCRC with market share reports which include grouping by clinical service line utilization by hospital professional services agreements, by majority of inpatient visits, total visits, and by diagnosis and charges.
- **Analysis of potentially avoidable volume**: These services will include reports on visits with ambulatory sensitive conditions, readmissions, and market share shifts.
- **Episode of care analysis**: These reports are going to include analyses based on all subsequent hospital visits after discharge, by diagnosis or disposition, and by census tract or neighborhood [61].

Future Work

Maryland's Integrated Care Network (ICN)

Numerous care coordination activities are already underway in Maryland. These activities are often led by hospitals, medical groups, payers, health departments, community-based organizations, and other groups. The state has identified the need for a population-level care coordination infrastructure to support the all-payer waiver program by: (1) an effective risk stratification approach to identify people with complex medical and social needs; (2) the development of health risk assessments to ascertain patients' needs; and (3) the formation of patient-driven care profiles and plans addressing the medical and social needs of patients [60].

In the near future, CRISP is going to play a critical role in the development of Maryland's "Integrated Care Network" (ICN) which will be used by the State to provide the centralized, real-time care coordination services. CRISP will essentially provide a data infrastructure to facilitate identification of individuals who would benefit from care coordination. This process will involve the following components: (1) develop procedures and policies to secure patient consent for the sharing of data for purposes of care coordination; (2) combine existing data sources for the purpose of identifying individuals who would benefit from care coordination; (3) secure new data sources, specifically the Medicare patient-level data, for the purpose of identifying individuals who would benefit from care coordination and chronic care management; (4) use advanced analytics to identify individuals who would benefit from care coordination; and (5) use alert mechanisms to connect these patients to the physicians and hospitals who care for them (eg, using CRISP ENS system to send alerts to primary care physicians when their high-risk patients are in the ER or admitted to the hospital) [60].

CONCLUSION/SUMMARY

The increasing cost of healthcare has accelerated the adoption of value-based care among US healthcare delivery systems, including adoption of ACOs. These value-based healthcare delivery models attempt to achieve Triple Aim but have experienced challenges in collecting and analyzing the information needed to improve the health of their patient populations.

There are no turnkey HIT solutions available for value-based healthcare systems. HIEs have the capability to fill in the population-wide informational gap for ACOs and play a pivotal role to enhance value-based care. An HIE can collect, analyze, and provide critical information about patients associated with all providers within and out of an ACO network.

The all-payer waiver program in Maryland has resulted in reforming Maryland hospitals to operate under a value-based global budget. One of the key factors to achieve such an ambitious value-based program in Maryland is its statewide HIE that offers a set of informational and HIT resources to assist value-based organizations such as ACOs to better manage their attributed population.

CRISP is the designated statewide HIE in Maryland which covers a diverse set of stakeholders ranging from hospitals to ancillary providers. CRISP provides a number of services that are deemed essential to the operations of ACOs in Maryland and, more importantly, to the broader inpatient all-payer waiver program. Some of these population health-IT services include: real-time encounter notification of significant events; centralized care coordination infrastructure; automated reporting of quality metrics; and population-based health risk stratification and predictive analytics.

DISCUSSION QUESTIONS

(1) List the essential health IT needs of value-based care delivery systems and discuss which of these requirements can be fulfilled with your statewide HIE services. If you don't have a statewide HIE, pick a state with an HIE and find which of its services can realize these needs. Identify what the technical and operational gaps are and how the HIE can solve them in short term.

(2) Discuss the potential services that HIEs can provide to ACO entities if interoperability was not a concern. Explain how such an assumption—full interoperability—can change the role of underlying health IT systems within each of the stakeholders (eg, EHRs used by hospitals).

(3) Identify the recent CMS quality measures for ACOs. Explore the potential data sources and services that HIEs can collect/offer to help the ACOs to calculate/improve these metrics. Determine which type of these ACO measures have a significant application in the HIE context and propose new ACO metrics that can be easily measured/operationalized by HIEs.

(4) Study the main financial reimbursement streams of CMS' Medicare Shared Savings Program (MSSP) for ACOs (eg, hospital readmissions). Then prioritize the most viable solutions that an HIE can provide to MSSP ACOs. Consider that a certain percentage of the shared savings of the ACO can be shared with the HIE. Identify which of the HIE services are more sustainable in the long run.

References

[1] Centers for Medicare and Medicaid Services (CMS). Hospital inpatient value-based purchasing program (Medicare program; final rule). Federal Register; 42 CFR § Parts 422 and 480. 2011;76(88):26490–547.

[2] Dartmouth-Hitchcock. What is value-based care? Available from: http://www.dartmouth-hitchcock.org/about_dh/what_is_value_based_care.html [cited August 9, 2015].

[3] Centers for Medicare and Medicaid Services (CMS). National Health Expenditure (NHE) fact sheet. Available from: https://www.cms.gov/Research-Statistics-Data-and-Systems/Statistics-Trends-and-Reports/NationalHealthExpendData/NHE-Fact-Sheet.html; 2015 [cited August 8, 2015].

[4] de Brantes F, Rosenthal MB, Painter M. Building a bridge from fragmentation to accountability—The prometheus payment model. N Engl J Med 2009;36(11):1033–6.

[5] Institute for Healthcare Improvement. The IHI Triple Aim. Available from: http://www.ihi.org/Engage/Initiatives/TripleAim/Pages/default.aspx; 2015 [cited August 10, 2015].

[6] Berwick DM, Nolan TW, Whittington J. The triple aim: care, health, and cost. Health Aff 2008;27(3):759–69.

[7] Rittenhouse DR, Shortell SM, Fisher ES. Primary care and accountable care—two essential elements of delivery-system reform. N Engl J Med 2009;361(24):2301–3.

[8] McClellan M, McKethan AN, Lewis JL, Roski J, Fisher ES. A national strategy to put accountable care into practice. Health Aff 2010;29(5):982–90.

[9] Centers for Medicare and Medicaid Services (CMS). Accountable Care Organizations (ACO). Available from: https://www.cms.gov/Medicare/Medicare-Fee-for-Service-Payment/ACO/ [cited July 9, 2015].

[10] Centers for Medicare and Medicaid Services (CMS). Summary of final rule provisions for Accountable Care Organizations under the Medicare Shared

Savings Program. Available from: https://www.cms.gov/Medicare/Medicare-Fee-for-Service-Payment/sharedsavingsprogram/Downloads/ACO_Summary_Factsheet_ICN907404.pdf; 2014 [cited August 4, 2015].
[11] Centers for Medicare and Medicaid Services (CMS). Federal Register Part II. Available from: http://www.gpo.gov/fdsys/pkg/FR-2011-11-02/pdf/2011-27461.pdf; 2011 [cited August 2, 2015].
[12] Centers for Medicare and Medicaid Services (CMS). Medicare Sharing Saving Program (MSSP) Application. Available from: https://www.cms.gov/Medicare/Medicare-Fee-for-Service-Payment/sharedsavingsprogram/Downloads/2016-MSSP-New-Application-Form.pdf [cited August 5, 2015].
[13] National Committee for Quality Assurance (NCQA). NCQA Accountable Care Organization accreditation. Available from: http://www.ncqa.org/Portals/0/ACO/ACO-web.pdf; 2015 [cited August 3, 2015].
[14] Muhlestein D. Growth and dispersion of Accountable Care Organizations in 2015. [Health Affairs Blog]. Available from: http://healthaffairs.org/blog/2015/03/31/growth-and-dispersion-of-accountable-care-organizations-in-2015-2/; 2015 [cited August 2, 2015].
[15] Centers for Medicare and Medicaid Services (CMS). ACO quality measures. Available from: https://www.cms.gov/Medicare/Medicare-Fee-for-Service-Payment/sharedsavingsprogram/Downloads/ACO-Shared-Savings-Program-Quality-Measures.pdf; [cited August 7, 2015].
[16] Centers for Medicare and Medicaid Services (CMS). National impact assessment of CMS quality measures report. Available from: https://www.cms.gov/Medicare/Quality-Initiatives-Patient-Assessment-Instruments/QualityMeasures/downloads/2015-National-Impact-Assessment-Report.pdf [cited July 22, 2015].
[17] Stoto M. Population health measurement: applying performance measurement concepts in population health settings. eGEMs (Generating Evidence & Methods to Improve Patient Outcomes) 2015;2(4).
[18] Sharfstein JM. The strange journey of population health. Milbank Q 2015;92(4):640–3.
[19] Kindig D, Stoddart G. What is population health? Am J Public Health 2003;93(3):380–3.
[20] Kindig D. Understanding population health terminology. Milbank Q 2007;85(1):139–61.
[21] Kindig D. Improving population health policy: What is population health? Available from: http://www.improvingpopulationhealth.org/blog/what-is-population-health.html [cited May 15, 2015].
[22] Hacker K, Klein Walker D. Achieving population health in accountable care organizations. Am J Public Health 2013;7(103):1163–7.
[23] Institute for Health Technology Transformation. Population Health Management: A roadmap for provider-based automation in a new era of healthcare. Available from: http://ihealthtran.com/pdf/PHMReport.pdf; 2015 [cited August 5, 2015].
[24] Lawrence D. How to forge a high-tech marriage between primary care and population health. Health Aff (Millwood) 2010;29(5):1004–9.
[25] Handmaker K., Hart J. Nine steps to effective population health management [Healthcare Financial Management Association]. Available from: https://www.hfma.org/9StepsPopulationHealth/; 2015 [cited August 7, 2015].
[26] Velusamy S.R. Analytics: the key ingredient for the success of ACOs [HTC Global Services]. Available from: http://files.himss.org/FileDownloads/HTC%20ACO%20Analytics.pdf; 2015 [cited August 3, 2015].
[27] Standards and Interoperability (S&I) Framework. What is the S&I Framework? Available from: http://www.siframework.org/whatis.html [cited August 12, 2015].
[28] Health Level 7. Fast Healthcare Interoperability Resources (FHIR) specification. Available from: http://www.hl7.org/fhir/; 2015 [cited August 11, 2015].
[29] U.S. Department of Health and Human Services (DHHS). American recovery and reinvestment act of 2009: Advance interoperable health information technology services to support health information exchange. Available from: http://healthit.gov/sites/default/files/advancedinteroperablehie-foa.pdf [cited August 9, 2015].
[30] U.S. Department of Health and Human Services (DHHS); Office of the National Coordinator for Health IT (ONC). Community interoperability and health information exchange cooperative agreement program funding opportunity announcement. Available from: http://www.healthit.gov/sites/default/files/communityinterophie-foa-4-10-15rev.pdf [cited August 11, 2015].
[31] Kharrazi H, Weiner JP. IT-enabled community health interventions: challenges, opportunities, and future directions. eGEMs (Generating Evidence & Methods to Improve Patient Outcomes 2014;2(3).
[32] Pricewaterhouse Coopers (PwC) Health Research Institute. Designing the health IT backbone for ACOs Part I: Hospitals look to meaningful use and health information exchanges to guide them. Available from: http://s3.amazonaws.com/rdcms-himss/files/production/public/HIMSSorg/Content/files/Code%20209%20PWC%20Designing%20the%20Health%20IT%20backbone%20for%20ACOs.pdf; 2015 [cited July 6, 2015].

[33] Certification Commission for Healthcare Information Technology (CCHIT). A health IT framework for accountable care. Available from: http://www.healthit.gov/FACAS/sites/faca/files/a_health_it_framework_for_accountable_care_0.pdf; 2013 [cited July 11, 2015].

[34] Dullabh P, Ubri P, Hovey L. The state HIE program four years later: key findings on grantees' experiences from a six-state review. Bethesda: NORC at the University of Chicago; 2014. [cited August 10, 2015] [Case study report]. Available from: http://healthit.gov/sites/default/files/CaseStudySynthesisGranteeExperienceFinal_121014.pdf.

[35] Chesapeake Regional Information System for our Patients (CRISP). The CRISP response to the request for application for a consumer-centric health information exchange for Maryland. Available from: http://mhcc.dhmh.maryland.gov/hit/hie/Documents/CRISP.pdf; 2009 [cited August 9, 2015].

[36] Chesapeake Regional Information System for our Patients (CRISP). CRISP Mission. Available from: https://crisphealth.org/ABOUT/General-Info; 2015 [cited August 10, 2015].

[37] Chesapeake Regional Information System for our Patients (CRISP). A plan for a citizen-centric statewide health information exchange in Maryland. Available from: http://mhcc.dhmh.maryland.gov/hit/hie/Documents/CRISP_FinalReport.pdf; 2015 [cited August 9, 2015].

[38] Chesapeake Regional Information System for our Patients (CRISP). CRISP Encounter Notification System (ENS). Available from: https://crisphealth.org/CRISP-HIE-SERVICES/Encounter-Notification-System-ENS; 2015 [cited August 12, 2015].

[39] Chesapeake Regional Information System for our Patients (CRISP). The Maryland Prescription Drug Monitoring Program (PDMP). Available from: https://crisphealth.org/CRISP-HIE-SERVICES/Prescription-Drug-Monitoring-Program-PDMP; 2015 [cited August 11, 2015].

[40] Chesapeake Regional Information System for our Patients (CRISP). CRISP Participating Organizations. Available from: https://crisphealth.org/FOR-PROVIDERS/Participating-Organizations; 2015 [cited August 12, 2015].

[41] Chesapeake Regional Information System for our Patients (CRISP). CRISP policies and procedures. Available from: https://crisphealth.org/Portals/0/Files/Policies%20&%20Agreements/CRISP%20Policies%20and%20Procedures%204-17-2014.pdf; 2014 [cited August 10, 2015].

[42] Chesapeake Regional Information System for our Patients (CRISP). CRISP policies and agreements. Available from: https://crisphealth.org/ABOUT/Policies-Agreements; 2015 [cited August 12, 2015].

[43] U.S. Government Publishing Office. Electronic Code of Federal Regulations (eCFR). Part 2—Confidentiality of alcohol and drug abuse patient records. Available from: http://www.ecfr.gov/cgi-bin/text-idx?rgn=div5;node=42%3A1.0.1.1.2; 2015 [cited August 10, 2015].

[44] Mirth. Industry solutions: exchange health information. Available from: https://www.mirth.com/Industry-Solutions/Exchange-Health-Information; 2015 [cited August 11, 2015].

[45] Audacious Inquiry (AINQ). Initiate master data management in HIE. Available from: http://ainq.com/case_study/initiate-master-data-management-in-hie [cited August 12, 2015].

[46] Galvez E. HIE bright spots: How ADT messages support care coordination (Part II) [ONC Health IT Buzz]. Available from: http://www.healthit.gov/buzz-blog/state-hie/hie-bright-spots-adt-messages-support-care-coordination-part-ii/; 2013 [cited August 13, 2015].

[47] The Direct Project. The Direct Project overview. Available from: http://wiki.directproject.org/file/view/DirectProjectOverview.pdf; 2010 [cited June 5, 2015].

[48] Audacious Inquiry (AINQ). Population health initiatives and data analytics enabled by the CRISP reporting system (CRS) provide actionable insights into healthcare trends and utilization. Available from: https://ainq.com/case_study/population-health-initiatives-and-data-analytics-enabled-by-the-crisp-reporting-system-crs/; 2015 [cited July 11, 2015].

[49] Rajkumar R, Patel A, Murphy K, Colmers JM, Blum JD, Conway PH, et al. Maryland's all-payer approach to delivery-system reform. N Engl J Med 2014;370(6):493–5.

[50] Sharfstein JM, Kinzer D, Colmers JM. An update on Maryland's all-payer approach to reforming the delivery of health care. JAMA Intern Med 2015;175(7):1083–4.

[51] Maryland Health Services Cost Review Commission (HSCRC). Improving care coordination and care management: supporting the all-payer model design by reducing avoidable use of health care, lowering spending, and improving health. Available from: http://www.hscrc.state.md.us/documents/md-maphs/wg-meet/cc/2015-03-31/2-Care-Coordination-Work-Group-draft-report-3-24-15.pdf; 2015 [cited August 10, 2015].

[52] U.S. Census Bureau. Small Area Health Insurance Estimates (SAHIE) Methodology. Available from: http://www.census.gov/did/www/sahie/methods/index.html; 2015 [cited June 10, 2015].

[53] Fielding NG. Triangulation and mixed methods designs: data integration with new research technologies. Mixed Methods Res 2012;6(2):124–36.

[54] Johns Hopkins University. The Johns Hopkins ACG System. Available from: http://acg.jhsph.org [cited July 24, 2015].

[55] Schuster A., Feeney D., Haile E., Afzal S. Readmission reduction incentive program: Overview of methodology and reporting [Health Services Cost Review Commission]. Available from: http://www.hscrc.state.md.us/documents/HSCRC_Initiatives/readmissions/Readmission-Reduction-Incentive-Program-Webinar-06032014-v2.pdf; 2014 [cited August 9, 2015].

[56] Maryland Health Care Commission (MHCC). Maryland all-payer model agreement. Available from: http://mhcc.maryland.gov/mhcc/pages/hcfs/hcfs_hospital/documents/chcf_all_payer_model_agreement.pdf; 2014 [cited August 12, 2015].

[57] Chesapeake Regional Information System for our Patients (CRISP). CRISP data utility overview draft [HSCRC Data and Infrastructure Workgroup meeting]. Available from: http://www.hscrc.state.md.us/documents/md-maphs/wg-meet/di/2014-03-04/5-CRISP-Data-Workgroup-Slides.pdf; 2014 [cited August 12, 2015].

[58] Agency for Healthcare Research and Quality (AHRQ). A community HIE (health information exchange) based hospital readmission risk prediction and notification system (Maryland). Available from: https://healthit.ahrq.gov/ahrq-funded-projects/community-health-information-exchange-based-hospital-readmission-risk [cited August 11, 2015].

[59] Maryland Department of Health and Mental Hygiene (DHMH). Health Enterprise Zones (HEZs). Available from: http://dhmh.maryland.gov/healthenterprisezones/SitePages/Home.aspx; 2015 [cited August 11, 2015].

[60] Chesapeake Regional Information System for our Patients (CRISP). CRISP data utility overview [HSCRC Data and Infrastructure Workgroup meeting]. Available from: http://www.hscrc.state.md.us/documents/md-maphs/wg-meet/di/2014-03-04/5-CRISP-Data-Workgroup-Slides.pdf; 2014 [cited August 12, 2015].

[61] Chesapeake Regional Information System for our Patients (CRISP). CRISP Care Management Support. Available from: http://www.hscrc.state.md.us/documents/md-maphs/wg-meet/cc/2015-02-27/3-CRISP-Care-Management-Support-v2-4.pdf; 2015 [cited August 10, 2015].

[62] Schuster A, Scott A. CRISP Reporting Service (CRS): introduction overview of schedules, reports, and access to reports. Available from: http://www.hscrc.state.md.us/documents/HSCRC_Initiatives/readmissions/HSCRC-CRISP-Hospital-Reporting-Overview-8212014.pdf; 2014 [cited August 10, 2015].

CASESTUDY

5

Health Information Exchange—The Value Proposition: A Case Study of the US Social Security Administration

Sue S. Feldman

University of South Carolina, Arnold School of Public Health, Columbia, SC

OUTLINE

MAJOR THEMES

This case study focused on the following major themes:

- Factors to consider when assessing blended value propositions in a public–private health information exchange.
- Extent to which organizational value propositions regarding health data-sharing change over time.
- Secondary use of data for uses other than diagnosis, treatment, or payment.
- Influence of governance structure on technical data-sharing and organizational collaboration.

INTRODUCTION

Stakeholder value proposition is not unifocal, but comprises multiple factors. Studies on the secondary use of medical information, and associated frameworks and taxonomies, fail to mention using these data for benefit determination, disability or otherwise. Furthermore, explorations into organizational value propositions typically locate the value of Health IT for health information exchange (HIE) in the area of diagnosis, treatment, and operations—even for providers whose clients may need SSA disability benefits within their lifetimes. Current literature lacks any high-impact value proposition regarding secondary uses of health information for disability determination. This case study addresses that gap, using a framework that examines blended value propositions within enacted collaborations for successful HIE between a public and a private organization.

Sociotechnical Systems Approach

A sociotechnical systems (STS) approach examines social/community links to technical processes [1]. STS design includes several levels of interactions including mechanical (hardware), informational (software), psychological (persons), and social (community). This inclusive approach aims to understand interdependent linkages among a hierarchy of social and technological components. These components interact with social motivations and accomplish a set of social goals that otherwise could not be realized.

Therefore, social motivations and benefits should be examined in a different light than is customary in the return on investment model commonly used for information exchange in business. This blended value proposition has been defined as the combination of social and economic value used to maximize total returns where "the core nature of investment and return is not a trade-off between social and financial interest, but rather the pursuit of an embedded value proposition composed of both" [2]. Emerson continues: "Societies cannot function strictly on the basis of their economic enterprise. It is social commerce that allows individuals and institutions to pursue the traditional financial returns sought by mainstream financial capital market players" [2].

An STS approach focused on systems that are both technologically sound and socially sustainable [3] has been applied to studying HIE, because of the multiple organizations, user types, hardware and software technologies, and sociopolitical motivations and goals involved in HIE composition. Relatively few studies have examined HIE networks in operation, but a sociotechnical approach was previously applied and shown appropriate for studying HIE [4,5].

Interorganizational Systems

An interorganizational system (IOS) is an IT-based system shared by two or more independent organizations for the purpose of information flows and strategic advantage [5,6].

Previous research on IOS focused on cross-organizational features of an STS [6,7]. While the implementation of IOS has been studied for decades across a wide array of industries, few studies have addressed the value proposition related to health care, and fewer still have considered the value proposition related to HIE [5]. However, consistent with HIE, an IOS creates a virtual value chain for instant encounters or transactions of information between non-predetermined participants [8]. An important consideration of this value equation is that the participating organizations' values may be unequal as well as interdependent [9].

Historically, the basis for collaborative efforts has been primarily economic, with the goal of information exchange being strategic advantage leading to increased earnings—an easily quantifiable metric [10–12]. Technical performance is crucial and quantifiable in information exchange, but the success of information exchange within interorganizational collaborations frequently hinges on less quantifiable factors such as shared leadership or aligned and dynamic value propositions [13–16]. Governance can also influence the facilitation and coordination of data exchange [17]: For example, knowing who has decision-making power was shown to increase accountability, foster a more cooperative environment, and decrease intra- and interorganizational tensions [18]. Yet, the formal governance structures typical of mature interorganizational collaborations may negatively affect newly established or emerging collaborations [19,20].

Value Proposition

Many organizational mission statements include both social and economic factors. In their book, *Ben & Jerry's Double-Dip: How to Run a Values-Led Business and Make Money, Too*, Ben Cohen and Jerry Greenfield describe their corporate social mission as being just as important as their economic mission, and perhaps even more exposed—given that economic audits are written in financial speak, whereas social audits are written in plain English [21]. However, Emerson suggests:

> We must move beyond the traditional belief that an organization's Economic Value is separate and at odds with its Social Value. While one might attempt to track the two (such as by examining the financials of the corporation and then reading the social audit completed by an outside observer), they are wrongly viewed as two separate aspects of the corporation's value proposition [2].

Various research studies have concluded that value propositions in collaborative efforts are supported by the ideal of public good, where social drivers can include elements extending beyond the organization and having a variety of influences for social good; however, such value is diffuse and not easily measured [22,23]. More recent studies note that an organization's economic needs may be driven by elements that comprise organizational fiscal health and are usually easily quantifiable [16]. Yet another perspective suggests that stakeholder value proposition is not a single-focus proposition, but rather an evolving blend of social and economic factors within a particular context [24].

Value propositions, therefore, may be blended and may change over time. Answering stakeholder value questions such as: "What's in it for me?", "Why is this important?", and "What is needed for sustainability?" is essential for collaboration, especially in health data exchanges and public–private collaborations [16,25]. To answer these questions and further understand value proposition changes, we must examine evolving social and economic value propositions within the larger context of a blended value proposition.

The highest-order intangible social benefits (human life) of health information sharing are succinctly stated by Porter and Teisburg [26]: "The social benefits of results information will be even greater in health care than in the financial markets, because the physical well-being of Americans is at stake." Social value considerations for collaboration extend beyond those that are actor-based or organizational in nature. In his book on infrastructure delivery in public–private collaborations, Mody [27] draws examples from the railway and transportation systems to suggest that social considerations, such as being able to deliver goods and information to the right place at the right time, might exceed those of economic returns and could exert greater significant pressure.

Social motivations may support economic motivations in some situations but be at odds with them in other situations, a fact that contributes to the need for value propositions to evolve over time in order to sustain the collaboration.

As with supply chain information sharing, health information sharing is a costly investment from which organizations expect an economic return. However, with health information sharing at a more nascent stage of development, upfront investments are likely to be very high and a sustained commitment to the collaboration is critical for successful outcomes and sustainability. The health care industry could learn a lot about sustainability from other industries such as supply chain management. For example, two recent studies suggest that factors contributing to positive outcomes and sustainability include co-creating value (relationships being an important component), strategy formation, and competitive advantage [28,29]. A parallel can be drawn with a recent HEAL NY case study of NY's investment to create an interoperable Regional Health Information Organization (RHIO), which cites "the need to convince stakeholders of the project's value" as a factor in financial alignment and sustainability [16].

In the past, the conceptual basis for exploring collaborative efforts was primarily economic, and the goal of information exchange was increased earnings [10–12]. However, recent literature suggests that the benefits of interorganizational information sharing can be diffuse and not limited to "the bottom line." For example, Aldrich [30] suggests that collaborating organizations now consider reasons other than economics as drivers for sharing information, and Brynjolffson and Saunders [31] note that the intangible benefits of interorganizational information sharing may be the untapped value proposition for interorganizational information collaborations. The idea that the value proposition may be a blend of intangibles such as social value, and tangibles such as economics, is compatible with the use of blended conceptualizations to understand health information collaborations.

Within the social and economic motivations underlying interorganizational collaborations are multiple dimensions of information sharing. The following are some important studies of HIE implementations examining the elements contributing to value propositions and how they change over time. Delone and McLean [32] note that exploring multiple dimensions can help align organizational needs and bring value to each organization individually and to the collaboration collectively. Malepeti et al. [33] suggest that value can be found in a wide spectrum of benefits, ranging from organizational fiscal health (changes in market share) to technical performance (getting usable data where needed). While technical performance is crucial in information exchange between organizations, the success of interorganizational collaborations and information exchanges frequently hinges on other factors such as: interorganizational alignment, shared leadership, and a blend of value propositions [13,14,16,34]. In the case of HEAL NY (the RHIO mentioned earlier), a study 2 years postimplementation revealed that concerns over technical issues increased, but so did the potential for misaligned persistent stakeholder value propositions [16]. And a more recent case study of Virginia statewide HIE implementation found that technical, organizational, and governance elements were critical success factors in collaborations and in realizing a shared value proposition [5].

Governance can influence how collaborations facilitate and coordinate data-sharing [17]. Governance, in terms of intra- and interorganizational authority (knowing who has decision-making power), has been shown to increase accountability, foster a more cooperative environment, and decrease intra- and interorganizational issues [35]. The nature of the relationships between decision-makers is also important in navigating complex governance processes and structures [36,37] and sharing decisions [38]. A 2010 case study examining the demise of CalRHIO (California Regional Health Information Organization) indicated that a lack of formal governance practices led to the need for subsequent overhaul and eventual restructuring [39].

To summarize: Governance may not be "one size fits all," and newly formed collaborations may be negatively influenced by the formal governance structures that characterize more mature interorganizational collaborations. This is especially true of collaborations involving governmental entities [19], which may need evolving governance that is responsive to change.

A framework depicting HIE relative to public agencies as consumers of electronic health record (EHR) data (supplied by private providers) is specific to personal (pertaining to the patient) and public (pertaining to disease prevention and health promotion) health uses but not to benefit determination, disability, or otherwise [40]. SSA was very innovative in establishing a public–private collaboration for using Medical Evident Gathering and Analysis through Health Information Technology (MEGAHIT) across an HIE to gather clinical data from EHRs for secondary use (ie, medical information not used for diagnosis, treatment, or payment).

Achieving successful public–private collaborations for HIE may require a shared understanding of what is valued by each collaborating organization and a recognition that, over time, the value proposition may shift. One could conjecture that, in some cases, value (like beauty) is in the eye of the beholder—in that each collaborator may have a different opinion of what constitutes value. Furthermore, the value proposition may change as organizational goals change. Therefore, both context and perspective are necessary to understand value propositions. Identifying the value proposition—in this context meaning the worth, importance, or utility of the information received through HIE—helps answer the question: "What's in it for me?"

A 2010 report underscores the observation that collaborations designed specifically for sharing health information may have misaligned motivations for sharing data, and more research is needed to clarify the value of HIE as related to stakeholders' motivations and perspectives [41]. For example, a public agency may be satisfied with finding value in sharing health information for the public good (eg, disease prevention and health promotion), while the private organization wants to understand the value proposition in terms of business value, with some degree of economic impact (eg, operational savings or cost avoidance) [16,42,43]. In the context of disability determination, SSA as a public agency may find value in faster disability determinations, which could provide economic benefit to the private organization through decreased uncompensated care losses. Understanding the value that SSA and disability benefit determination collaborators find in the overall process may provide information that can facilitate sustainable heath information exchange.

Research findings on public–private information exchange suggest that unsustainable value propositions (eg, no economic benefit) and poorly defined governance are key reasons for failures [25,42,44]. Thus, it is critical to consider that, while the initial value in HIE may have been the technical exchange of data, that value evolves over time and organizational and governance factors begin emerging as critical factors.

Aligned and evolving value propositions related to successful HIEs have yet to be empirically established, but information from other industries suggests that a strong relationship exists between understanding value propositions and sustained success. For example, a recent study examining a variety of service industries (eg, automotive) suggests that initial value may have been in the mere exchange of goods, but over time the value moves to use of the goods [45]. As applied to HIE, the initial value may have been in the technical exchange of data but that value evolves over time, and organizational factors—such as use and usefulness of the data to impact organizational fiscal health—begin to emerge as critical factors.

The Agency for Healthcare Research and Quality (AHRQ) released a vision and strategy document discussing a strong relationship between HIE sustainability and value proposition [46]. The report also identifies the potential for federal programs to contribute to HIE sustainability and comprehensive information exchange but does not discuss this contribution in the context of SSA. Thus, the opportunity presents itself to better understand stakeholder value propositions in health data exchange within a high-impact area of disability determination.

Conceptual Framework

Enactment theory proposes that a rationale is ascribed to outcomes [5,47]. Fountain's Technology Enactment Framework (TEF) applies enactment theory to IT to suggest that more than the technology produces outcomes; rather, organizational factors combined with the technical factors provide a rationale that is embedded *within* each collaborating organization; it is *how* the technology is enacted that influences outcomes [5,17]. Schooley's Time Critical Information Systems (TCIS) framework suggests that the core components of a public–private collaboration involve more than governance and IT, and also include interorganizational relationships [34]. Robey et al. [48] note that we can no longer examine IOSs as if they were a snapshot of a moment in time, but must revise existing theories to reflect technical evolution.

Based on the previous frameworks of Emerson [2], Fountain [17], and Schooley and Horan [15], this case study uses a Blended Value Collaboration Enactment Framework shown in Fig. 1 [5]. The framework suggests that, while the output may be seen in terms of quantifiable system performance, the HIE value proposition is influenced by a combination of factors—technical, organizational, and governance—within and between organizations. The value proposition may be motivated by social or economic considerations.

Within each organization (labeled as Organization A, B, etc.), multiple dimensions influence the Output and subsequent Value. These dimensions are shown as technical and organizational (unique to each organization), which are supported by governance structures and motivations for collaboration within each organization. The value propositions for organizations A, B, etc. are considered to be social or economic, or a blend of the two. The balance beam denotes the dynamic nature of the motivation and allows for motivations changing or evolving over time. As the collaboration evolves (lower axis) the Output and resulting Value (HIE value proposition) result from *what* drives the collaboration and *how* the multiple dimensions of collaboration are enacted. This conceptual framework illustrates that as time passes (denoted by T_1, T_2, and so on), changes occur, and that these events recur (as opposed to occurring at only one moment in time). This Blended Value Collaboration Enactment Framework guided the methodology of this case study. The framework is especially valuable for its consideration of the recursive nature of *how* collaborations are enacted and that

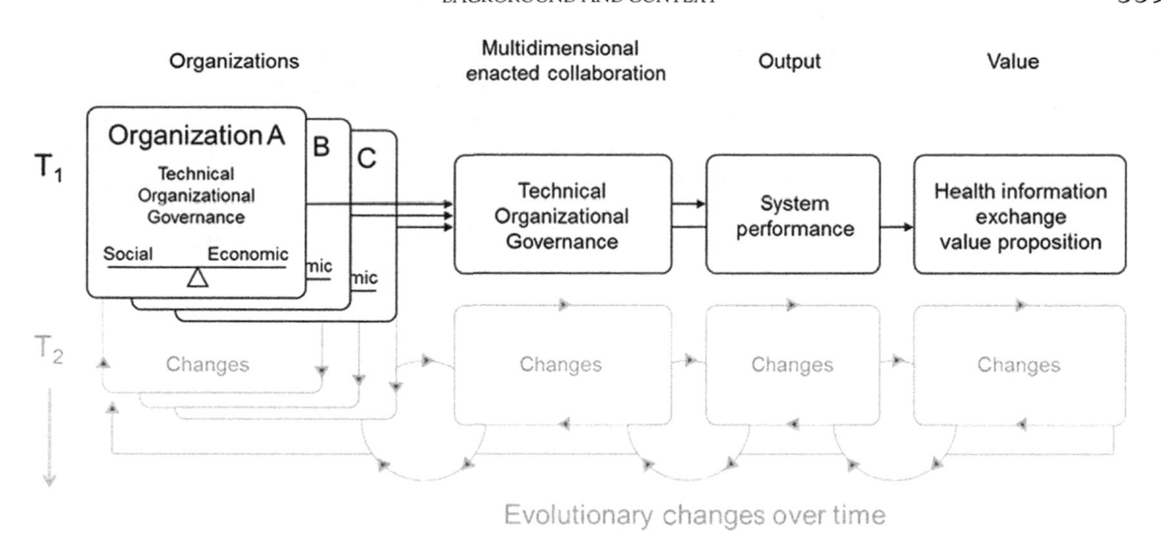

FIGURE 1 Blended Value Collaboration Enactment Framework, first published in the *Journal of Medical Internet Research* [5].

changes occur over time—both within each organization and between organizations, influenced by the perceived value proposition.

BACKGROUND AND CONTEXT

This case study involves the collaboration between three entities: the Nationwide Health Information Network (the transport mechanism), MedVirginia (the HIE providing information), and the US Social Security Administration (the Federal agency requesting information).

Nationwide Health Information Network

One of the earliest initiatives of the Office of the National Coordinator for Health IT (ONC) was the Nationwide Health Information Network (NwHIN), designed to be a "network of networks" and the nation's HIE [49–51]. Recently rebranded the eHealth Exchange,[1] NwHIN consists of a set of technical standards, web services, and policies that facilitate secure and interoperable information exchange across multiple entities using the Internet. Participants in the NwHIN must go through a technical certification process as well as a governance review process to ensure their multiorganizational, regional, or national network of facilities can meaningfully exchange data with the other participants while adhering to established policies to protect data as it is exchanged for a range of use cases.

MedVirginia/Bon Secours

MedVirginia, Virginia's RHIO, is an HIE in Richmond, Virginia, that began in 2001 with a

[1] When this case study was conducted, the NwHIN was managed by ONC. It has since been transitioned into the private sector and renamed eHealth Exchange. To preserve the integrity of the case study, references to NwHIN and ONC are retained.

vision of creating communities of care making Richmond the most health data-connected community in the nation. By 2005, using the Internet, MedVirginia launched a HIPAA-compliant portal giving clinicians access to lab, pharmacy, and other patient health information at the point of clinical care; any secondary uses of this information were unrealized potential whose value had not yet been considered.

MedVirginia provides services for physicians and hospitals in the Bon Secours Health System, and four Bon Secours hospitals were involved this study. On February 28, 2009, MedVirginia and SSA began using NwHIN to transmit patient health information for disability determination, using an SSA-developed heath IT solution called MEGAHIT. This project was the first instantiation of a much larger initiative that was later expanded with funds from the American Recovery and Reinvestment Act (ARRA). Before collaborating with SSA, MedVirginia's data-sharing focused on clinicians, diagnostic laboratories, pharmacies, etc., primarily for purposes of diagnosis, treatment, and payment. The uncompensated care cost recovery in this case study is that of Bon Secours and not of MedVirginia.

In February 2010, MedVirginia received one of SSA's 14 ARRA-funded awards to expand the initial use of MEGAHIT across NwHIN for collecting medical evidence for disability determination. This meant that more of MedVirginia's current providers could participate in MEGAHIT and provided a unique opportunity, as well as the means, to examine the evolution over time of factors contributing to value propositions.

US Social Security Administration

The US Social Security Administration (SSA), the nation's primary disability benefit provider, is among the largest US users of medical record information, particularly for determining disability benefits [52]. Disability applications begin when a claim is filed with SSA (Internet, telephone, in person) at a local field office. The field office then sends a signed form (Authorization to Disclose Information to the Social Security Administration (Form 827)[2]) to the state Disability Determination Services (DDS) office, which generates an authorized request to the claimant's health care provider(s) for supporting documentation (medical evidence) to be used in deciding the merits of the claim. This begins an arduous process of requests and re-requests for medical evidence. Re-requests are often needed because many responses are incomplete, some are inadequate, and many remain unanswered, resulting in delays and increasing disability determination costs. Fig. 2 illustrates the disability application process.

SSA uses health IT solutions to expedite delivery of medical records for disability determination and has dedicated some of its ARRA funds to incentivizing providers to exchange medical information for disability determination. In the context of disability determination, health IT advances (such as the use of MEGAHIT) provide a secure and interoperable transport mechanism for transporting medical record data to SSA. SSA's goal is to use MEGAHIT (which includes business rules for automated processing) across NwHIN, enabled by existing Internet technology, for HIE for disability determination. Doing so changes the lens through which we see HIE and brings into focus the high-impact, high-value motivations for secondary uses of existing EHR data. Using MEGAHIT through NwHIN has both social and economic motivations: time savings in disability determination and uncompensated care cost recovery, respectively.

[2] SSA Form-827 is an Authorization to Disclose Information to the Social Security Administration (SSA). The purpose of this form is to obtain medical and other information needed to substantiate the merits of a disability claim and render a disability determination.

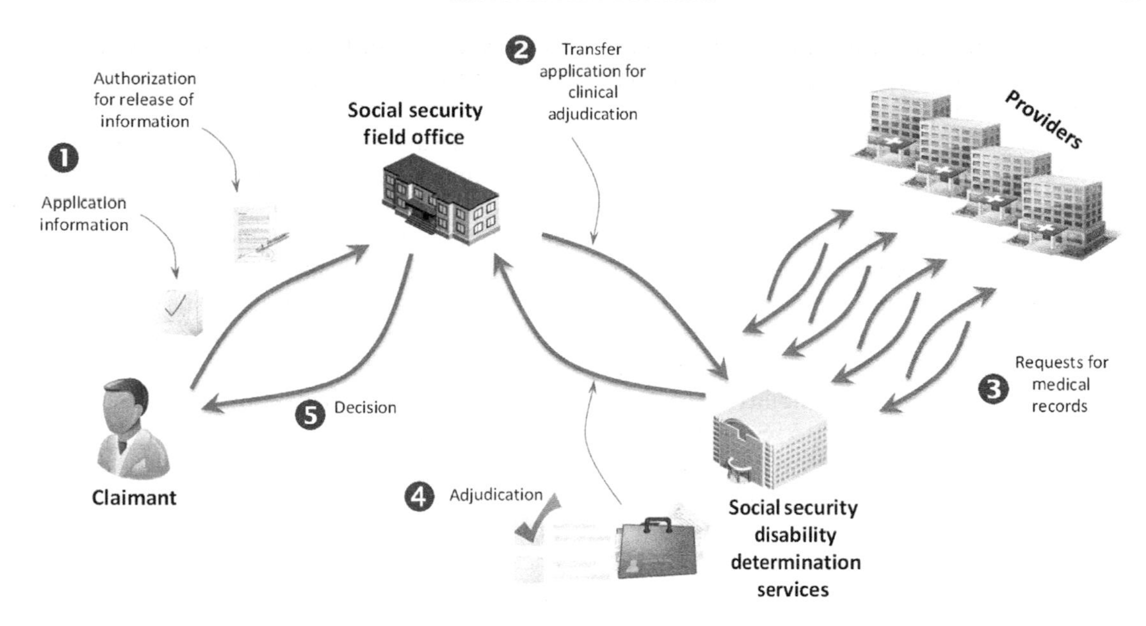

FIGURE 2 Disability determination process. *Adapted from the Social Security Administration.*

In the context of disability determination, public–private collaborations for HIE offer opportunities to understand the multiple dimensions and evolving organizational motivations of sharing health data information. This opportunity is especially unusual in that the public organization (SSA) is not typically considered a health care provider and is therefore frequently left out of the collaboration loop of sharing health information. Therefore, examining this collaboration for disability determination changes our image of viable collaborators and consumers of EHR data in HIE and provides a unique opportunity to understand changing and evolving value propositions for sharing health information in a public–private collaboration.

CASE STUDY MAIN CONTENT

The Challenge

Relying upon principally manual methods for developing (requesting, receiving, and analyzing) medical evidence for disability determination is an inefficient process [53,54].[3] A Government Accountability Office (GAO) report suggests that SSA disability claims take too long, the backlog is too large, and the processes are out of step with technological advances [55]. Such factors lead to decreased access to health care,[4] delayed receipt of cash benefits, and increased uncompensated care costs. Note that gains in health care coverage provided through the Affordable Care Act have led to a 21%, or $7.4 billion, decrease in uncompensated care costs

[3] When medical records are collected by SSA, they become medical evidence. This process is part of the medical evidence development process (http://www.ssa.gov/disability/professionals/bluebook/).

[4] In most states, a favorable decision for SSDI includes Medicare (after a 2-year waiting period).

[56]. However, Medicaid expansion is not mandatory and several states have not participated. States *not* engaging in Medicaid expansion are estimated to decrease uncompensated care costs by only half as much as do those states participating in Medicaid expansion. Thus, access to health care services made possible through SSA disability benefits remain an important value proposition for health care providers.

Some speculate that, if there is no substantial impact on the processes underlying SSA's disability program, SSA's disability trust fund could run out of money; a 2015 SSA report suggests insolvency by 2016 [57]. With over 3 million new disability applications annually and more than 15 million medical records associated with these applications, the MEGAHIT program has the potential to improve the process of medical evidence development and eliminate human and fiscal waste [58].

Opportunity

The inefficient process of medical evidence development for disability determination stands to benefit from the technological advances so well suited to routine and predictable processes: requesting, gathering, and analyzing information [54,55,59]. However, SSA does not collect medical evidence in a vacuum, but depends on health care providers to supply the medical evidence. HIEs have emerged as logical candidates with whom SSA could collaborate to collect medical evidence for disability determination.

The Case: Examining Social Versus Economic Value Propositions

SSA underwent two reorganizations during the course of this study. The first reorganization "institutionalized" health IT: Instead of health IT being its own division with a division director, responsibilities were spread across the agency. The second reorganization relocated the accountability for health IT from the Office of the Deputy Commissioner of Systems (DCS) to the Office of the Chief Information Officer (OCIO). Each time, the value of MEGAHIT needed to be resubstantiated, causing delays and miscommunications. Such situations can fracture developing or already accepted value propositions.

Organizational value propositions may be located across several dimensions rather than in a single dimension. Furthermore, organizational value propositions (whether socially or economically motivated) change over time and much of this change can be prompted by the organizational direction. The value in blended value propositions, as described here, is the ability to provide balance within a collaboration. This balance proved beneficial during SSA's reorganization, when key elements of the collaboration were weakened.

The social–economic–dimensional value blend is illustrated in Fig. 3. The value proposition is indicated along the social value (x) and economic value (y) axes, with a line equidistant from both axes indicating an equal-value blend. The dotted arc provides a reference for changes that occurred for each organization between the first and second instantiations of MEGAHIT. Each organization's location on the diagram is based on the case study findings and represents each organization's value blend associated with the first and second instantiations of MEGAHIT. The nature of each organization's focus (with respect to dimension) is also indicated—tech = technical, org = organization, and gov = governance—reflecting observations in the literature that collaborations should focus on multiple dimensions [32].

As interpreted from the findings of this case study:

- SSA began MEGAHIT for the social value from a technical dimension and migrated toward finding economic value while retreating slightly on the social value scale, but remains below the equal-value line.

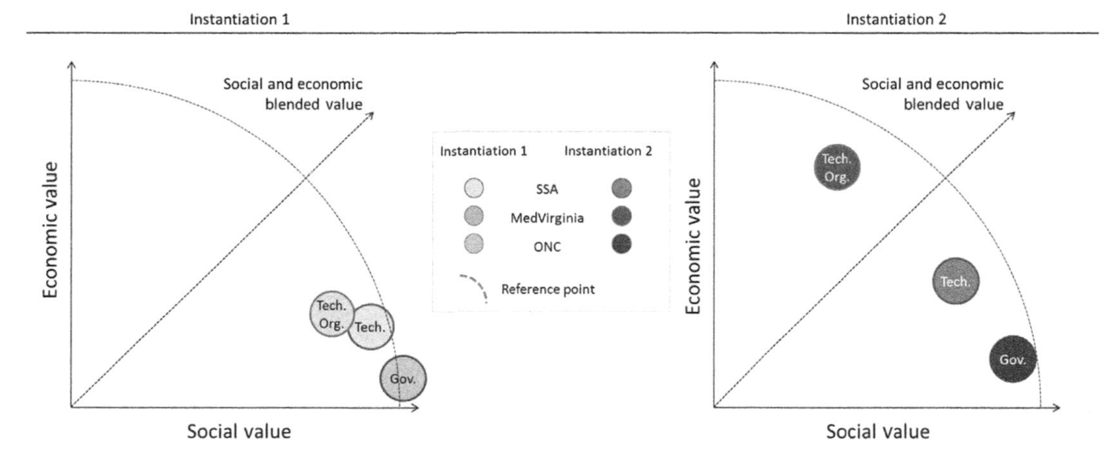

FIGURE 3 Social–economic–dimensional value blend by organization.

- MedVirginia began MEGAHIT from a social value focus from technical and organizational dimensions and has migrated toward an economic value proposition (retaining the focus on technical and organizational dimensions); however one notes that MedVirginia is now closer to the equal-value line, indicating a more balanced blended value proposition rather than being weighted heavily toward either the social or economic value zones.
- ONC began NwHIN from an almost purely social value proposition and is beginning to think about the business case that might accompany NwHIN sustainability.

Note in Fig. 3 that all three organizations, regardless of how far to the right they were on the social value scale in the first instantiation, show a leftward shift (ie, slightly less social value) in the second instantiation. Likewise, all three organizations migrated toward a higher economic value, with MedVirginia crossing the equal-value line so economic value exceeds social value.

One could speculate that, as time evolves, MedVirginia will find a balanced position on the equal-value dotted line in Fig. 3, representing a more balanced social–economic value proposition. Likewise, the evolution of MEGAHIT, both in terms of time and collaborators, is likely to see SSA seeking some economic impact as well.

The Case: Examining the Blended Value Collaboration Enactment Framework

The findings of this case study are a result of analysis from 41 key participant interviews and extensive document analysis and illustrated within the Blended Value Collaboration Enactment Framework (see Fig. 4). In Fig. 4, advances are indicated by a "+" and setbacks are indicated by a "−".

Social Security Administration

SSA experienced both advances and setbacks during the project. In terms of advances, (indicated in Fig. 4 by +), the findings suggest great progress toward increasing the number of listings or medical conditions for which business rules were established within MEGAHIT. Increasing listings provide earlier disability determination on more conditions. This increase enables MEGAHIT to provide

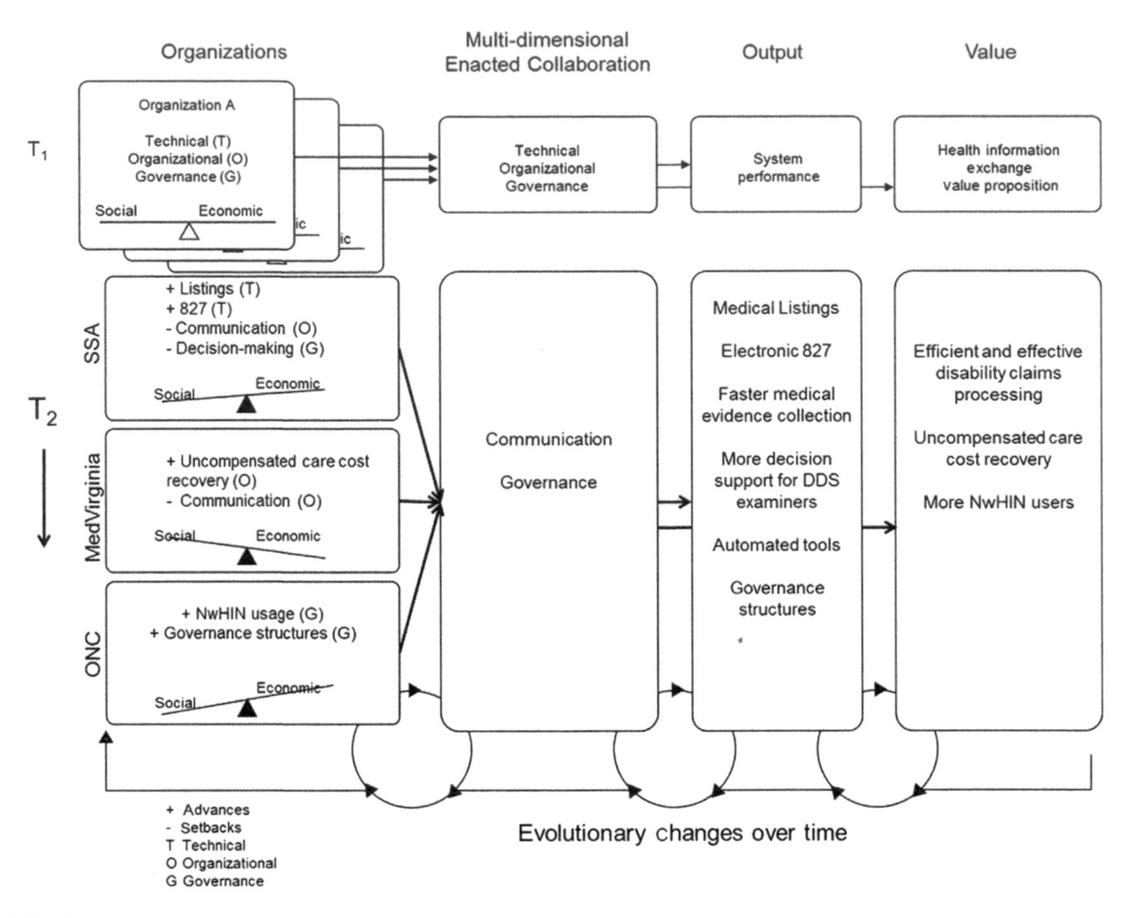

FIGURE 4 Blended Value Collaboration Enactment Framework as applied to this case study.

preliminary analysis on more conditions and represents SSA's ability to save overall case processing time and make faster disability determinations, thereby getting benefits to claimants sooner.

Findings regarding case processing time suggest that there was a 33% reduction in how long it took to process cases. Faster processing can potentially provide faster benefit payments and increased access to care for the claimant and affect the provider's "bottom line" in terms of uncompensated care cost recovery. This is an example of a social–economic blended value proposition in which SSA gets benefits to claimants faster (social) and the provider gets paid faster (economic). Findings also support the view that 827 has been a bit of a conundrum, both as a faxed document in early prototype phases and, later, while trying to find a standard to accommodate "at will" viewing by the provider. The move toward an electronic 827 represents great progress.

As discussed by interviewees within and outside of SSA, the main contributor to setbacks (indicated in Fig. 4 by –) was communication issues related to multiple changes in Program Directors, staff, and positioning of the program within SSA; these issues stalled decision-making. The presentation of a blended value proposition in this area is interesting, as the time delays may have different economic impacts on the public agency and the private agency. While MedVirginia experienced some frustrations, they stayed motivated by continuing similar work with VA and DoD, knowing that time invested with those two agencies held economic value. These results are consistent with the literature, which suggest that a public agency may be satisfied with the social value proposition, but a private organization must find a business value, as measured by economic impact, to support the organization's social mission [16,42,43,60].

MedVirginia

MedVirginia, as an HIE, provides another lens through which to evaluate HIE. The current situation is that HIEs (as entities) and HIE (as an activity) are government incentivized (through ARRA funding). Thus, HIEs must struggle to find a sustainable model with the appropriate blend of economic support and governance structure [25,39,61]. Survival is associated with HIEs that respond to changes brought about by evolving *technical*, *organizational*, and *governance* dimensions [16]. This collaboration between SSA, MedVirginia, and ONC involved many changes within the three dimensions, requiring that MedVirginia be responsive without being reactive. Most notable among the changes were the communication delays reported due to reorganization within SSA. As noted in the literature, communication is critical throughout all phases of a collaboration [62]. Likewise, consistent with the TEF, the output is less about the technology and more about *how* the technology was enacted [17].

While respondents at MedVirginia did not feel that the communication delays due to reorganization within SSA affected the technical processes of the collaboration, they said it did influence their ability to *execute* the technology. The findings show that, early in MedVirginia's collaboration with SSA and ONC, MedVirginia was very heavily motivated by intangible assets such as seeing if the technology to use MEGAHIT *could* work and being the first in the nation to use it. However, as time went on, MedVirginia needed to tip the scales more toward the economic end. Economic considerations for MedVirginia lie in why a provider should subscribe to them as an HIE—their value lies in being able to respond to MEGAHIT queries (for which they are paid $15 each), potentially getting the claimant benefits sooner, and potentially increasing uncompensated care cost recovery to the subscriber, in this case Bon Secours. Across the four Bon Secours facilities participating in this case study, and over the one-year period of time, Bon Secours realized $1.9 million USD in uncompensated care cost recovery. For MedVirginia to keep evolving as an organization directed toward remaining a sustainable HIE, they will have to create and maintain a balanced value proposition.

ONC

This study was conducted within a larger and changing national health IT context in which governance structures related to NwHIN are evolving. The information in this study provides a better understanding of the evolving governance structures for broader uses of NwHIN as a transmission vehicle for HIE. The main benefit for ONC resulting from the efforts between SSA and MedVirginia was usage of NwHIN. Prior to this collaborative effort, NwHIN was in a test environment with only theoretical uses. SSA and MedVirginia put NwHIN into production; SSA continues to drive value in NwHIN participation for organizations and regional and statewide HIEs.

SUMMARY

The literature is clear about the need to align medical evidence development practices with current technology and the potential benefits thereof [20,54,55,59]. Less clear, however, is the value proposition for collaborating organizations to engage in information sharing for secondary purposes, such as disability determination. This study examined three organizations—SSA, MedVirginia, and ONC—to gain insights into the multiple dimensions (technical, organizational, and governance) of the collaboration and the associated evolving value propositions. MEGAHIT also provided a context within which to examine the key elements of *how* the collaboration was enacted over a period of time, using the Blended Value Collaboration Enactment Framework.

The findings and the literature suggest that value may be located in different places for different organizations and at different times in their lifecycles. For example, uncompensated care cost recovery is of great interest to care providers, but not for medical records clearinghouses whose only focus is getting the record from point A to point B and being paid for that transmission. Thus, for clearinghouses, value may be located solely in the organizational dimension (human resource and/or capital equipment outlay, etc.). As more diverse organizations exchange clinical information across NwHIN, with SSA or other federal agencies, alternative value streams are likely to emerge.

This case study examined uncompensated care cost recovery as a use case for the value proposition of HIE, within the context of SSA disability determination. Table 1 summarizes key findings related to this context. The Blended Value Collaboration Enactment Framework was used to understand the collaboration between three organizations—SSA, MedVirginia, and ONC—and to gain insight into the factors influencing their collaboration and the associated value propositions.

TABLE 1 Summary of Case Study Findings

- Reduced case processing times leading to faster benefit determination
  - 32% time savings
  - 50 days saved per disability applicant
- Faster favorable benefit determination
  - 33% time savings
  - 52 days saved per disability applicant
- Changing value propositions over time
  - Original value proposition socially motivated
  - Value proposition eventually stronger toward economic motivations for two organizations (SSA and MedVirginia)
- Uncompensated care cost recovery resulting from faster favorable determination
  - $1.9 million over 12 months

Modified from Ref. [63].

Acknowledgments

Fig. 1 was first published in the *Journal of Medical Internet Research* [5]. The figure is open-access distributed under the terms of the Creative Commons Attribution License (http://creativecommons.org/licenses/by/2.0/), which permits unrestricted use, distribution, and reproduction in any medium, provided the original work is properly cited with original URL and bibliographic citation information.

DISCUSSION QUESTIONS

1. Describe the short- and long-term benefits and consequences of Medicaid expansion related to uncompensated care cost recovery.
2. Describe other secondary uses of clinical data.
3. Describe how HIE could facilitate the exchange of clinical data for other secondary uses (consider other state, federal, or international uses such as a State Department of Health, the Federal Aviation Administration or the World Health Organization). In your description, map out social versus economic drivers for participation and governance structures needed to facilitate streamlined information exchange.
4. In developing and implementing HIE, health care entities learned from the banking and transportation industries. Describe potential outcomes from health care that other industries might implement.

References

[1] Whitworth B, Ahmad A. Socio-technical system design The encyclopedia of human-computer interaction, 2nd ed Hershey, PA: Information Science Reference; 2013.

[2] Emerson J. The blended value proposition: integrating social and financial returns. Calif Manage Rev 2003;45(4):35–51.

[3] Whitworth B. The social requirements of technical systems. Handbook of research on socio-technical design and social networking systems. Hershey, PA: Information Science Reference; 2009.3.

[4] Unertl K, Johnson K, Gadd C, Lrenzi N. Bridging organizational divides in healthcare: an ecological view of health information exchange. JMIR Med Inform 2013;1(1):e3.

[5] Feldman SS, Schooley BL, Bhavsar GP. Health information exchange implementation: lessons learned and critical success factors from a case study. JMIR Med Inform 2014;2(2):e19. Available from: <http://medinform.jmir.org/2014/2/e19/>.

[6] Cash JI, Konsynski BR. IS redraws competitive boundaries. Harv Bus Rev 1985;63(2):134–42.

[7] Williams CB, Fedorowicz J, editors. A framework for analyzing cross-boundary e-government projects: the CapWin example. In: Proceedings of the 2005 national conference on digital government research. Digital Government Society of North America; 2005.

[8] Benjamin R, Wigand R. Electronic markets and virtual value chains on the information superhighway. Sloan Manage Rev 1995.

[9] Riggins FJ, Mukhopadhyay T. Interdependent benefits from interorganizational systems: opportunities for business partner reengineering. J Manag Inf Syst 1994:37–57.

[10] Levine S, White PE. Exchange as a conceptual framework for the study of interorganizational relationships. Adm Sci Q 1961:583–601.

[11] Blau PM. Power and exchange in social life. New York, NY: John Wiley & Sons; 1964.

[12] Wright DS. Federalism, intergovernmental relations, and intergovernmental management: historical reflections and conceptual comparisons. Public Adm Rev 1990:168–78.

[13] Markus ML. Power, politics, and MIS implementation. Commun ACM 1983;26:14.

[14] Geels FW. From sectoral systems of innovation to socio-technical systems insights about dynamics and change from sociology and institutional theory. Res Policy 2004;33(6–7):897–920.

[15] Schooley B, Horan T. End-to-end enterprise performance management in the public sector through interorganizational information integration. Gov Inf Q 2007;24(4):755–84.

[16] Kern LM, Barron Y, Abramson EL, Patel V, Kaushal R. HEAL NY: promoting interoperable health information technology in New York State. Health Aff 2009;28(2):493–504. PubMed PMID: ISI:000264445100025.

[17] Fountain JE. Building the virtual state: information technology and institutional change. Washington, DC: Brookings Institute Press; 2001.

[18] Phillips N, Lawrence TB, Hardy C. Interorganizational collaboration and the dynamics of institutional fields. J Manag Stud 2000;37:1.

[19] Mintzberg H, Jorgensen J, Dougherty D, Westley F. Some surprising things about collaboration—knowing how people connect makes it work better. Organ Dyn 1996;25(1):60–71.

[20] Feldman SS, Horan TA. The dynamics of information collaboration: a case study of blended it value propositions for health information exchange in disability determination. J Assoc Inf Syst 2011;12(2):1.

[21] Cohen B, Greenfield J, Maran M. Ben & Jerry's double-dip: how to run a values-led business and make money, too. New York, NY: Fireside; 1998.

[22] Sen AK. Rational fools: a critique of the behavioral foundations of economic theory. Philos Public Aff 1977:317–44.

[23] Alter C, Hage J. Organizations working together. Newbury Park, CA: Sage Publications; 1992.

[24] Arthur W. The nature of technology: what it is and how it evolves. New York, NY: Free Press; 2009.

[25] Miller RH, Miller BS. The Santa Barbara County care data exchange: what happened? Health Aff 2007;26(5):568–80.

[26] Porter M, Teisberg E. Redefining health care: creating value-based competition on results. Boston, MA: Harvard Business School Publishing; 2006.506.

[27] Mody A. Infrastructure delivery: private initiative and the public good. Washington, DC: World Bank Publications; 1996.

[28] Ramaswamy V, Gouillart R. Building the co-creative enterprise. Harv Bus Rev 2010:100–9.

[29] Flint DJ, Golicic SL. Searching for competitive advantage through sustainability: a qualitative study in the New Zealand wine industry. Int J Phys Distrib Logistics Manage 2009;39(10):841–60. PubMed PMID: 47117776.

[30] Aldrich H. Organizations and environments. Palo Alto, CA: Stanford Business Books; 2007.

[31] Brynjolfsson E, Saunders A. Wired for innovation. Cambridge, MA: MIT Press; 2010.

[32] Delone WH, McLean ER. The DeLone and McLean model of information systems success: a ten-year update. J Manag Inf Syst 2003;19(4):9–30.

[33] Malepati S, Kushner K, Lee JS. RHIOs and the value proposition: value is in the eye of the beholder. J AHIMA 2007;78(3):24–9.

[34] Schooley BL, Horan TA. Towards end-to-end government performance management: case study of interorganizational information integration in emergency medical services (EMS). Gov Inf Q 2007;24(4): 755–84.
[35] Phillips N, Lawrence TB, Hardy C. Interorganizational collaboration and the dynamics of institutional fields. J Manage Stud 2000;37(1):23–43.
[36] Sullivan H, Skelcher C. Working across boundaries: collaboration in public services. Baskingstoke: Palgrave Macmillan; 2002.271.
[37] Greenwald HP. Beery W, NetLibrary I, editors. Health for all [electronic resource]: making community collaboration work/Howard Greenwald and William Beery. Chicago, IL: Health Administration Press; 2002.
[38] Hergert M, Morris D, Contractor FJ, editors. Trends in international collaborative agreements. Lexington, MA: Lexington Books; 2002.
[39] Ruaber C. CalRHIO closes, but board to help state on IT; 2010 [cited January 15, 2010]. Available from: <http://sanfrancisco.bizjournals.com/sanfrancisco/stories/2010/01/11/story7.html>.
[40] Bloomrosen M, Detmer D. Advancing the framework: use of health data—a report of a working conference of the American Medical Informatics Association. J Am Med Inform Assoc 2008;15(6):715.
[41] eHealth Initiative. National progress report on e-health 2010; 2010. Available from: <http://www.ehealthinitiative.org/sites/default/files/file/National%20Progess%20Report%20on%20eHealth%202010.pdf>.
[42] Adler-Milstein J, McAfee AP, Bates DW, Jha AK. The state of regional health information organizations: current activities and financing. Health Aff 2008;27(1):W60–9. PubMed PMID: ISI:000257188400055.
[43] Kohli R, Grover V. Business value of IT: an essay on expanding research directions to keep up with the times. J Assoc Inform Syst 2008;9(1):23–39. PubMed PMID: ISI:000255118300002.
[44] Walker J, Pan E, Johnston D, Adler-Milstein J, Bates DW, Middleton B. The value of health care information exchange and interoperability. Health Aff 2005;19:W5–10W5.
[45] Vargo S, Maglio P, Akaka M. On value and value co-creation: a service systems and service logic perspective. Eur Manage J 2008;26(3):145–52.
[46] Rosenfeld S, Koss S. Evolution of state health information exchange-a study of vision, strategy, and progress. Rockville, MD: Agency for Healthcare Research & Quality; 2006.
[47] Weick K. Small wins. Redefining social problems. New York, NY: Springer Science+ Business Media; 1986.29.
[48] Robey D, Im G, Wareham JD. Theoretical foundations of empirical research on interorganizational systems: assessing past contributions and guiding future directions. J Assoc Inform Syst 2008;9(9):497–518. PubMed PMID: ISI:000261357800001.
[49] Department of Health & Human Services US. Nationwide Health Information Network (NwHIN); 2013 [cited February 21, 2013]. Available from: <http://www.healthit.gov/policy-researchers-implementers/nationwide-health-information-network-nwhin>.
[50] Gravely SD, Whaley ES. The next step in health data exchanges: trust and privacy in exchange networks. J Healthc Inf Manag 2009;23(2):33–7. PubMed PMID: 19382738. Epub 2009/04/23. eng.
[51] Rishel W, Riehl V, Blanton C. Summary of the NHIN prototype architecture contracts. Washington, DC: U.S. Department of Health and Human Services; 2007.
[52] Social Security Administration. Nationwide Health Information Network Forum. Washington, DC, December 15–16, 2008. Report No.; 2008.
[53] Horan TA, Daniels SM, Feldman SS. The prospective role of personal health records in streamlining and accelerating the disability determination process. Disab Health J 2009;2(3):153–7.
[54] Tulu B, Daniels SM, Feldman SS, Horan TA, editors. Role of Health Information Technology (HIT) in disability determinations: when medical records become medical evidence. Washington DC: American Medical Informatics Association; 2008.
[55] United States Government Accountability Office. Social security disability: collection of medical evidence could be improved with evaluations to identify promising collection practices. In: Subcommittee on Social Security, Committee on Ways and Means, editors. Washington DC: GAO; 2008.
[56] Morse S. Uncompensated care costs shrink under Obamacare, especially in Medicaid expansion states; 2015 [cited April 20, 2015]. Available from: <http://www.webcitation.org/6ZjOg1iGe>.
[57] Social Security Administration. DI Trust Fund, a Social Security fund; 2015 [cited May 3, 2015]. Available from: <http://www.ssa.gov/oact/STATS/table4a2.html>.
[58] Astrue MJ. Testimony before the Senate Finance Committee; 2007. Available from: <http://www.ssa.gov/legislation/testimony_052307.htm>.
[59] Feldman SS, Horan TA. Collaboration in electronic medical evidence development: a case study of the Social Security Administration's MEGAHIT System. Int J Med Inform 2011.
[60] Chaudhry B, Wang J, Wu S, Maglione M, Mojica W, Roth E. Systematic review:impact of health information technology on quality, efficiency, and costs of medical care. Ann Intern Med 2006;144(10):E12–22.

[61] Frohlich J. In Search of … Health Information Exchange; 2010 [July 30, 2010]. Available from: <http://www.ihealthbeat.org/perspectives/2010/in-search-of-health-information-exchange.aspx>.
[62] Fountain JE. Central issues in the political development of the virtual state. Castells M., Cardoso G., editors. The network society: from knowledge to policy, 2005. Washington, DC: Johns Hopkins Center for Transatlantic Relations; 2006. p. 149–69.
[63] Feldman SS, Horan TA, Drew D. Understanding the value proposition of health information exchange: the case of uncompensated care cost recovery. Health Syst 2012.

Index

Note: Page numbers followed by "*b*," "*f*," and "*t*" refer to boxes, figures, and tables, respectively.

D

F

G

H

T

U